KIKO

HIDDEN POWER
ELECTRIC MOVES

A *Revolutionary* Discovery
about Traditional Martial Arts
for the Fight & *Beyond*

Hayashi Tomio

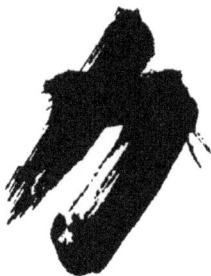

ISBN 978-0-9792697-6-9

Published by Wind School
16 Braidburn Way
Morristown, New Jersey 07960

Book Design by Kathleen Otis
Original Photos: Chris Goedecke,
Illustrations: Tigana

Printed in the United States of America

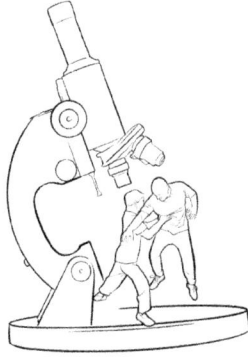

We need a new scientific paradigm if we are to understand the nature and function of Ki, consciousness, spirituality and our own deeply intuited subjective inner landscapes.

Hayashi Tomio

八卦游俠の騎士

DEDICATION

This book is dedicated to the *Knights of the Bagua*, all those men and women who embrace the tripartite relevance of the mental, physical and spiritual dimensions of martial life in a common cause toward evolution of the individual and planet as a whole.

In particular, my deep appreciation goes to Stone, Tian Zhua, Dharma Wheel, Prince Five Weapons, Wayfarer, Shielding Cobra, Standing Bear, Silver Tiger, Raging Bull, Wise Counsel, Eight Trigram Furnace, Inner Kata Queen, Stream Enterer, White Falcon, Sha Wujing, Diamond Wave, Black Snake Fireworks, and Arakawa Mitsugi for granting permission to represent some of Nagaboshi Tomio's teachings.

Without their support, enthusiasm, and curiosity for their art, I might not have sustained the momentum to press into such rich martial frontier.

TABLE OF CONTENTS

PART 1
KI FINDS ME

PART 2
INITIATION

PART 3
INSPECTION

MIND MATTERS

OBJECTS

TECHNIQUE

PART 4
Questing for Answers

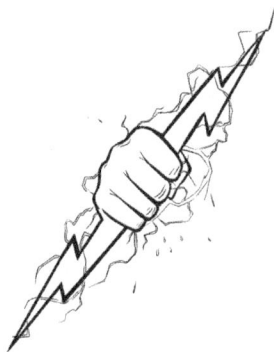

A REVOLUTIONARY DISCOVERY

If you could step back from all the traditional Fighting Forms of the world and all their diverse levels of overt application, if you could look beyond all their external values and merits, you would see something inherent within the very structure of the Forms themselves, a masterful comprehension of the body's bioelectric architecture designed to magnify and replenish the force of every move and movement set on multiple planes. So brilliantly embedded is this internal subsystem that it has gone virtually undetected by all but the thinnest community of modern martial professionals. The precise patterns within these compositions reveal a calculated alchemy of breath, mind, body motions and posturing merged with an awareness of geomagnetic field and cosmic cycle influences that when properly activated can lead one down an evolutionary path to a new species of martial humankind; the *Hikari O Ayatsuru Tsukaite*, the *Light Wielders*, whose expanded consciousness and elevated awareness will use their own Biofield's influence as a dynamic third limb.

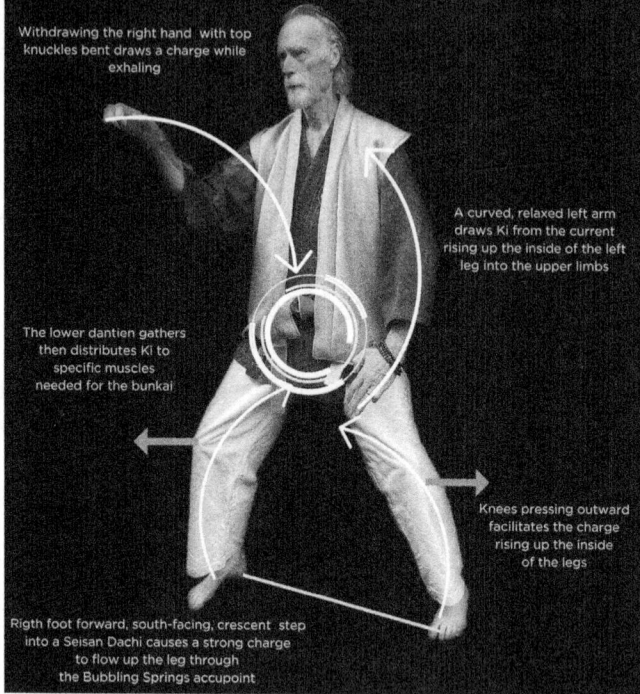

Take Charge!

Embedded within the Traditional Fighting forms of Asia
lie powerful hidden formulas for manipulating
the body's electro-magentic field currents
for impressive strength gains

Withdrawing the right hand with top knuckles bent draws a charge while exhaling

A curved, relaxed left arm draws Ki from the current rising up the inside of the left leg into the upper limbs

The lower dantien gathers then distributes Ki to specific muscles needed for the bunkai

Knees pressing outward facilitates the charge rising up the inside of the legs

Rigth foot forward, south-facing, crescent step into a Seisan Dachi causes a strong charge to flow up the leg through the Bubbling Springs accupoint

The essential fighting forms of Asia reveal an underlying energetic substructure supporting and amplifying all manner of martial technique. We all have the potential to elevate these mostly dormant principles from their visceral origins to conscious, impressive and repeatable strength feats. If we discover that Ki consists of a strong electro-magnetic and/or photonic base, future students will be learning to control their body's Biofield to enhance their disciplines.

Testimonials

Twenty-two experts share their Kiko experiences

Those martial artists not working with their Ki are amateurs.
A. Hugh, 70 years' martial experience

With my best effort, I could barely budge my partner from his Kiba dachi pushing from his side. He outweighed me by eighty pounds. Following Hayashi's instructions, I was told to relax and use a Reverse Cat (Hook stance) properly positioned. When I pushed, my partner hurtled backward at least four feet. **T. Smith, 39 years' martial experience**

I was unable to hold my stance during push hands with a particular person until Hayashi told me to imagine I was wearing a leather jacket. I don't know why, but my partner could not uproot me.
R. Nakashima, career Tai Chi teacher

When conducting a slow wrist takedown, I had difficulty rotating my partner's wrist against his resistance. I was asked to bounce my Ki to the floor then direct it into my partner's left shoulder. The results were amazing. My partner was unable to offer any resistance whatsoever.
T. Zhua, 40 years' experience

Being a large man, I've been very effective using my size against most students, particularly in standing grappling exchanges applying grips and locks or resisting them. Strangely, I noticed the tide changing when a long-term training partner, one hundred pounds lighter, demonstrated a surprising advantage over me using Kiko. His power to weight ratio defied comprehension. My only recourse was to meet him on that same plane. I've since become a Kiko advocate.
B. Giangrande, 37 years' experience

I find myself able to uproot individuals from their stances using Hayashi's process called Gating. It's freaky how well it works.
B. Vivas, 15 years' experience

I was shocked by Hayashi's strength using the Motobu fist in a Neihanchi stance. He shrugged me off his back with incredible force. I went flying three feet away, even though I outweighed him by thirty pounds and was trying my best to prevent him from rotating. I also had a high dan-ranked Kyokushin teacher try to resist my press down of his middle block. It was tough to even budge him using my natural strength. After I gated and pressed, his arm flopped over as if it had no strength whatsoever. Lastly, at a social gathering I was approached by a martial

artist who got a bit testy. At one point I demonstrated my one-inch Kiko punch. He lifted completely off his feet and slammed into the counter behind him. Even I was shocked how powerful my strike had been.
J. Austin, 50 years' experience

Most young martial artists today do not realize that modern martial arts have separated from their yogic (internal) principles at the turn of the century. As an example, no one prior to Hayashi had ever been able to stop me from thrusting my right arm forward with them resisting with both hands in a strong posture. Hayashi held me with one hand. I couldn't even get my arm out of the chamber. This level of 'technical' knowledge has disappeared in the mainstream martial arts.
A. Mitsugi, 65 years' experience

Hayashi's insight into the Kiko aspects of kata are brilliant. They were developed over 25 years of responsible research which resulted in subtle changes in body movement and position that greatly enhance the practitioner's energy (ki) and power. These discoveries can inform and improve the kata experience in any style. I experienced some of the effects firsthand. I highly recommend, this book to every serious practitioner of the Martial Arts. **D. Shapiro, 39 years' experience**

I had flown to southern Texas for a vacation with a former member of our dojo who was studying Bagua. He was built like a fire plug and a skilled fighter. At some point we started horsing around when he asked me to push him. Recalling Hayashi's instructions, I pushed. He went flying. He was dumbstruck. He told me no one prior had ever been able to budge him from his posture. **T. Marotti, 51 years' experience**

While on an out of state business trip, I discovered several associates also studied martial arts. At one point I asked them to try and overpower my wrist. They could not budge my arm with their best efforts. Coming from an engineering background I was skeptical of Kiko at first, but admittedly, it's amazing how the techniques work.
N. Buccherri, 25 years' experience

I am 91 years old. I can make my arm feel like a steel rod using the Kiko techniques I learned from Hayashi. Equally amazing, is how much more aware I've become of both my physical and mental potential since study-ing Kiko. **E. Leithead, 12 years' experience**

The two of us, both big men, had trouble slow escaping from each oth-er's cross-hand wristlock using a move from the Neihanchi kata. Hayashi recommended we visualize a counter-clockwise ring rotating around our gripped wrist. We were utterly surprised at the ease of the release. It

didn't seem real given the fact that neither of us could break the other's grip without great effort.
B. Tighe, 22 years' experience. C. Bracco, 7 years' experience

I tried a shoulder strike with a dojo member with and without Kiko. My non-Kiko attempt was marginal. When I applied Kiko, I was shocked at the result. My partner went flying backward, stunned at the force of my blow. Another time, at a party for friends and family, some of the guys wanted to arm wrestle. One of the ladies joined in. She didn't have a chance. I told her to try again. Just before she and her male challenger started, I tapped his liver meridian with my foot. She beat him hands down—no contest. Such is the disruptive power on another's electrical field with slight touch. **R. Andrade, 34 years' experience**

I was one of the first senior students to work with Hayashi in the early years of his Kiko research. Early on, I noted in amazement, how slight adjustments in hand and finger positions led to significant strength shifts in the body. One of the more extraordinary revelations came years later—the ability to shut down another's energy purely by thought projection alone. **J. Noonan, 53 years' experience**

The highlight of Kiko for me has been its usefulness as an energy management tool and the constant reassurance that the correct details, factors that mainstream martial artists rarely consider, make a significant impact. Kiko helped me to realize that competence and power are the result of lots of little things done well, which can swing the balance of power in your favor. **T. Maloney, 20 years' experience**

I was extremely skeptical of Kiko at first. Even though the results of test after test worked, I still thought it was just the power of suggestion. One day, my teacher and I were both surprised when a test failed. Shifu looked at my stance and announced that I had negated the results by having my back foot turned outward. That's when I realized Kiko could not just be based solely upon self-suggestion, for we had both expected the technique to succeed. I could also never tell if a Kiko technique would actually make me stronger. The game-changing moment came one day; I was going to try and break my partner's stance using Kiko in a Naihanchi bunkai. In one attempt, before pushing him, I felt I would bounce right off, but when I shifted my breathing, and my awareness shifted, I knew that I would barrel through him like he wasn't even standing there. **D. Winograd, 25 years' experience**

After earning my black belt, I was invited to become a member of the Sanchin Seven, a senior group of students studying the internal aspects of Sanchin Kata. This was like nothing I had ever done before.

The strength difference in technique properly applied was remarkable.
S. Rago, 37 years' experience

As a small female practitioner, I have seen dramatic increases in strength when correctly organizing both my physical and Subtle Body through Kiko. This has allowed me to execute techniques effectively against men much heavier and stronger than myself. Slight reorganizations of breath, visualization, or seemingly insignificant physical movements prior to the execution of a technique have led to consistent and formidable results. Particularly intriguing: Simply imagining energy moving in a particular direction in the moments before attempting to push a partner has made the difference between feeling I've hit a brick wall and being able to send someone fifty pounds heavier than myself hurtling across the room. **A. Lyons, 20 years' experience**

It became unmistakably clear after a few simple tests that holding a cell phone versus not holding one had an overall weakening affect upon my physical strength.
C. E. Goedecke, brother of the author, no martial experience

I was initially very excited to be introduced to Kiko principles and techniques, so much so that I was hoping to find some valid scientific means of testing the why and how such significant outcomes occurred. The question that looms for me is how effective such techniques would be in a real world, violent encounter. I look forward to this question being answered in the future. **N. Armitage 40 years' experience**

I was seventeen, standing at my high school locker, when Anthony, the school tough, spun me around to grapple. As I turned, I placed my hands on his chest and pushed. To my surprise he flew backward across the hall and crashed into the adjacent lockers. It wasn't until I began studying Kiko four decades later that I understood the reason for the remarkable strength and ease of my push that day. Although some people may have a spontaneous moment in which everything connects, Kiko is the art that makes sense of it all. **J. Murphy 25 years' experience**

I had done about fifteen Sanchins concentrating on my hands, my breath, and packing Ki into my dantien. My hands became unbelievably hot, even though I was training outside in 35 degree weather. I also used to have trouble breathing through my nose. Kiko breathwork remedied the issue. The alignment of breath, body motion and intent really helped me to organize internally and brought home the impressive magnitude of power possible to obtain through Kiko study.
E. Camarata, 23 years' experience

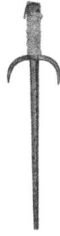

Marking the Trail

This book places a series of trail markers amidst the vast and intricate passages of the Martial Ways. These markers fall neither at the beginning nor at the end of the journey. It is my hope they open new trailheads for some of you into truly pristine martial backcountry.

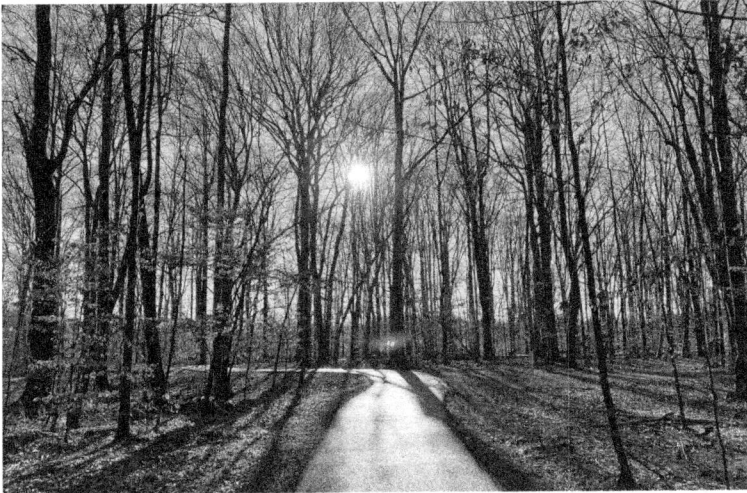

Walk with Me

When asked how I prefer to be addressed in my professional capacity, I tell people to simply call me *Hayashi*. It is my given Buddhist name. I find this informality avoids unnecessary barriers. Although I hold the formal title of *Shifu*, I've long known that everyone has something to offer, even the novice. The key is to become porous to our surroundings, for wisdom can reside in the most inconspicuous of places and one must be ready to grasp it when the opportunity presents itself. Nothing could be truer than the main subject of this book, *Kiko*. Kiko is an *electrifying,* art-with-in-an-art sitting right under our noses—but so few catch its scent, hence, the subtitle, *Hidden Power - Electric Moves. Effortless power* generated by the body's bioelectrical system hides behind the thinnest of mental veils. With the right explanations, which I hope to present, anyone reading this book can experience a significant and instant boost in their overall strength for any task, martial or otherwise. Although Kiko is unique to the fighting arts of Okinawa, its value weaves through every martial art taught in the world.

A Bodhisattva Warrior monk pointed out that there was a time in the classical history of the martial arts when the *Sensei* was regarded as a person who taught the *physical* mechanics of one's art while the *Shifu* was the teacher adept at instructing in the art's *non-physical, spiritual* or *Energy* mechanics. I endeavor to live up to that monk's description. This book is an extension of my aspiration as a *Shifu* with the above distinction to share what I have learned about the martial Ways, human power, subtle human energy, and spiritual action in the pursuit of martial excellence, and how you can access your own untapped powers.

The revolutionary discovery about traditional martial arts lies in an emerging awareness about the interpenetrating energy fields science has discovered exist in and around our bodies, and how past masters used these fields as evidenced in the construction of their fighting forms. This book will bring what I believe was once a visceral feeling into conscious light in a way that anyone interested in this subject can apply to their own practices.

What led me to this subject? I will start with my background.

I was ushered into the U.S. imported, traditional Asian martial culture of the late 1960's before commercialization had a death grip on its future. The training was tough, straightforward, and heavily infused with a military air from the returning servicemen who had claimed their coveted black belt overseas and begun to teach in their hometowns. The art was presented as a no-frills, ballistic-centered discipline with its mysterious addendum—*Kata*, a warrior dance we magically hoped would make sense.

Zoom ahead fifty-five years. I have since lived a full-time, martial art teaching life. My formal introduction into Okinawan karate began in 1968 at age seventeen at the International School of Judo and Karate in suburban Summit, New Jersey. We informally called our dojo, *Bank Street*, named after the side street the school was accessed. Bank Street was one of the pioneering martial arts schools in the U.S. It opened in 1962 initially offering judo instruction. Karate followed like a gangbuster in 1965, eventually nudging judo out. The Bank Street dojo permanently shuttered in 1982 due to a fire in an unrelated first floor business, but not before leaving its indelible footprint in its untold martial history.

Bank Street's teaching roster included some of the North East coast's top Judo and Karate sensei; Shimamoto Mamoru, All Japan Judo Champion; Yoshisada Yonezuka, (1937-2014) head coach of the U.S. Olympic Judo Team. Robert Murphy (1937-2007), Isshin Shorin Ji Ryu Okinawa-Te founder; Gary Alexander, Isshinryu Plus founder; Edward Doyle, Goju headmaster under the American Gojuryu master Peter Urban, and William Scott Russell, founder of the Isshin Kempo system.

I am both a second and third generation American martial artist. The first generation studied directly with Asian teachers. My formal teaching career began at twenty years of age as a wet behind the ears, junior instructor in 1971. Since then, I have had an extraordinarily long and unbroken profession which has allowed me to teach unobstructed nearly every day for over half a century.

My three teachers at Bank Street in succession were Robert Murphy, Frank Brita, one of Murphy's senior black belts, and lastly, and most influential, W. S. Russell, author of *Karate: The Energy Connection,* (Dell, 1976), also a student of Sensei Murphy. Russell founded Isshin Kempo (IK) as an extension of Okinawan Isshinryu. IK was officially recognized a martial system in 1970 by Albert Church (1930-1980), a noted Shorinji Tetsukempo Kamishin Ryu master from South Carolina.

Isshin Kempo has since evolved into a close quarter, Hard/Soft fighting art excelling at both ballistic and standing grappling technique. We use all the Isshinryu kata of Tatsuo Shimabuku. We consider Isshin Kempo, Isshinryu's *Internal* sister art for we have discovered some amazing principles embedded within its fighting forms, the main subject of this work.

Usually, it is all too familiar to hear about students moving from teacher to teacher. In my case, it was my sensei who moved on, replaced by different headmasters, each with different skill requirements. Fortunately, my martial education moved in a logical arc from long range, Shorin-based, Hard style karate, to short range, close quarter, Hard/Soft, Isshin kempo.

Several men distinguished themselves nationally as teachers in their respective disciplines after training at Bank Street while I served as a senior instructor; Tony Franco, became a noted East Coast Hung Gar expert, and Tom Bisio, became an international competitor. Today, he remains a respected author, healer, Xingyi and Taijiquan authority.

W.S. Russell's early boxing background led him to challenge the way karate kata was being performed in the 1970's, the hay days of American martial arts. Aligning with Brue Lee's critique, Russell felt that our martial katas were being performed unrealistically and grossly under-interpreted. Noting that karate students seldom fought like they executed their kata, he sought to close this gap with a stronger connection between its traditional Forms and its *jiu-kumite* (free fighting). Russell was an articulate, charismatic teacher who presented diverse ideas from his relationships with Robert Murphy (Isshin Shorinji ryu Okinawa Te), William Chung (Hung Gar), Gin Foon Mark (Southern Praying Mantis), and Edward Smith (*Hokushin Aiki Bujutsu*).

I found time between my teaching responsibilities to add intensive study of Yang style Tai Chi Chu'an with master Sidney Austin (1925-1993), then a senior student of the noted Taiwanese master Jou Tsung Hwa (1917-1998). I continue to evolve my knowledge of the monastic side of martial arts with Shifu, Arakawa Mitsugi, a Japanese-trained Aiki Budo expert and Bodhisattva Warrior Monk from Tennessee, currently head of the *Wu Hsin Tao*. I studied Aikido briefly in the 1970's with *Shihan* Rick Stickles (1950-2015). Sensei Stickles was one of the first Caucasian Aikido teachers in the U.S., a senior student of Yoshimitsu Yamada, a direct disciple of Aikido's founder, Morihei Ueyshiba. I studied an esoteric form of the Sanchin kata under the guidance of Aston Hugh, an East Coast martial art kata expert with over seventy years' experience. Hugh is adept in Isshinryu, Goju, Tai Chi, and *Liu He Ba Fa* (Water Boxing).

Late in my career, in 2009, I became a Bodhisattva Warrior monk in the Chen Yen Shingon Mikkyo Mi Ching sect of Buddhism after studying the teachings of the British martial scholar and Kempo master, Nagaboshi Tomio (1946-2005) and exchanging ideas with his successor, Shifu Arakawa Mitsugi

The Chen Yen Shingon Mikkyo Mi Ching is a liberal sect of Southern Chinese Esoteric Buddhism, originally created for Buddhist bodyguards during the Ming dynasty. My personal ideology fit well with the Chen Yen School teachings. Aside from its practical self-defense aims, we use martial kata and kumite as a means to further personal development. The difference between what I do and teach, and mainstream martial training, lies partly in our practice of kata as a self-unraveling meditation to reveal one's essential nature. Esoteric martial Buddhism takes training beyond the fight toward specific inner experiences through the regulation of the breath, body posturing, visualizations and other internal foci to bring about radical shifts in consciousness.

It has never been the goal of the martial arts to perpetuate fighting. Its central aim has been to quell violence, establish peace, and exhibit its potential in the competitive arena. The martial arts offer individuals the means to bring all these ends about. In the monasteries of Asia this goal seeped into their mental and spiritual aspirations. The idea emerged to take the fight to the *enemy within*—our own discordances. We've never needed this dual-bladed tool as much as we do today; the ability to intelligently fight imbalances with the aim to establish peace. All martial arts stand upon a foundation of empowerment, and for those of *Right Aim,* teach their adherents how to direct their powers ultimately to a life of the *Triple Harmonies*; harmony within oneself, harmony with the environment, and harmony with the Heavens. At its highest realization, the authentic self that emerges from the pursuit of the three Harmonies is where I believe the pinnacle of human power lies.

Kiko and The Dō

Modern people train themselves to ignore anomalies.
Dr. Lewis Mehl-Madrona

Two decades into my teaching career I unexpectedly stumbled headlong into *internal* karate-dō principles, what Chinese martial artists refer to as *Neigong,* and some old-world Okinawan masters called *Kiko*.

These Kiko revelations radically altered my ideas about the underlying nature of *all* formal martial disciplines regardless of culture or generation. I believe Kiko is where the true *spirit* of the martial arts dwells, a position I will unravel in this book. Its principles were once highly prized by the monks of Shaolin and remained secret from mainstream practitioners. According to the late Kempo expert, Nagaboshi Tomio, prior to 1900 the study of the most advanced forms of Kempo were known to only a few

noble families and their trusted students. It was practiced in se-
crecy after having to swear many vows and was regarded as highly dangerous. In this study, there were no grades or ranks, only
masters and students. Nor were there competitions. Kumite and
Kata were strictly controlled. Any fights engaged were continued
to the death. The manner in which one trained and understood
the art reflected such an approach and was restricted to those
who had knowledge of the Chinese classics, religious literature,
and their related traditions.

Today, such teachings are mostly lost to time, relegated to
small pockets of teachers as evidenced by the scarcity of knowledge and clear dialog about their workings. I say this because
there has been almost no attention on why the limb configurations and actions of many Asian movement sets were selected
with the exception of narrow spikes of focus given to a Form's
hidden *bunkai* or *kyusho* technique. Within most Hard style curriculums, Kiko knowledge is entirely absent, yet its wisdom remains
firmly rooted, though stubbornly buried, in its essential Forms.

I never thought I'd be discussing Quantum physics as a martial teacher, but at the turn of the 20th century a scientific theory emerged about the nature of reality that not only challenged
modern scientific theories, but turned many on their heads. Quantum physics offered a pleasant aeration of many classical scientific dogmas.

As a result of this pioneering science, a minority of body professionals have come to realize that within the body's biomechanical laws seems to lie a previously unseen platform of *bioenergetic*
laws. This Kiko subflooring, in my opinion, forms the foundation of
real human power. I contend some high-end martial art masters
knew about this subtle infrastructure and incorporated its quantum mechanisms into their combative systems.

Martial artists reading this book may be hearing about the art
of Kiko for the first time, even though they may be long term practitioners of Okinawan Karate or other fighting arts. In the pages to follow I will outline the major Kiko principles I discovered
that underly all our physical movements and movement arts. Kiko
compliments known biomechanical principles like our right and
left hands, yet, few martial artists will experience this dimension
within their training.

This book also shares my personal journey over the last half
century into and through martial life as it was supplanted in West-

ern culture, and, in particular, my engagement with the interlacing of its three primary pillars; the practical, therapeutic, and meditative dimensions. Kiko weaves through these three realms with the Dō serving as its interlinking thread.

Few students question why the movements of their particular systems are assembled and taught the way they are; why *these* basics, *these* fighting sequences in *this* order, *this* selection of Forms, *this* pacing? Should they question, they may become perplexed by the sheer variety of existing methods and occasionally, the vagueness of the answers. In my opinion, martial arts have advanced with significant aspects of its core nature missing from modern curriculums, with few of its teachers the wiser. The West has perpetuated a martial pedagogy, worshiping only what is readily seen. What we can't see, we can't teach, and we can't practice because, for all practical purposes, it doesn't exist. I want to shed some light on a vital aspect of traditional, kata based martial arts that I never saw, and that many within our martial community still don't see. I call it Kiko.

沖縄気功

What is Kiko?

Kiko is an old word found in Okinawa's *Hogen* or *Uchinaguchi*, (Okinawan language) dialect. Its literal meaning is "to hear" or "to listen." Today, depending on the context and the dialect of Okinawan language being used, "Kiko" can have different meanings. In Okinawan culture, the term "Kiko" is also commonly used in the practice of the traditional form of Japanese energy work known as "Ki" or "Qigong." This is a category of training found amongst a broad collection of contemporary Asian systems and practices aimed at activating and exercising the body's *internal* forces. In this context, "Kiko" refers to the ability to both sense and manipulate the flow of Ki (energy) within the body and surrounding environment.

Okinawan Hogen is a dying dialect today limited to certain regions and communities in Okinawa. Therefore, the meaning and usage of the word "Kiko" in Hogen may not be widely understood or recognized by younger generations or non-native speakers of the language.

From my vantage, I find Okinawan Kiko standing in a class of its own, particularly in the fact that it is embedded in the kata of the Island's fighting systems. Within the structure of the essential fighting forms of Okinawan lies a brilliant power infrastructure in the selection and sequencing of its techniques. Most Qigong today deals primarily with energy flow in regard to health and well-being, far less so in terms of its martial *chikara* (power/force). Rare is the teacher able to articulate Qigong's complexities and dimensionality in their Hard style martial systems.

According to the British kata adept, Ian Abernathy, the West's adoption of Asian fighting Forms has only scratched their surface; "The katas contain a vast amount of martial knowledge; *Atemi-waza* (striking techniques), *Kyusho-jitsu* (attacking vital points), *Tuidi* (releasing techniques), *Te-gumi* (grappling), *Kansetsu-waza* (dislocating joints), *Shime-waza* (chokes & strangles), *Gyakyu-waza* (counters), *Ne-waza* (ground fighting), *Nage-waza* (throws & takedowns) etc."

Running beneath all of the aforementioned technical categories, lies a subsystem so fundamental that when activated will *electrify* all the above expressions. Up until now however, this system has remained locked in the gut as a visceral reality, out of sight, hence, out of mind. However, there does exist a lens through which anyone can witness Kiko's behavior. This lens is the capacity of heightened senses, when directed where and how to look, to consciously experience its mechanisms. Talking about Kiko, or seeing it demonstrated, pales to experiencing it for yourself. Therefore, this work only points the way.

A typical Qigong practitioner, martial or otherwise, or an acupuncturist would not be able to easily determine whether one's right wrist was more resistant to a wrist lock, or that a particular manner of stepping or breathing could easily uproot another's grounded stance merely as a result of a specific bodily (or mental) posture *prior* to the action.

The tip of Okinawa's Kiko iceberg is most evident in its *Tuite* and *Kyusho* (vital point striking) systems based upon meridian theory, which we can now say has a root in quantum physics. Martial Kiko is the study of Ki to amplify our technique either by physical or mental means, or a combination of the two methods.

To give the term contemporary relevancy I define Kiko as *Energy Breathing*—the movement of invisible, intrinsic, tide-like, interpenetrating energy currents. To make sure I could take this liberty, I consulted my *yudansha*, Diamond Wave, who provided the following analysis of the above kanji.

> The first part (沖縄) is Okinawa. The second, with the first character being *ki* as in energy, our understanding of ki, and the second being the first character in kung fu. The reason the compound is so familiar is that 気功, pronounced kiko with a long o, is literally 'qigong' in Japanese. So, the kanji for kiko are, rather fittingly, "Okinawan qigong". To translate the kanji in the "qigong" part, they're "spirit/energy" (ki) 気 followed by what my dictionary lists as "achievement, merits, success, honor, credit", but I'd describe the nuance as "achievement through hard work/cultivation" (ko) 功.

> I think the existing characters cover the idea [of energy breathing] you have in mind, but here's a long tangent about linguistics to explain.

> "Energy work" is a good translation for this kanji, but there is lots of room for interpretation in the existing characters. The character we use for ki (気) can indicate air (for instance, 空気 is atmosphere in the sense of ambiance, 天気 is weather, etc.). 気 is derived directly from one of the traditional Chinese characters for qi (氣) where the 气 is a radical indicating breath/steam and the 米 indicates rice, such that the compound would suggest a nourishing energy. Sometimes it's treated as energy derived from nourishment ("the steam coming off rice"), but I think it could also function more like "breath = rice/nourishment" as a nod to those monks who survived by "eating qi" or foregoing food and treating the qi from the air as nourishment.
> I think the character for ki (気) itself is where we find the "breath" in the kiko/qigong compound (気功). It's essentially a double entendre for "energy work" and "breath work", because ki (気) suggests energy coming from the breath.

> My other related thought is that I can't readily find a second character pronounceable as "ko" which would suggest breath, so if kiko has been translated as "spirit breath/spirit breathing/energy breathing" etc. in the past, it probably still used these kanji. The ko (呼) in the common word for breath "kokyuu" 呼吸 isn't actually the part that indicates breathing, rather it's a kanji that means something more like "call" or "invite", while the kyuu (吸) suggests inhalation. Moreover, the single character word for breath

27

(息) is pronounced "iki" on its own or "soku" in a compound, and the compound 気息 (*kisoku*) just means "breathing".

I take further freedom to upgrade the Kiko definition to *quantum movement*, moving a collective of atomic forces outside of normal perceptive range. I believe that Kiko emerged from the observations and intuitions of some premodern Asian masters of the behavior of the human Energy Body to become a study for deriving personal power from manipulating our Ki. We can move Ki without moving our physical bodies but we cannot move our physical bodies without moving Ki.

I understand there are Kiko, *Chinkuchi*, and *Aiki* experts who refuse to use the term Ki due to its lack of scientific proof. This reminds me of an indirectly related comment from a spiritual healer, *"You don't have to know the name of the thief to know that your house was robbed."* We have witnessed valid behaviors historically labelled as Ki-based despite precise modern scientific rationales currently remaining speculative. Science has some catching up to determine the cause of outcomes I have consistently observed that do not fit our biomechanical models.

Kiko is the art of cultivating and directing subtle human energies for the trifold purpose of increasing mental and physical power, health, and personal and spiritual growth.

Kiko's principles can be found embedded in all the essential Fighting Forms of Okinawa, although many of these forms need to have 'the rust and dust' removed to restore their potent formulaic luster. You would think something so profound, underpinning all human activity, would be the talk of the day. Yet, Kiko appears to be known to only a small fraction of the world's martial community.

I am aware that Kiko holds much broader, life-enhancing implications. However, the main focus in this book will be on Kiko's *martial* use. Here, its principles are most evident today in *Kyusho*, pressure point technique, but Kiko's wider context appears absent in practices outside of a minority of Internal schools.

The word 'subtle,' in the context of subtle energy, requires an acute sensitivity for detecting shifts in our surrounding invisible fields and their effects upon us. It takes time to turn the mind's eye inward deep enough to grasp the power and importance of a Kiko system and acute enough to actually feel one's Biofield. At present, Kiko remains an unexplored novelty to the bulk of Western practitioners.

I consider Kiko the fifth and highest level of training within five essential layers of martial Formwork. Those five layers are; Tools, Tactics, Strategy, State of Mind, and Intrinsic Energy flow. Kiko, the last layer, is the most difficult level to master because it requires both a high degree of intelligence and a heightened body sensitivity. This makes Kiko less accessible to the general martial population, evidenced in how little the current profession- al community understands the potential depth behind their own techniques. Kiko is the art that bridges matter and spirit through the conscious infusion of *spirit* (quantum laws) into one's fighting technique.

Lastly, I must dispel the myth that Kiko guarantees one will trump a non-Kiko practitioner. Kiko is not an excuse to abandon hard, physical training. Kiko is an enhancement to external prac- tice, another training tier. When Hard style (biomechanical) prin- ciples are combined with Soft style (bioenergetic) principles, you have a *complete*, authentic, and powerful art.

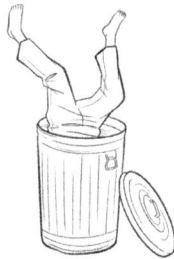

Trashed

I must comment on those few videos of Hard style professionals pummeling internal experts in open challenges. It is a mistake to think that internal work guarantees victory in the ring. External competency is a force to be reckoned. I wondered why these internal practitioners did not fall back on their external skill sets, until I realized, they likely overestimated their Soft technique. Thinking that Ki manipulation will solve every issue is akin to the Feng Shui novice who believed that placing a red couch in the south corner of his living room would bring him a new job. As a wise Feng Shui master quipped, "Work on your resume first!" Earning a black belt doesn't defeat your bullies. Proper applica- tion of your skills does.

Of all the dimensions I have explored, Kiko yielded the keenest insight regarding the essence of the Martial Ways. I never imag- ined the sheer depth and breadth of knowledge that went into the composition of the essential Asian Fighting Forms. Kiko cast the clearest light on why martial technique and its kata were conveyed in such exacting detail. Even though Kiko seemed an elusive study initially, once I experienced its effects in practice, I was hard pressed to deny its viability and importance to any fighting system.

I am tossing the subject of Kiko into the martial arena to challenge, refresh, restore, and raise the bar of excellence we professionals strive for. But I am not a holy crusader madly driven to convince you of Kiko's merits. I wrote this book primarily to make Kiko's presence known by opening a trailhead into the subject and to chronicle the story of my own martial journey and revelations along the way. What you do with this information remains your path to unfold.

I can tell you with certainty that every physical movement you perform will cause internal currents to move in a precise fashion leading to a range of consequences in both immediate and successive martial motions. I have witnessed in the simplest of moves, the most profound reactions.

Because I had no consistent formal guidance into Kiko study save for my dogged persistence to know more and my unrelenting intuition and personal investigations, the language I will use to describe Kiko will not entirely be that of a formal, Asian-trained martial internalist.

Only after I had both aged and matured in my art, did the spiritual significance of martial arts take on more relevance in my life and Kiko's grand value loom into view. I never entered the martial arts to fight. I joined to learn how to avoid conflict and, if necessary, to protect myself intelligently. Within the skill sets the martial arts offered me, I found both my manhood and my place in my community, and have since secured a peaceful existence. I also found a means to grow and maintain my wonderment for the dynamism of everyday life. The Dō of the traditional martial arts couldn't be expounded upon enough in my opinion, for it broadens the scope of martial training well beyond the physical arena and its, sometimes, restrictively narrow focus solely on personal combat for those wanting a more comprehensive presentation. Don't get me wrong. I choose the fighting art's lethality—along with its enlightenments. I believe that martial technique taught without its underpinning spiritual tenets and a firm philosophical platform conveys only half the martial story. Martial arts taught exclusively as a physical pursuit represents a fraction of the benefits the traditional arts offer. The *Upanishads*, one of the oldest spiritual works in Indian culture, reinforces this notion by stating that neither the body nor the mind alone can bring us to the apex of our potential. We need the alchemical mix of both. The far less travelled frontiers of consciousness, mind, and spirit await the willing adventurer.

The essence of the martial arts, as wisely understood by the Okinawan masters, lies in the concept of the *Sanchin* or *Three Battles*; the three primary struggles or frictions we encounter in life as we try to harmonize head, heart and spirit toward a life of authenticity, peace and well-being.

I hope you find some refreshing potential in this book to broaden how you think about your art. This subject might also answer some long-standing questions as to why martial *kihon* (basic technique) and its Form work (Jp. *kata*, Ch. *Hsing*, Korean, *Poomse* or *Hyung*) can vary so widely from school to school, and why the old masters were so adamant their technique and Forms were practiced to their full depth with such precision.

I have divided the book into four parts. Part One tells my story of how my foray into the internal nature of martial life began. Part Two is a brief overview of critical revelations uncovered during my thirty years of on-going research which profoundly influenced my physical and mental well-being. Part three dives into each of the observations in more detail. Part Four answers pertinent questions students have asked over the years relevant to the subject of this book. (Unattributed quotes throughout this work are the authors).

PART 1

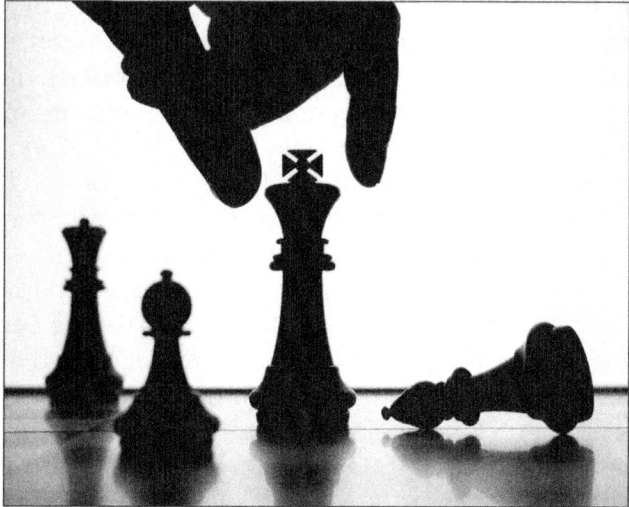

Ki Finds Me

*The universe has its own plans
of which we are sometimes players, sometimes pawns.*

Exceptional Power

I am a straight-shooting teacher. I have observed that what you believe is what you see, and what you see is what you get. Train hard and intelligently and you will go far in these arts. But training that challenges your foundational beliefs can completely alter your martial trajectory into truly pristine frontiers.

As a young karate teacher in 1971, I was marginally aware of the subject of *Qigong*, Internal, or *Ki* work. The idea of some 'invisible' or 'secretive' energy never grabbed my mind in any significant way. I assumed that any serious practitioner would develop his or her *inner* power as a normal byproduct of hard, committed practice. I never had a face-to-face encounter with anyone claiming to be an Internal expert or use Subtle Energy on me in my early years of training. I do, however, recall three events where I encountered unusually powerful martial technique that did not match my idea of power-to-weight performance. Because these three events left a strong impression upon me, and may have been the early catalysts sparking my later research, they merit explanation.

The first event occurred in 1971, during an adult karate class at the Bank Street Dojo. This particular night, Sensei William Scott Russell, an articulate 6'2", 185 lb., twenty-seven-year-old, Caucasian teacher of Welsh descent, decided to demonstrate what we in the class later deemed, the *slow punch*. This radical young sensei, seven years my senior, casually asked us what we thought of the force behind the punch he would demonstrate in the air. Russell had exceptional hand speed. Disappointingly, he tossed out a vertical fist strike so matter-of-fact that, honestly, I didn't think much of it at all. He then walked over to me, told me to brace myself and struck me in the abdomen with that same *matter of fact* slowness. I was exceptionally fit. I could take a strong fist blow to my torso. Not that punch. To this day, I still recall my abdominal muscle separating like I had been hit with a sledgehammer.

It took me several years to duplicate Russell's feat. I wouldn't say it was a hidden power, or the result of Ki. I came to understand it as the consequence of a relaxed, uninhibited, well-trained and focused strike, an enviable goal for any martial student

My second encounter with unusual power came seven years later. I had taken up additional study in Yang style Tai Chi Chuan with the noted New Jersey master, Sidney Austin. Austin had invited me to train after I had arranged for him to appear on *Talent Today*, a live, Manhattan cable TV interview. He and I, along with his teacher, Jou Tsung Hwa, were each given a twenty-minute slot to demonstrate our skills. As compensation for his media exposure, Sidney, a big-boned, soft-spoken, mild-mannered, career teacher, offered me one free year of Tai Chi lessons. I accepted, with the idea that his soft, Tai Chi training might complement my Hard karate practice.

One day Sidney chose me to demonstrate his slow-moving, two-handed Tai Chi push. How bad could a slow-motion push be? It had to be easier to absorb than Russell's belly buster. I didn't pay much heed to the wrestling mat vertically affixed to the wall roughly two feet behind me. When Master Austin pushed, I lifted completely off the ground and slammed into the wall with such force I nearly had the wind knocked out of me.

Here was another event done slowly, yet demonstrably powerful and impressive. Again, it took me a bit of time, but like Bruce Lee's one-inch punch, a punch, a push, a pull, isn't done solely with the arms but with the whole body to add significant weight to the action. Anyone with focused, consistent training can accomplish these two feats when they learn to put their body behind their strikes.

My third encounter with exceptional power came while attending a pressure point seminar with the Pennsylvanian, Kyusho expert, George Dillman. Dillman has travelled the world displaying his impressive skills and has created a highly effective community of pressure point experts. He struck me in the forearm with a quick, short chop. Although Dillman did not knock me unconscious, as he often did with his prime subjects, his light *shuto* buckled my legs and momentarily reset my brain. For such slight impact, Dillman's strike had profound consequences. It was a strange irony that as my mind shut down from his 'tap', it simultaneously woke me up to the enormous power inherent in our arts.

As a sidebar, although I find pressure point study fascinating. I side in thinking with the British martial author, Nathan Johnson, Fundamental problems exist working with its efficacy. First, point work can be dangerous to play with, especially if you are an older adult over forty, according to Dillman. I recall a conversation with a noted high-dan, Gojuryu expert who shared that while attending a strike-point seminar he was knocked unconscious and never felt right afterward. Months later, he suffered a heart attack. Although he could not prove his heart attack was directly related to that seminar event, he attributed it to that single, disruptive strike to his body that day.

The second observation is that pressure point strikes do not always produce equal results, and sometimes have no effect at all on certain individuals. Pressure points are not easy to execute in a freestyle interaction against someone skilled in blocking, striking or grappling. A talented martial artist, lacking pressure point knowledge may not only deflect most strikes but can be lethal in their own right with well-directed blunt force trauma and deft grappling skills. Lastly, and rarely talked about, the reason I bring up this sidenote, is that Kiko forms the underlying platform for effective pressure point study. A Kiko expert can 'seal' meridians against a variety of point attacks. However, pressure point strikes are impressive when they work.

If Ki was behind the technique I experienced, I did not see it. I felt that anyone engaged in earnest training would likely release this mysterious force in their martial technique over time. Therefore, I didn't look any further than my own three-to-six-hour daily workouts. As for my lack of knowledge about Ki, I was a typically trained Hard stylist. The idea never interfered with my busy teaching career in any way. I instructed hundreds of students weekly, year after year for decades, turning out excellent martial artists despite my Ki-*less* curriculum.

All that changed the day I became aware of what I began to call my *Energy Body* and its deceptive power potential. A single event working with the Frogman turned my art completely upside down.

Frogman and the Elusive 'Effortless Power' Paradigm

In 2012, I published, *Internal Karate: Mind Matters and The Seven Gates of Power*. In this book I shared a brief story of a benign training event that caused a major shift in my career both as a teacher and avid, multi-decade student. The story to follow explains how and why over the ensuing years I began a personal quest to investigate what I began to call the *Art of Kiko*.

As a young man of seventeen in 1956, Joe Noonan joined the Navy and became a Frogman, precursor of the modern Navy Seals. He received top secret clearance and was sent abroad onto a new class of spy ship. Two decades later, nearing his forties, Joe accompanied his son into one of my martial art classes and took to the art like a frogman to water. From that point on, Joe faithfully arrived at my private studio every Thursday evening for thirty years to plunge the depths of martial arts with me. He eventually earned the Warrior name, *Stone,* as he became a permanent fixture in the dojo.

On this particular day, Stone and I had begun drilling several simple wristlock escapes, a staple in many martial art schools. Our drills were straightforward. We would grab each other's wrists and rehearse various escapes and counter-locks. Most jujitsu adepts know that the most common wrist releases use clockwise or counter-clockwise moves to break a grip, rather than the layman's impulse to rip their hand away with brute force. During one breaklock maneuver, Stone clenched my right wrist firmly in his right hand in a common, cross-hand grip; right grabbing right. Strangely, I escaped as if he barely held me. I commented that he ought to grip tighter next time. His reply startled me; "I was holding as tight as I could," he said.

Stone gripped me a dozen more times. Each time I tried what I believed was the identical motion, a tight clockwise arc chopping over the ulnar side of his wrist. I encountered his typical, firm resistance. I could not duplicate the elusive ease of my prior escape.

Clearly, the Frogman and I had experienced a strength anomaly. We agreed that my ease of escape was likely the result of some overlooked detail. So, we did what any good sleuths would do. We began to break down every physical nuance that might have influenced the anomalous outcome and tried the escape again and again, until we got it. I should add, we tried every nuance *we were aware of.* With hindsight, we had limited awareness. I don't mean this in any self-deprecating way. At that time, the Frogman and I had thirty-seven years of martial experience between us. We were experts at our craft with a very good technical grasp.

We eventually concluded that either Stone had lost strength, or I had magically gained some mysterious extra power. We even joked that I stole his strength and added it to my own. But honestly, we didn't have a clue why my escape had felt so effortless. Clearly something unusual had happened. Little did we know that we had crossed a major technical threshold into the vast terrain of internal martial study, the elusive art of Kiko.

That day with the Frogman, when I realized something out of the ordinary had occurred, I became interested in the concept of Ki. If Ki was behind the ease of my wrist release, I wanted to know how it connected to my martial technique. Could I find a clear, practical use for Ki that would elevate my martial art? If so, what degree of this energy's behavior might have been known to the early masters of India, China and Japan? Naturally, I focused my inquiries around the variables surrounding a physical conflict.

When threatened, assaulted, or engaged in intense competition, all our physical abilities are immediately summoned and challenged. In these situations, most people will undergo a broad range of physiological changes to prepare them for their heightened level of response. The senses sharpen, particularly sight and sound. Respiration amps. Breathing usually quickens and rises into the chest. The endocrine system swings into high gear dumping adrenaline into the blood stream. Large blood vessels dilate to shunt more blood to the limbs. The circulatory system cuts blood flow to non-essential organs and diverts oxygen and sugar to the primary muscles for fight or flight. The gastrointestinal system stops digesting, in some cases it forces the stomach to purge its contents. Emotions like fear or anger intensify. Healthy fear warns us. Healthy anger produces the necessary muscular charge to fight back or run like hell. The mind becomes hyper alert. There is no biological part of the human matrix unaffected by a serious threat or challenge to our person.

If every part of our being focuses on and diverts attention, information, and energy to our self-preservation when threatened, why wouldn't our Energy Body, our Ki, contribute to this process? And if it did—*what* and how did it contribute? My gut told me that our Energy Body does not remain inert, benign, or unaffected under such circumstances. I believed it comes to our defense as well.

Currently, science isn't sure if our Biofield, their term for Energy Body, adds to the event above, takes something away, or just produces background static. Science has done *zero* investigation into the effects of the Biofield or Ki Field on the human Flight or Fight response—*zero!*

Convinced that Ki, or my Energy Body added significantly to my physical power, I sought to prove it with hands-on practicality.

It made no sense to me that during the multi-thousand-year history of martial arts, *no one* noticed what their Ki, Energy Body, or Biofield might have added to their combative abilities. I also did not believe that modern civilization suddenly sprouted an Energy Body which older cultures lacked. If anything, ancient cultures had stronger Energy Bodies because they were closer to a purer, more pristine nature. As you will learn, nature is a force we can borrow from. It's more likely the reverse circumstance was true. Nature was far more central to the cosmology of the ancients giving them a much better grasp of its influences than modern technocratic societies. We may have our ever-advancing academic and scientific knowledge, illuminating what early cultures couldn't see, didn't understand, but perhaps, directly sensed. But we live in an increasingly synthetic, digitized, and physically-pacifying world. We may be able to 'see' a Ki field with high-tech instruments, but we are in our infancy in how to work with it outside of studying alternative Energy therapies like Qigong, Reiki, or Internal martial arts.

Evidence tells us that some prior cultures knew how to use their subtle energies as an extension of their overall power base. We have plenty of documentation of its functioning and behavior in Asian medical, martial and spiritual literature.

One thing is sure, the moment the concept of Chi, Ki, or *Prana*, (the equivalent term used by the yogis of India) burst into Asian consciousness, this immaterial, some insist palatable, force took its place in human history. Ki's non-physical nature-field was observed long before Western science bagged and tagged it as the Biofield. In my mind, Ki was the Asian umbrella term for behaviors observed in various disciplines that fell outside of the hard sciences of the day.

Martial Kiko emerged from the acute observations by past masters of the behavior of the human Energy Body in conflict with other human bodies to derive additional power from this invisible field. Kiko is the art of cultivating and manipulating the human Biofield to get our needs met.

For the ancient warrior, Kiko was a means to direct extraordinary power to defeat an opponent. The only problem, still extant, is that Kiko teachers remain a scarce commodity. Martial Kiko's cultivation and use requires not only a competent guide, but a committed, intelligent, sensitive and persevering student, attributes which the average person from any time period did not have a good deal of, or easy access to.

The term Kiko must not be confused with the Japanese word *Keiko*, which means, *practice*. I am referring to an old-world Okinawan martial term for *chi-kung*, more specifically, martial chi-kung. Kiko is the art of manipulating the Human Energy Field (HEF) to effect noteworthy strength changes in both yourself and/or your opponent/partner. Activating Kiko principles will make you markedly stronger and/or your partner significantly weaker. I have conducted thousands of tests with students of all ages from multiple martial disciplines demonstrating these principles with repeated success. I assert that the patterns of the primary kata or Fighting Forms of China, Okinawa, Korea, India and Japan are all Kiko-based.

Kiko is different from simply 'being strong' from biomechanically-induced strength training or posturing. First, strength is not a constant variable. It can wildly fluctuate with the flow of Ki into and out of your muscle tissue, which you can consciously control. Your bicep, for example, is only as strong as the energy and mental resolve you bring into it. If the nerves to your bicep were severed, no matter how large, those muscles will not contract. Likewise, as you will see, without Kiko activated, you might completely fail to break out of another's grip. With Kiko properly applied, you might escape *effortlessly*. This observation alone makes the subject worth investigating.

Rather than a step-by-step manual for applying Kiko, I offer readers a personal tour into the many rooms of the Kiko mansion to whet your appetite to explore this subject further.

The Hunt Begins in Earnest

Through trial, error, and deductive reasoning, Stone and I investigated our effortless power enigma, hoping to repeat my 'too-easy-to-be-true' wrist escape.

We eventually duplicated the feat. But we couldn't comprehend why it had felt *effortless*. We weren't striking, tapping, rubbing or pressing any acupoint(s)—*to our knowledge*. We weren't aware of doing anything different in our execution from all the hundreds of other practices we had done. So why had I escaped so easily from Stone's grip? We weren't looking for a mystical or magical justification. We were two practical-minded martial disciples seeking a sound explanation. It was obvious that something outside of our awareness had triggered a powerful escape.

Our first platform for investigation was to look closely at the micro-mechanics of the body. We revisited stances, leveraging angles, distance, breath, sidedness (right versus left side), timing, and other positional possibilities; the time of day, lunar cycles, clothing. I started journaling my observations and the outcomes of our experiments in detail in 1994. We broadened our scope of technique to include the patterns of the Okinawan kata for further clues. Isshinryu karate, my source discipline, has been described as a 'time capsule' of significant Forms whose essence sheds light on the whole panoply of Okinawa's karate kata.

Despite breaking down our technique to a fine degree using the above template, we came to a puzzling realization. Nothing in our biomechanical repertoire fit the reason for the phenomenon we had experienced.

Manifold Entrances

What you move toward, you enter. How you enter has consequences.

Each of us comes into this world with many potential powers. The first step in every journey will direct you toward one of manifold entrances to these powers. Each power represents one room in the great mansion of the Self. The *Dō* of martial arts sets the disciple on the quest to claim each room—each power. The most active ingredient in anyone's personal evolution is *self-awareness*. Each entry point represents a degree of self-awakening. Which door you enter first is inconsequential. There is no predetermined order. When your heart is right, your karma will lead you appropriately. Entry into one room does not end your journey but rather, grants you access toward increasing capabilities. Interacting with any one room of your interior is to interact on some level with all the rooms, for something understood implicitly in one room can be understood in the others as well.

This idea of crossing a threshold is a metaphor for becoming aware of different dimensions within yourself for greater self-expression in the world. Awakening each of your powers will give you more vitality and purpose.

Coming Into Existence

You were born gifted with the power to exist in multiple dimensions of life. From the moment of your birth onward it is up to you to maintain your existence with your *power to feel*.

Claiming your creative/destructive capacity in the world of matter.

The *power to act* gives you the choice to build up or tear down. As you pass through different life stages you are given the ability to destroy, dismantle and reconstruct the old to make room for the new.

Defining your self-identity activates your *power to discriminate*. Coupled with your *power to feel* and to *act* is the ability to align your head with your heart to merge the two in harmony with your desires and goals.

Claiming your voice gives you the power to *truth tell*. Being honest with yourself and capable of hearing the truth when it is spoken, allows you to speak, hear and act with forceful clarity.

Claiming your intellect and intuition leads to knowledge and insight for negotiating the world. This is your *power to see* and to *understand*.

Awakening your spiritual sensitivities gives you *the power to realize* and leads to wisdom and harmony with the surrounding world.

We get a fair sense of our physical strengths and weaknesses by the various tasks and challenges life presents us and by our comparisons with others engaged in similar events. You might say R has faster kicks, or T has twice the grip strength. I can see that my overall coordination is far better than most men, and my footwork complexity is equal to a man twenty years my junior. But B can outrun me and S has higher kicks, etc.

Our brains record and remember these distinctions. And most of us have also observed over time that our bodies will adapt to changes in our physical circumstances. As my martial training upgraded my coordination and general health, my physique followed suit. My musculature became more defined. My techniques grew markedly faster, more accurate. My grip strength improved and grappling skills sharpened. Along with physical changes, the gains in my martial confidence began to seep into other areas of my life.

But none of the above observations, nor my cultivated physical abilities, applied the day the Frogman had gripped my wrist and I had escaped with uncanny ease. It was as if we had suddenly been transported into an alien environment where generally held beliefs in a human's physical abilities did not apply.

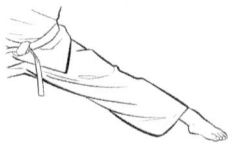

A Foot in the Door

Had a momentary lapse of attention resulted in Stone's loss of strength? Had we missed a subtle shift in the angle of our arms or wrists? It wasn't at all in our thinking that the affect could have been produced by a wide range of as yet, *unimagined* variables; something previously eaten, what we were wearing, how we were wearing it, our foot positions, a quality or time of the day, the shape of the room we were in, a function of mind, like a subliminal self-suggestion. Perhaps, it was a shift in our breathing patterns, the direction we were facing, imperceptible pressures in our body. Our list ran long.

Looking back, we had our heads too tightly stuck in our martial sand box. For most of the above-mentioned variables seemed irrelevant to me. Truthfully, I should say, unconscious. We were two martial artists doing martial technique sensing there must be something martial we were not seeing. So, we redoubled our focus on that single point of engagement, Frogman's right hand gripping my right wrist.

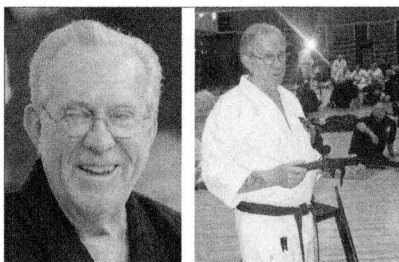

Sensei Joe Noonan (Stone), 2006, 2015

Over time, we discovered that many of the variables I mentioned above, and others yet unmentioned, could have played a role in what had occurred. We had entered the labyrinth of an unfolding adventure with only the slightest clue of where it would lead us. This quest presented a slowly emerging picture of how body, mind, and Energy Body (Spirit) performed as an integrated unit both in our normal daily events and during those rare moments when we find ourselves embroiled in serious conflict.

I want to qualify my use of the word 'spirit' in this context. Spirit has a broad range of interpretation that when extended far enough can be defined as a Vital Life Force, or the will of God. I am taking only one feature, Spirit's most empirical or practical manifestation, its electrifying infusion into the musculature.

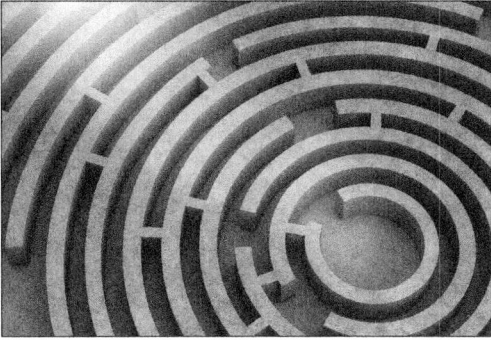

Martial Labyrinth

Stone and I started off well equipped for a deductive foray into our technical mystery. I had been teaching professionally for nearly a quarter of a century, and Stone was a senior dan-ranked member in our School's inner circle.

The average martial student learning a bread and butter, small circle wrist escape might get a total of several minutes of verbal instruction on how to do the release. After that, it is rote practice, maybe followed by a brief explanatory tune up. In many schools there isn't much verbal explanation. This learning atmosphere harkens back to old school Asian instruction. Technicalities were to be discovered through practice, not in the talk about the practice. You learn by feel or what one Behavioral psychologist calls *System 1*, that part of our mind that uses an innate sensing to quickly conclude how something is to be done. Amongst martial art teachers, the general notion is that if you practice a technique long enough, you will instinctively figure it out (or quit in frustration).

But the above statement has long since been disproven in our dojo. You might practice a basic move or a Fighting Form for twenty years and never once dip your little toe into its Kiko nature. By the end of this book, you should discover new insights about your stable of punches, kicks, blocks, takedowns and locks.

Since 1970, Isshin Kempo has been evolving as a highly refined technical school with a tried template in which to measure martial techniques—decades of collaborative, professional experience. Stone and I meticulously dismantled the grip escape. Like allopaths introducing one allergen at a time searching for the cause of a patient's allergic reaction, we introduced one technical variable after another then tried the escape again, and again, *ad nauseum*. At the very least we would end up with a wickedly good understating of how a small, clockwise circle of the gripped hand works and doesn't work. In the cup half-full/half-empty *koan* we were going for the whole cup—the big picture.

By analogy, few individuals will ever successfully reach the summit of Mount Everest after a basic, one-week mountain climbing course. Most mountaineers concur you will need a minimum of one year of specialized training. What follows is not a beginner's course on wrist escapes.

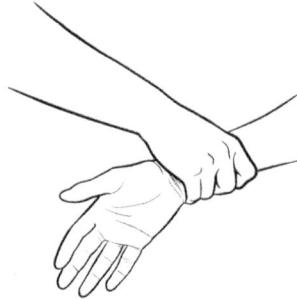

From the perspective of the one being gripped we considered a Mount Everest height of variables; the size of the circle escape, (i.e., a small vs. large circle); whether the gripped hand kept the wrist straight or bent when circling. If bent, the angles of bend available to the joint. Whether the bend used the forearm flexors or extensors, degrees of tension or relaxation in the forearm, hand and fingers, including combinations of finger tension or relaxation. (The reason for this being that two separate nerves in the hand divide finger control between the bottom two and top three fingers). The distance of the gripped arm's elbow from the waist, measured as one fist away, or more or less than one fist away.

This last factor brings up a side note about strength. It is a gross misassumption to believe that physical strength is simply relative to body/muscle size.

Strength is relative to organization, not size.
The most organized player wins.

Strength is *always* specific to the task at hand. You know you are strong at some things but not at others. In the martial arts there is a biomechanical reality that as your arm moves further away from your torso, it becomes weaker against blocks and locks leveraged at the wrist and elbow joints. This overlooked concept confirms that strength is not relative just to the size of a muscle, but to the position of a limb as well. An arm becomes stronger when closer to the torso, weaker when further away from it. Why? Because as your limb nears the torso you can couple torso strength with your limb action.

A person whose arm is gripped while it is extended the maximum length from their body will find it much more difficult to escape a wrist grip. Keeping one's arm close to the torso can reverse this situation, making it easier to pull off an escape. The average person is not conscious of this simple, biomechanical principle.

Back to more variables; whether prior to circling, the forearm moved slightly or grossly in any other direction, given that the forearm can move in a 360 arc. The proximity of bodies measured in foot length distances, i.e., one foot length away from the other, two foot lengths, etc.; the angle of hip and torso to the other's hip and torso; Whether the gripped arm's wrist lay on the opposite side of one's spinal column or the same side; The degree of tension or relaxation in the body overall: Specific parts of the body tensed or relaxed other than the arms in question; the chosen stance. Assuming it was a natural stance, shoulder width, we still noted whether our feet were straight, or slightly turned inward or outward. We observed whether our feet pointed straight at the others, or fell to the inside or outside of their foot position. The breathing pattern, whether inhaling or exhaling during the escape. The pace and depth of the breath; slow, medium, fast; breathing high in the chest, mid-body or lower abdomen. The position of the middle joints of the arms and legs; locked or unlocked and to what degree; the position of the neck tilted down toward the grip, upright, or facing straight ahead. The position of the eyes, whether opened, half-opened or closed.

We looked at our state of mind from the standpoint of three possible intentions; *"I can escape from his grip. I can't escape from his grip. I wasn't sure if I could escape from his grip."* We evaluated the escape from the perspective of being self-distracted (the mind preoccupied with given mental task like doing a simple mathematical equation while escaping), or other-distracted (focusing on something external to draw attention away from full concentration on the escape). We considered mental factors like faulty memory, not being sure how the escape worked, to being very sure how it worked. We also visualized a range of outcomes before actually escaping, versus not visualizing any outcome prior, then trying to escape.

There were countless variables, including those I mentioned earlier that we hadn't considered that might play a role as we realized we were unearthing a trove of valuable data.

So far, I have only mentioned the variables tested from the side of the one being gripped. We had to take all these same variables and apply them to the one doing the gripping. The combinations were infinite. Consider breathing alone; What if the gripper is breathing out as I am inhaling, or vice versa, or any combination of upper, middle and lower breathing at different speeds? The senior yudansha, Dharma Wheel, quipped, "It's like playing a four-dimensional chess game."

What were the chances we could deduce the formula of our effortless escape? What is the probability anyone else is going through this same degree of testing in their martial school? I believe slim to none. Western culture is a society of instant gratification. If a gross circling action of the wrist will break a grip even from a strong assailant or competitor 75% of the time, who cares about the above finesse? I do. I wanted to know if the system I had learned had been created by masters aware of *effortless power.* I wanted to prove these masters either knew or didn't know about the internal side of their martial arts. How was I going to confirm this if these men had long since passed away? I was going to look for the answer in the archives and artifacts of their techniques and Kata.

In the everyday world, any martial art is *relative.* Even the absolute worst technique might do the job if the assailant or competitor is too clumsy to counter it and the technique hits a sensitive target. The issue reminds me of the radio host who asked a noted meditation teacher, *"Why do terrible teachers exist?"* His response*, "to accommodate terrible students."*

To arrive at a profound understanding of any martial art, it's better to have a guide than wading through an enormity of trial and error to get there on your own. Videos and books are *static* teachers. They can only get you so far. It's better to have a good teacher than a bad one. It's better to have a great teacher then a good one. But fate isn't always so kind. You get what you deserve until you feel you deserve better. It's that simple.

Frogman and I were getting what we deserved – the challenge to find a better explanation, the hallmark of progress. My karma was ripe for this challenge.

We eventually duplicated the effortless wrist escape. But I could not say we used the *same* formula. It turns out there are multiple ways to accomplish the same outcome with Kiko. But when we succeeded, in our mutual *satori*, we knew that we had stepped into the treasure room of the masters. To this very day, Kiko treasures continue to pour out of our research. Our conclusion; any martial technique from any system is far more powerful when Kiko is applied. In Kiko we find *authentic* power.

Kiko underlies all the above-mentioned skills, all martial art technique and fitness protocols, regardless of culture or purpose. Kiko adds extraordinary power to every one of the above-mentioned dimensions.

The main reason so few see this aspect of their arts is due mostly to a single phenomenon; the overt or biomechanical functionality of a martial art has become such a fixed dogma it has concealed its bioenergetic principles and functionality. The curiosity of the common-minded person is easily discharged when the topical rationale is given, even though the real marrow may lie untouched inside the bone of the obvious answer. It's uncommon for martial artists to ask questions outside of the box presented by their teachers. And most martial systems are big boxes with lots of playthings to engage and distract a disciple on the trail of the martial sages. You need uncommon curiosity to uncover a not so obvious art within an art. You also need a courageous, adventurous and strong spirit to step off the beaten path into the wilderness of your own art.

PART 2

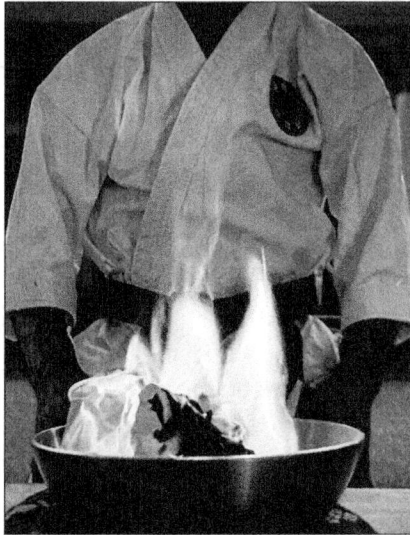

INITIATION

Touch red paint, become red.
Chinese proverb

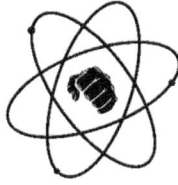

Sixty-Nine Critical Observations

Regarding the Human Energy Body (Biofield, Ki)

In an attempt to widen the Martial Ways, I present a curated overview of sixty-nine revelations encompassing decades of personal investigation into the internal nature of martial practice. This work spans the immediately practical to the broadly philosophical and metaphysical. Each facet supports the others to frame out a holistic training template in line with monastic lineages. Throughout this book I will use the terms *Energy Body*, *Biofield* and *Ki* interchangeably. These three terms represent the personal, scientific and historic labels I have adopted for my own use when navigating Kiko's alluring and occasionally, misty terrain. Kiko is the study, application and implications of the Energy Body, Biofield, or Ki as an intimate part of human nature and for the purposes of this work, as it relates to martial life.

I have grouped some observations into general categories, though they should not be construed to reflect a fixed hierarchy of values. You can enter Kiko study through any number of access points. In Part 3, I will expound upon each of these observations in more detail, adding practical examples and personal stories.

Observation 1
Everyone possesses an Energy Body (Biofield, Ki)

Observation 2
A visceral sensitivity to their Energy Body likely caused some fight masters to embed Kiko principles and techniques into their fighting forms.

Observation 3
Martial biomechanics complement martial bioenergetics and vice versa.

Observation 4
Normal is not always natural.

Observation 5
Your Energy Body can be physically manipulated to greatly enhance strength by the proper alignment of the limbs and torso in both static and moving actions with a methodology I call *Hard Gating*.

Observation 6
Each traditional stance will activate one of five Elemental Phases in the Energy Body.

Observation 7
Because respiration is a mechanical as well as an electro-chemical action, its musculoskeletal dynamics form part of Kiko's Hard Gating system.

Observation 8
Aggressive moves toward you by another generally sends a Ki wave ahead of their action.

Observation 9
Kiko integrates our non-physical nature with our physical structure.

Observation 10
Your kinetic pattern defines your Energy personality.

Observation 11
Large quantities of Energy drawn into your body can cause an effect known as *Induced Ki Flow*. Large energy outflows can cause its opposite effect, *Reduced Ki Flow*.

Observation 12
Your Energy Body can move independently of your physical body.

Observation 13
The average martial artist is unaware of the complex interactions of their Energy Body during training. Most Biofield effects are registered below awareness.

Observation 14
Your Biofield is affected by proximity to the radiating fields of animate and inanimate objects.

Observation 15
Persons in proximity will exchange energy and information on seven distinct levels.

MIND MATTERS

Observation 16
The Energy Body can be manipulated *mentally* through intention and visualization in a method I call *Soft Gating*.

Observation 17
Intention drives Ki

Observation 18
Mental *chi nate*, (throwing energy) is supported by imagination and visualization.

Observation 19
Your Biofield patterns are reflected in your foundational beliefs, forming a mental *Platform* upon which your physical and psychological behaviors spring.

Observation 20
Examining your beliefs can unleash your full powers by revealing limiting or obstructed Ki flow.

Observation 21
Skepticism is Soft Gating.

Observation 22
False gatekeepers may block your advance through misdirection due to their limited knowledge or restrictive convictions.

Observation 23
All manner of negativity *causes* suppression,
drag or friction on your Ki flow.

Observation 24
Mind and body co-depend on correct energy and information
to function properly.

Observation 25
Mind and body share governance of your Energy Body via
conscious and unconscious intent.

Observation 26
You can instantly install Biofield templates
of past successes or failures.

Observation 27
Depending upon the circumstances, your mind, physical body
or Energy Body can dominate your actions.

Observation 28
Your Energy Body always seeks to maintain internal homeostasis
consistent with your state of consciousness.

Observation 29
Ki is regulated through voluntary and involuntary processes
and outside influences.

Observation 30
The Chinese internal energy model recognizes
three primary power centers

Observation 31
The body's three power centers distribute their charge
as the need arises.

Observation 32
Society is reorienting the upper dantien
to be the dominant energy center.

DIRECTIONALITY

Observation 33
Physical strength is influenced by the direction one faces.

Observation 34
The role of directionality in modulating physical strength may
have influenced the composition of key kata so its performers
moved along the strongest Ki pathways.

SIDEDNESS

Observation 35
The lack of understanding how sidedness influences martial
technique has led to widespread misassumptions, distortions
and improper use of common martial technique.

Observation 36
Your Biofield functions differently on the left
and right sides of your body.

Observation 37
Physical movements on the left side of the body generally
initiate an 'energy-in' action while movements on the right
side generally initiate an 'energy-out' action depending upon
the direction faced.

KATA

Observation 38
Soft Gate principles and techniques were not included in Western Hard style martial curriculums.

Observation 39
Solo kata performance may require a slightly altered movement
pattern than its application against a partner.

Observation 40
As evident in their postural arrangements, all essential Kata store
a record of Hard Gate, Energy Body principles.

Observation 41
Each and every kata is a five-in-one form

Observation 42
Okinawa's premiere Form, the Sanchin Kata, presents both
a brilliant tactical combat framework and
an Energy-cultivating meditation.

Observation 43
Kiko activates Kata's Yantric (sacred) nature.

Observation 44
The concepts of *Mantra, Mudra* and *Mandala* reveal the intimate
interrelationship of Energy Body functioning with all forms and
levels of reality

Observation 45
Kiko gives rise to the Form and No Form schools

OBJECTS

Observation 46
All objects vibrate and thus possess an Energy Body

Observation 47
Everyone and everything in proximity is engaged in an ongoing,
dynamic communication by means of their radiant Energy fields.

Observation 48
Kiko includes the *Feng Shui* of the immediate environment

Observation 49
The relationship of your Energy Body to the living and non-living can be reduced to three core affects; positive, neutral or negative.

SYMBOLS

Observation 50
The Chinese Bagua symbol may have been a visual diagram for understanding aspects of Biofield/Ki functioning.

SCIENCE

Observation 51
It is theorized that atomic and subatomic communication takes place via electro-magnetic, acoustic and photonic signaling.

Observation 52
Electro-Magnetism and/or Biophotonic communication likely defines one of Ki's many dimensions.

Observation 53
Some people are naturally more attuned to Ki's linear, electrical flow while others are more connected to its spiraling magnetic flow.

Observation 54
Not all meridians functioned equally.

Observation 55
An exchange of electrons between people may explain the strength differential when the Biofields interact.

Observation 56
Your Energy Body has five primary *orientations* or *attitudes* the Chinese refer to as *Elements* or *Phases*.

Observation 57
Your Energy Body is always attempting to synchronize with the Energy fields of your immediate environment and the Universal Cosmic System.

Observation 58
We live in two worlds.

Observation 59
The *mezzocosm* (middle world) is the junction between matter and spirit. It reveals the entanglement and complimentary nature of particle and wave, and marks a critical threshold of awareness in one's training.

Observation 60
Kiko practice is oriented toward three interlocking goals; heightened practical use, enhanced therapeutic effect, spiritual and evolutionary advance.

TECHNIQUE

Observation 61
Directing the mind to systematically attend to micro and macro-orbits around the body vitalizes the Energy Body for more potent movement.

Observation 62
Correct proportionality in limb positioning is part of the Energy Body equation.

Observation 63
Each limb can move up to a maximum of four primary directions simultaneously, out of a total of eight directions.

Observation 64
The eight limb directions can be combined into four paired sets.

Observation 65
Four of the eight limb actions are Yin. Four of the eight are Yang actions. One of the four is a primary function fueling the remaining three.

Observation 66
Understanding how to overcome any one of the four Yin or four Yang pairs allows you to identify and overcome the other three.

Observation 67
The two major formulas for diminishing another's Energy Body are *underwhelming*, drawing the charge off someone, or *overwhelming*, sending a fast, increased charge into them.

Observation 68
Duration (the time a limb or the body can hold a charge) is part of Energy Body functioning.

Observation 69
We are the world. The world is shifting.
We are the essence of this shift.

PART 3

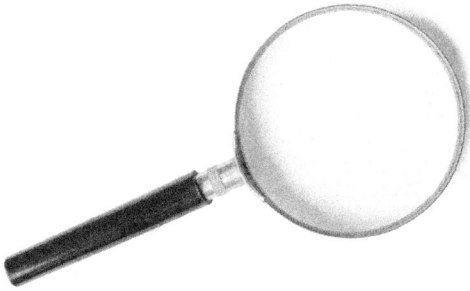

INSPECTION

Discovery is seeing what everybody else has seen,
and thinking what nobody else has thought.

Albert Szent-Gyorgyi

1* Everyone possesses an Energy Body (Biofield, Ki)

In a few decades, scientists have gone from a conviction that there is no such thing as energy fields in and around the human body to an absolute certainty that they exist.
James Oschman, Ph.D., Energy Medicine

To unravel my story of why I consider Kiko a *hidden* path to power, and its intimate relationship with the martial arts, I must begin with an overview of the human Biofield. This term is synonymous to what through the ages has been called the 'human energy field, subtle energy, Energy Body, aura, Light-Body, Soul, Essence, to the Indians, *Prana*. To the ancient Greeks, pnuema. To Pacific islanders; *mana*. To the Chinese; *Chi, Qi*, Japanese; *Ki*, Vital Life Force, Universal life force.' To Western philosophers, *energia*, *elan vital*, and Willhelm Reich's Orgone energy.

Any description of human nature and martial practice must today include this interpenetrating Energy Body or Biofield. The term biofield was coined by scientists at the National Institute of Health (NIH) in 1994 to describe a dynamic energy field that surrounds and interpenetrates our physical body.

What is the Human Biofield?

There is no scientific consensus on a precise definition of the human Biofield or its overall bioeffects. Most research has focused on the field's electromagnetic properties, although we know the body also emits low-level light, heat, acoustical energy which may or may not be inclusive of, in the eyes of scientific community, the hypothetical Ki.

William A. Tiller, Phd., is one of the world's leading scientists on solid-state physics and psychoenergetics. Tiller points out that only a fraction of the electromagnetic spectrum is detectable by our eyes. Likewise, our ears only detect a fraction of the sound spectrum. This suggests we only sense a narrow band of reality. The normally unsensed bands are perceived by very few.

It is due to the highly sensitive individuals who claim cognition of this field's presence that Kiko exists conceptually. Energy healers say they can "touch" another's Energy Body without touching their physical body. Such individuals are referred to as possessing a sixth sense, or using their 'Third Eye, an intangible faculty that allows them to feel, manipulate, even decode, the Biofield's relevancy to health, strength and/or foresee future events. Highly advanced martial artists throughout time appear to be able to manipulate this field to overcome opponents.

Current instrumentation tells us that our Biofield is composed of measurable electromagnetism. The Biofield has also been described as a *Bioplasma* with varying viscosities and densities like a diffuse magnetic fluid. Western science's inability to determine the Biofield's exact composition is due to the lack of instrumentation sensitive enough to describe and/or measure it. How do you measure the composition of a subtle Energy you don't understand? Yet, old world martial art and other movement disciplines, especially ancient, Indian or Vedic cultures have described the behaviors of this energy in great detail.

Several thousand years ago in India, observations were made about energy vortices at key locations along the spinal column as part of the body's energy anatomy. This gave rise to the Sanskrit term, *chakra*, (wheel), referring to the spinning and spiraling action of these vortices. This observation was critical enough to be worked into the culture's yogic, medical and warrior arts. Not coincidentally, each chakra corresponds to clusters of nerves or plexuses believed to communicate energy and information via photonic, magnetic and/or electro-chemical pathways.

Margaret Moga, Phd., defines the chakras as mini-fiberoptic balls, functioning like organic computers, routers and information processors for all organs in seven areas of the body comprising part of our body's third circulatory system. These fiberoptic systems, known as Bonghan channels, were discovered using microscopic photography.

Manipulating our Energy Body is not defying any laws of physics. It's using these laws in an uncommon manner.

A pioneer in Biofield research, Eileen Day McKusick, describes the Biofield as a toroid (doughnut-shaped) sphere surrounding and extending from the body about 5-6 feet to the sides and 2-3 feet at the top and bottom; bounded by a plasma membrane similar to the protective boundary encasing earth's upper atmosphere. My own anecdotal description, based upon decades of testing, concurs that our body is surrounded by an immaterial, yet malleable, airy-like field, concentrated around the torso and highly manipulable from 1-3 feet away.

Our Biofield or Ki does not function separately outside of the rest of us. It is an integral part of our non-material nature. Just as our thoughts are not bubbles that disengage from our minds and float into nothingness once thought, our Biofield is highly engaged with all our biological processes in ways science has yet to fully comprehend. There are Energy practices within some ancient warrior cultures relatively unknown to Western science. In Tom Bisio's book, *A Tooth From the Tiger's Mouth*, the author reveals an entire methodology of medical practices for healing martial art injuries and imbalances once exclusive to China's martial community.

Cartesian Martial Science Challenged

In the early 20th century, the emerging scientific field of Quantum physics challenged our understanding of the fundamental nature of the universe. Advances in technology allowed us to glimpse into the previously unknown working of atomic and subatomic reality. This led to several significant observations. One, everything in the universe is made entirely of energy consisting of particles and energy waves. Secondly, our world of hard matter is actually 98% empty space. Our physical body is 98% empty space.

How can solid matter seem so tangible yet be so vacuous when we see and touch solids at every turn? Physicists tell us the answer is *vibration*. Atomic and subatomic particles are moving so fast they create the illusion of solid forms.

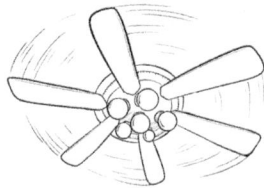

Imagine a ceiling fan that could be set to an increasing speed without breaking. Soon it becomes a blur of whirling blades. At some point the blades spin so fast they appear to harden into a non-moving block of matter. This is the nature of our materium, our hard matter world, according to the Quantum scientists.

It seems odd that our normal perceptions grant us full and easy access to the world of form and substance, but little access to the immaterial world, save for the intangibility and elusiveness of own thoughts, feelings and emotions.

All matter has a frequency pulsing at different speeds. These frequencies give us the softness of gases and liquids. The world's least dense solid is a graphene aerogel with a density of just 0.16 mg/cm^3; Hydrogen gas is the least dense substance in the world. By contrast, Nuclear Pasta, a material deep inside the heart of neutron stars, is considered the strongest substance known.

Our emotional states produce different vibrational signatures. Happiness, joy, love, treating others with kindness, meditation, mindfulness practices, yoga, martial arts, fresh foods, fresh water, essential oils, crystals, energy work modalities, time outdoors in the sunshine, positive thoughts, all raise our frequency. Conversely, negative emotions like fear, guilt, grief, anger, create low vibratory signatures.

A mere two percent of subatomic particles and waves whirl in a vast sea of Dark Matter comprising our universe. If Quantum physicists insist that we look at both particle and wave for a complete picture of reality, then I insist the time has arrived for us to incorporate the unseen component of our natures and make waves in our martial art practices by taking a hard look at our own invisible energy waves, for all our martial maneuvers generate different frequencies.

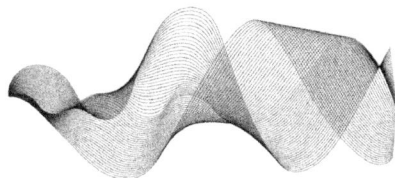

If you wish to understand the universe,
think of Energy, Frequency and Vibration.
Nikola Tesla

Body Frequency

Frequency is defined as *the number of occurrences of a repeating current flow per second*. The frequency of any phenomenon with regular periodic variations is measured in hertz (Hz). This term is commonly used in connection with alternating electric currents, electromagnetic waves (light, radar, sound, etc.). 1 Hz is one vibration cycle per second. One megahertz (MHz) is one million vibration cycles per second). The hertz (Hz), was named after the German Physicist, Heinrich Rudolf Hertz, the first person to prove the existence of electromagnetic waves.

The subject of human frequencies is little known, studied, and understood by modern Western science, even though we have compelling evidence that early Indian and Chinese martial masters were aware of their body's vibratory behavior. Only a small number of scientists worldwide have focused on understanding human energy fields. According to the Biophysicist, Beverly Rubic, measuring the biofield, understanding its role in life, is more difficult than the study of more concrete phenomena. This is why funding for research into Ki has been extremely scarce, resulting in few scientific advances in Biofield research. Rubic feels the Biofield remains a frontier science ripe for exploration.

In 1992, the microbiologist, Bruce Tainio, built the world's first frequency monitor, called the Calibrated Frequency Monitor (CFM). Tainio determined that the average daytime frequency of the human body ranges from 62-68 MHz, independent of one's mass or height. Tainio explains that each of us vibrates at millions of cycles per second with frequencies as unique as our fingerprint. When you sense bad vibes from another you are responding to a frequency out of sync to your own.

Differing frequencies can cause objects to bounce off of each other. This bounce is called *resistance*. Consider the terms we use when talking about others: "I am *attracted* to her. I am *repulsed* by his actions." Consider our martial language; I *repelled* his attack or, I drew him in. We could just as easily be talking about the action of dipole magnets attracting or repelling one another.

According to Tainio, healthy body frequency is 62-72 MHz. He showed that the lower the frequency, the poorer the body's constitution. Drops below 58MHz compromise the immune system. I hypothesize this lower frequency will cause a drop in physical strength. Conversely, things and actions that raise our vibrational frequency enhance our health.

Tainio created the human body frequency scale below to show how different parts of us vibrate at different frequencies. Here are a few of his calculations:

Human Frequency Range

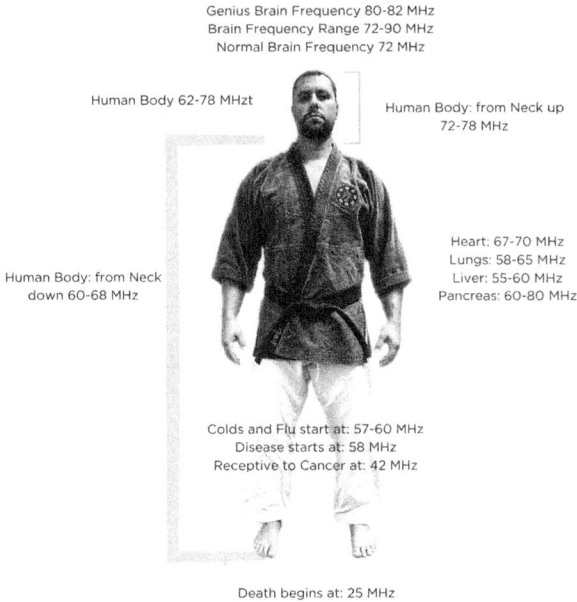

Genius Brain Frequency 80-82 MHz
Brain Frequency Range 72-90 MHz
Normal Brain Frequency 72 MHz

Human Body 62-78 MHzt

Human Body: from Neck up
72-78 MHz

Heart: 67-70 MHz
Lungs: 58-65 MHz
Liver: 55-60 MHz
Pancreas: 60-80 MHz

Human Body: from Neck
down 60-68 MHz

Colds and Flu start at: 57-60 MHz
Disease starts at: 58 MHz
Receptive to Cancer at: 42 MHz

Death begins at: 25 MHz

Collectively, our body produces a frequency range between 58-82 MHZ. This frequency is emitted by our organs, physical structure, and mental and physical activities.

As you will learn, we can consciously control our Biofield frequency via intention and/or physical movements to cause strength changes in our body and the bodies of those in proximity to us. The martial art masters of old were likely aware of this signaling mechanism on a visceral level, which I believe they relied upon to construct or compose their fighting arts.

The biophysicist, Beverly Rubik, points out that research on the human Biofield has focused mainly on medical therapies, with speculation that it may act directly on molecular structures, or transfer bio-information carried by very small energy signals interacting directly with the energy fields of life.

Living organisms respond to extremely low-level nonionizing electromagnetic fields, ranging from cellular and subcellular affects to emotional, and behavioral changes. My position is that one of the behavioral effects is on human strength, and thus critical for understanding martial Kiko.

If all of us possess an innate dynamic biologic field, involved in maintaining the integrity of our whole organism, regulating its physiologic and biochemical responses, integral to our development, healing, and regeneration, what other hidden qualities might we discover about this field? I hope to present compelling evidence that our biological field is responsible for raising or lowering our physical strength.

Indigenous healing systems like Ayurvedic and Chinese medicine, and modern modalities such as chiropractic, rest upon the concept of a vital force central to healing. Indigenous terms going back thousands of years may have been referring to the present-day concept of the Biofield, which is, in part, based on the electromagnetic field theory of modern physics and/or Fritz-Albert Popp's theory of Biophotonic communication (Observation 52). Subtler energy fields, as yet unknown, may also exist.

One distinction currently made between traditional and modern views of the vital force, is that the Biofield rests on measurable, evidence-based physical principles, while traditional and esoteric concepts like Ki remain bound in the metaphysical. Who is to say the metaphysical realm isn't a more inclusive or higher principled dimension?

Putting this debate aside, the ancient concept of Ki and the modern concept of the Biofield share similar assumptions, that a life-infusing form of energy flows throughout the body and that illness (and/or strength loss) arises as a result of blockages, excesses, or irregularities in its flow.

If practitioners of Biofield therapies, which incorporate notions of a universal life force, as in acupuncture, Reiki, Qigong therapy, and other types of energy healing performed today, can assess imbalances in the human Biofield via touch or intuition, is it a great leap to believe that we could detect and affect strength shifts by the same means of touch, movement and/or intention?

Current Theories Behind Human Energy Projection

The idea of a person being able to project energy to affect another person is often associated with various spiritual and metaphysical theories. The four most common ones being:

The Law of Attraction: This theory suggests that we can manifest our desires into reality by attracting them through the power of our thoughts and energy. According to this theory, projecting positive energy towards someone can help them attract positive experiences into their lives.

Energy Healing: This theory suggests that everything in the universe is made up of energy, and that imbalances in this energy can lead to physical and emotional problems. Practitioners of energy healing believe that they can channel their own energy or outside energy to balance the energy of others, promoting healing and well-being. Qigong falls into this category, but only in the martial arts does this theory explore such energy for its reverse effect, the power to destroy or incapacitate others.

Quantum Physics: This theory suggests that everything in the universe is interconnected through a web of energy and information. Therefore, it is possible to influence this energy and information through our thoughts and intentions to impact the physical world.

Chakra Theory: This theory comes from ancient Indian spiritual traditions and suggests that the body is made up of seven energy centers, or chakras, that govern different aspects of our physical, emotional, and spiritual well-being. Practitioners of chakra healing believe that they can use their energy to balance these chakras, promoting overall health and well-being.

The above theories are not universally accepted by the scientific community. Nevertheless, many people find them useful frameworks for understanding the world and their place in it. In my opinion, there is little separation amongst these theories. Their boundaries interpenetrate one another. For example, Energy healing could easily be a use of quantum physics described through a chakric lens motivated by an intuition activating the Law of Attraction. Many other configurations of these theories can be construed.

Why Science doesn't know more about the human Biofield or Ki

The concept of Ki or Chi is a fundamental concept in traditional Chinese and Japanese medicine and martial arts. However, as an empirical phenomenon that can be measured and observed through scientific methods, Ki remains a subject of controversy, debate and research. Studies attempting to investigate Ki's existence and its effects on human health and well-being remain mixed and scientific evidence for its existence is limited. Some studies have suggested that practices such as Qigong and acupuncture may have positive effects on certain health conditions, such as chronic pain and anxiety, but it is not clear whether these effects are due to the manipulation of Ki or other factors such as placebo effects. Overall, while research into the phenomenon of

Ki remains ongoing, the scientific community has yet to reach a consensus on its existence or mechanisms of action.

Most of our science about the human Biofield comes from conventional medical testing with the heart making the greatest contribution to the electromagnetic nature of the Biofield. The brain's electrical field emission is considerably weaker.

There are no Biofield instruments generally approved by the research community. The lack of valid measurement tools and energy markers remains an obstacle to progress in Biofield science. And a central question in regard to Biofield research is how, or if, the Biofield responds to changes in consciousness.

2* A visceral sensitivity to their Energy Body likely caused some fight masters to embed Kiko principles and techniques into their fighting forms.

The Intuitive Experts

Intuition is a felt sense, a non-linear awareness. It's not derived from any logical, sequential, deductive, or inductive line of reasoning the mind comprehends. It's a 'knowing without knowing,' awareness. Some of us just know things.

Perhaps, because we just don't inhabit our bodies, we are our bodies, some people just know how to move efficiently and powerfully. I believe the early masters were intuitive, in the flow, Kiko experts. Being closer to nature and the animal world these ancients knew the correct way to move. There are individuals who can feel or sense magnetism not unlike empaths describing seeing auras or sensing an ethereal field around a body. The theory is the more capacitance in your body the more likely you will become sensitive to this finer layer of self, as you literally become more coherent. The next step would be to control this Energy field.

Most of the historical evidence of internal mastery points to its successful disciples 'just doing it'. These disciples are told if they practice for decades, one day, maybe, they will get the feel of it. This may be one reason we have so few instructors able to articulate the internal nuances of their martial arts and why it has remained locked in the visceral realm. Only a minority of modern experts seem able to explain their internal skills using step-by-step logic. Further proof of this lack of esoterica is borne out by the scarcity of literature on the intricacies of Internal practice. For every one book written on internal martial arts we have a hundred penned on its external character.

Ki, Chi, Qi are Asian catchall terms for a phenomenon whose science has not fully matured but whose behavior has been keenly observed for thousands of years within certain spiritual, medical, and martial cultures. As previously mentioned, if Ki consists of a strong electro-magnetic and/or photonic base, then we could say that future martial Kiko students will be studying their Biofield's electro-magnetic and photonic influences on physical strength.

The Western world's primary contribution to the martial arts has been its information technologies, which have brought more of us into a wider community of enthusiasts and given us access to hitherto inaccessible aspects of these arts. This increased exposure offers us more precise pathways for entry into and through advanced martial concepts, theory, and technique. On the other hand, this same technology has dumped an avalanche of knowledge for us to chunk down, burying many under its sheer information overload. Too much information comes fraught with its own problems.

3* Martial biomechanics complement martial bioenergetics and vice versa.

Leverage is not the only key.
Sometimes 'Ki' is key.

There are biomechanical, leveraging, and timing tricks that can give anyone an advantage in applying or escaping from grips and locks. The techniques I've been working with do not fall into any clearly defined biomechanical model. For example, what principle lies behind the following exchange; Subject A stands across from subject B by a foot or so. Both subjects assume a natural relaxed posture. Subject A does a base test of Subject B's right wrist strength, determined by A trying to twist B's wrist with B resisting. Subject A is then asked to imagine rotating an invisible field around his torso, clockwise or counter-clockwise prior to testing, then retest. Subject A is told not to announce his chosen imagined direction of rotation. In one direction, Subject B tests 30-100% stronger resisting the wrist twist. In the other, 30-100% weaker.

Where is the biomechanical principle, when you add in that neither party knows what the experiment is trying to determine?

Kiko should be viewed as an enhancement not a substitute for biomechanical skills. Kiko presents a finer layer of technical study atop the necessary fundamental skills required for mastery of any martial art or physical discipline. I remember telling Stone during our unraveling of the Kiko enigma that if the reason turns out to be a form of psycho-mechanics like self-suggestion, "It's an impressive trick we need to learn."

Without Kiko principles the full face
of authentic martial arts will generally remain misunderstood.

From the late 1960's-90's I never came across any Western-based, Hard Style martial system that offered its practitioners a step-by-step methodology to interpret their Fighting Forms through the Kiko lens. Yet, I observed countless times that students standing in identical martial postures, or executing identical technique, could have markedly different outcomes which I now believe was due in part to Kiko's influence. The smallest or simplest shifts in moves, mentally and/or physically, can cause a profound difference in strength.

A critical distinction for grasping Kiko requires we divide martial movements into two broad categories; biomechanically sound technique and bioenergetically sound technique. These systems complement one another like the two halves of a table. A middle ground claimed by both sides has led to much ambiguity and skepticism. For what distinguishes a biomechanical technique from a bioenergetic one? The confusion lies in the open-endedness of these systems with the latter being mostly metaphysical too date. This topic is not a fixed line in the sand. The fluid nature of these concepts constantly changes their boundaries. As Western science advances its knowledge about optimal body mechanics, and Eastern intuitive science gains further awareness about the body's Energy fields, this line will continue to shift, and ideally merge.

Middle Ground
claimed as either Ki-
based or Biomechanical

Western evidence-based principles ➤ ‒ ‒ ‒ ‒ ‒ ‒ **Asian intuited principles**

Scientific and metaphysical
advances are closing
the gap between Western and
Asian disciplines

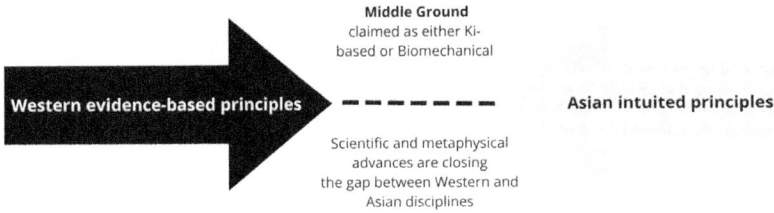

I suspect it is easier for Western culture to attribute everything martial to scientifically established biomechanical principles because of the West's orientation and emphasis on evidence-based science and logic. Likewise, it may have been easier for earlier subsects within Asian martial culture to peg everything to Ki because of their intuitive, spiritual-based acuity and keen anecdotal observations.

Martial actions that are biomechanically correct, but bioenergetically incorrect, often result in inferior technique. The opposite however, is not true. This reveals a hierarchy of principles supporting the premise that one's underlying energy flow is paramount for overall success. I could analogize the situation to a racecar kept immaculate on the outside but whose engine is unattended and hence, underperforms. Reverse the condition, with the vehicle's body rusted but the engine in superb shape. Which vehicle will more likely to get you to your destination?

I have worked with students with well-defined physiques but whose body behavior or headspace is in a disorganized, suboptimal shape. Your externals need to be aligned with your internals to generate substantial power.

Bioenergetic technique can defy, overwhelm, or resist a biomechanically correct and stable body structure or technique.

The Buddhist *Heart Sutra* strikes at the essence of Kiko in its opening observation of reality; Form is emptiness. Emptiness is form. 'The form that is no form is the true form'. The no form or formless quality of the Energy Body (Biofield) is where I believe the true foundation of our physical power lies. This is why significant power is still available when the internals are correct but the externals, incorrect.

I was explaining the Hard Gates for pulling to a black belt named Raging Bull. (I use the term Hard Gates to refer to purely physical actions of the body to move Ki). We faced one another with left foot leads and locked our right wrists to base test our pull strength. We measured about even. I asked Raging Bull to Hard Gate for a pull; breath in, pelvis back, knees drawn slightly inward. As long as I remained neutral-gated, he easily uprooted me. When he Hard Gated for a push; breath out, pelvis forward, knees pressed outward, I easily uprooted him. Since the pushing Gates distribute the wrong charge, this outcome was expected. You wouldn't think such slight alterations in this posture would add any further strength to the action. Hard Gates can feel counter-intuitive to some. At one point, after I had demonstrated a strong pull against him, Raging Bull replied, "Of course, you Hard Gated for the pull."

What Raging Bull didn't know was that as long as my underlying Ki flow was correct, it didn't matter how I postured. To demonstrate, I assumed a Hard Gate posture for a push, the opposite of what he'd been taught for an effective pull. To his surprise, I easily pulled him out of his stance. This is an advanced Kiko technique, part of the No Form or Formless School of internal power development (Observation 45). The Form Schools require the Hard Gates to be exact and the mind relaxed so not to interfere with the outcome. The No Form Schools require knowledge of how energy flows to accomplish certain tasks with the mind actively and correctly circulating Ki. Under this condition the physical posture is secondary.

The biomechanical versus bioenergetic topic ignited into sharper focus after I was contacted by the British, Gojuryu expert, Tom Hill, in 2010. Sensei Hill believed in and had experienced Ki's healing powers first hand. Hill wanted to believe in martial Ki but had only found its supposed application to be the result of shifts in body angles and pressures. Hill claims he had cut through the moves of every Ki master he met, or he called out the disguised biomechanical principle they were using.

I believe sensei Hill exposed some charlatans. It is also probable that his Ki was stronger than theirs. Hill and I wrangled over our divergent perspectives like the tenacious karateka we trained to be. Whatever we labeled each of our rationales, we got results.

We need more debates like this to firm up our international base of martial knowledge.

A significant power increase in all category of martial technique is accomplished through an accord amongst three complementary mediums; the physical, the mental, and the Bioenergetic. The failure I see most often occurring among these systems is discord when the internal structure is out of sync with the surface structure. This is a typical problem in kata performance. In the West, formwork is understood exclusively as a musculoskeletal organization. Lessons on how to exploit inner energy currents remain a rarity.

The reasons are obvious. First generation Western experts encountered five significant hurdles studying Asian martial disciplines. 1. The language barrier. 2. Asian culture's orientation to their martial arts. 3. The potential depth inherent in Asian Fighting Forms. 4. The lack of time spent with their teachers before commercializing their skills back home. 5. Reticence on the part of some Asian teachers to impart this information to non-Asians. Once the martial arts became a commercial venture, we see further divergence and degrade from any Kiko lessons.

Aesthetics And Ki

Aesthetics can provide us with an innate guideline for proper Ki flow. You don't have to be a martial artist to appreciate a sharp, well-executed fighting form or a crisp snap punch or thrust kick. Martial aesthetic conveys the beauty of power through an integrated and fluid physical form. Most of us possess a natural instinct that draws us to what looks or feels pleasing. This instinct is rooted in our awareness of an object, action, or setting's *energetic* balance. The mind is keen to pick up correct energy flow even if on a subliminal level. "It just looks good, sounds good, tastes good...," is what we say when someone or something feels right. Words often fail to express the feeling. Of the three primary values we look for in any martial technique; speed, power and proper Form, Form must be given the most emphasis because correct Form is the externalization of organized internal currents leading to its aesthetic. Only proper form fully activates martial technique. Speed and power, noteworthy attributes, do not represent the essence of proper Form. When the inner principles are intact there is a natural harmonization with the underlying energy flow in bodily expression. When the insides are attuned to the outsides, we have the emergence of aesthetic; the beauty, appreciation and pleasing appearance of frictionless power.

4* Normal is not always natural.

Is the life you lead normal or natural? Are they the same ideas? Is your body posture normal or natural? Are your martial practices normal or natural? Is your preferred state of existence, normal or natural? You must consider these questions to gain control over your Biofield.

> I asked a group of university students to stand quietly and feel their shoulders without making any changes to their posture. Immediately, several students adjusted their shoulders, exactly what I did not want them to do. I then presented the concept of normal versus natural. Consider the range of positions for your collarbone and scapula. You could sink your chest, spread your scapula and draw your collar bones forward. Or, reverse the posture and draw your scapula together by pulling you collar bones backward, lifting, opening and expanding your chest. Somewhere between these two extremes lies a midpoint. Where does your collarbone or clavicle fall; front, back, or center? Where is your midpoint? If your current posture is hunched or your chest thrust out, is that a normal or natural posture?

Normal is what you have become conditioned to be or accept. Natural is what your posture, actions, or thinking would be without any culturally imposed limitations.

Where do you place your feet, knees, hips, shoulders, mind, doing martial formwork or executing various techniques? Kiko considers mid-point joint positioning a neutral energy state where you neither gain nor lose Ki. It might be normal for you to walk hunched over, or with your chest puffed, but this is not natural. Shift your posture and not only will you feel different, your Energy Body will respond to the change. Natural posturing should cause an uptick in your overall strength and health.

> Take a moment to stand and relax. Release every muscle you don't need to hold yourself up. Let yourself go totally to gravity. You will

likely discover a host of subtle tensions in the process. Imagine you could balance your entire skeleton without any muscular effort. This would be an ideal state. Releasing unnecessary tensions or tightness frees up Ki flow. If you could relax all your body's extraneous tensions where would the freed energy go? That is, if you were expending 200 calories in unnecessary muscular tension every day because of poor posture, what would happen with that energy if you could retrieve it by standing upright? I will tell you. That energy goes into making you well. And that wellness will go into making you stronger.

Western society's cultural mores have affected the human posture in ways that may be normal living in the U.S. but unnatural to the way your body wants to stand, versus the way you (your parents, your ego, your culture) thinks you should stand. Normal is the 'norm,' the generally agreed to or chosen (conscious or unconscious) posture. But your normal may or may not be natural. The only way to find out is to decouple what may be a conditioned posture from how you might stand if you didn't think you had to stand in a particular way, as in your mother telling to sit up straight, or your father telling you push out your chest, hold your head up, etc. I performed kata for twenty-five years thinking I was doing the moves correctly. I was not under the Kiko spotlight. By every agreed standard, my katas were excellent.

Physical posture is propped up by our attitude. Therefore, we must ask, if our attitude about posture is normal or natural. Do you think your posture would change if you had more or less self-confidence, a better or worse self-image?

The Three Chested Posture Meditation

I use this exercise to help students feel the correlation between attitude and physical posture. This exercise can lead to a firmer grasp of your foundational strength. Foundational strength is the intrinsic power base you have without any prior training. While standing, you will 'try on' three different chest postures defined as over-inflated, just-right inflated and underinflated. As you try each one out, note the way you feel in each position.

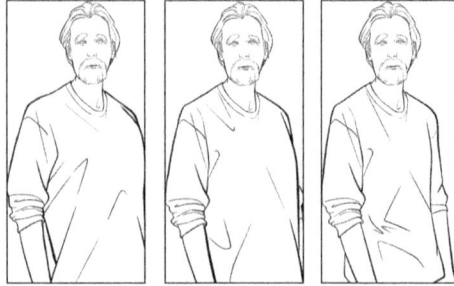

Posture 1: Stand with your chest pumped up, pushed out, scapula pulled back, head held high.
Posture 2: Find the mid-point for your neck, chest, and shoulders between the extremes of Posture 1 and 3.
Posture 3: Stand with your chest collapsed, shoulders pulled forward, back slightly hunched.

Which posture feels ideal? Which gives you a sense of power? Which of the three postures closely represents your own physique? Investigate the psychological nuances and feelings elicited holding each posture.

We can further divide the equation of normal vs natural into physical versus mental posturing. Body posturing is easy to grasp. Slouching may be normal for a depressed person, but it's not natural for a well body, or for a body to permanently stay this way. Straighten and you will feel better. Anxiety and worry are natural outcrops of an inner imbalance that we are made aware of through our feelings, but it is not natural to maintain anxious, agitated or restless states indefinitely. We were meant to be vital, virile, upright and calm beings. I find most people don't have a clear template for maximizing their vitality. They hold onto anxious or negative behavior because they don't know how to surrender it. Their minds are set on 'run the anxiety program,' or run the 'be like mom or dad program.' Our attitudes affect us and are reflected in our posture. Attitude and posture affect martial performance in more ways than you can imagine. Some street wise cops have an uncanny ability to detect perpetrators tells from the slightest of physical cures.

When fear is the result of an unconscious program running in your head, imbedded before you had a say in things, adulthood is a good time to unwind these fears, stop the inner voice claiming you aren't confident, aren't strong. This mental action is called *maturing*.

The instructions for getting us back to a natural state can be found in the world's initiatory communities. The more authentic martial disciplines have long been known to provide this transitional resource.

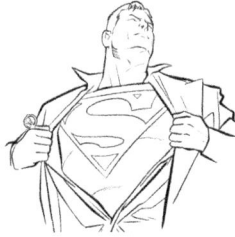

Natural or Supernatural?

What is our strength legacy as humans? I believe many people possess a latent, underorganized inner superbeing. Sadly, I've witnessed individuals assign away these suppressed superior abilities to their fantasy superheroes, convinced they are just average Clark Kents or Lois Lanes who then live vicariously through these media fictions. I embraced a 'humans aren't superbeings' mentality for a quarter of a century. I had no idea that Kiko could supersize my talents. I've spoken with Tai Chi practitioners, Qigong and Reiki masters unaware of the hidden strength side of their own disciplines due to their exclusive focus on health, not raw power.

The subjects I tested didn't have to believe in Ki when I taught them Hard Gate formulas (Observation 5). In some presentations, I never mention Ki or Kiko at all. I just ask participants to stand a certain way, relax, then attempt a particular strength challenge. I only ask initiates to have an open mind, to suspend any belief or disbelief in mystical powers and just look at the results. You don't have to understand why your strength jumps 30%-100% using Hard Gates. You just have to posture properly and relax. That's all there is to it. Simple but significant.

You cannot activate a potential you are unaware exists.

Just as there are many Hard Gate formulas that work, there are many incorrect actions that can ne-gate the results and thus rob you of energy. This is why I believe the more knowledgeable masters were, and are, sticklers for perfect Form.

I was rewatching an old video of a former athletic and skilled assistant teacher test for his black belt during my pre-Kiko years. I could sense the drag in his kata performance. It made me think of a driver applying the brakes while pressing the accelerator at the same time. The subtle buildup of friction was almost palpable.

In my book, *The Soul Polisher's Apprentice*, I talk about 'Masters of the How' versus 'Masters of the Why'. Masters of the How are the craftsmen with the ability to expertly duplicate what their teachers taught them—but usually, that's all. I've seen hundreds of videos of modern experts duplicating their teacher's kata to a T. But mimicking someone's kata doesn't give one any better clues why these movement sets were composed the way they are. Masters of the Why are the true artisans. When you understand the whys of your discipline, you can create your own success formulas.

5* Your Energy Body can be physically manipulated to greatly enhance your strength by the proper alignment of the limbs and torso in both static and moving actions with a methodology I call Hard Gating.

The Hard Gates: Kiko's Nuts and Bolts:

Enter into any martial art school and you are instantly initiated into warrior culture through the unique kinetic language of combative movement. Each school will frame out and pace the learning of its motive vocabulary differently. But in every school, regardless of discipline, you will learn precise ways to move in distinct physical categories encompassing strikes, blocks/parries, stances, takedowns, locks/holds and releases from locks/holds, as well as appropriate attitudes to forcefully convey these methods.

My focus has been on the martial behavior and application of Ki. I wanted to know how to further maximize my strength via body positioning. Placing my foot on a particular angle to increase the contractibility of my arm muscles would not be readily accessible knowledge to the average, Western-trained martial artist, nor today's exercise physiologists and fitness gurus.

From my experience, we have two methods for moving Ki. I label them as the *Hard* and *Soft Gates*. The Hard Gating singular system looks at the effects of precise physical actions and posturing on the movement of Ki for enhanced physical strength. A Hard

Gate activation is a much finer biomechanical action than current-ly applied in most fighting art curriculums. In Hard Gating, we take a deep look at movement and the positioning of the joints. Since our limbs have joints at different length junctures, executing any technique usually results in multiple Hard Gates being activated. Joint positioning can be put into three simple categories:

1. Fully rotated in one direction,
2. Fully rotated in the opposite direction,
3. Midway between the two end points.

(*Bilateral joint positioning is duplicating the same posture with the opposite limb simultaneously).

We can attach a relative value system to these positions:
1. The action or position increases strength,
2. The action or position decreases strength,
3. The action or position is neutral, neither significantly increasing or decreasing strength.

Standing with the feet parallel, shoulder width apart, is con-sidered a neutral, Hard Gate position. This is also referred to as a natural stance because this bilateral limb positioning produces a two-way signal to the musculature to distribute Ki equally be-tween Yin and Yang channels. A shift of any joint will send an in-voluntary message through the musculoskeletal system resulting in either a charging or discharging of Ki to the signaled muscle(s). A charged muscle will contract faster and harder. A discharged muscle will contract slower, with less force.

For most, this function occurs beneath general awareness. However, like breathing, this system can be brought into aware-ness, giving anyone more control over their Energy Body. The conscious regulation or distribution of Ki by way of precise body positioning and/or intention is what defines Internal from External martial training.

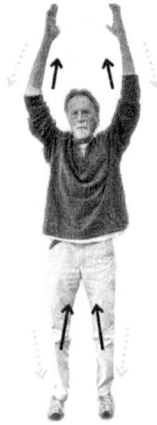

The Chinese Model of Qi

The Chinese internal martial model would view a neutral foot position as distributing Ki equally between Yin and Yang channels. The terms Yin/Yang used here refer only to the direction of Ki flow. Yin/Yang energy, in this context, is the same energy moving in opposite directions. I call these currents, *Strength Channels*, because they carry a charge to the musculature.

According to acupuncture theory, Ki flows through invisible, yet precisely defined, energy pathways called *meridians* running inside and close to the surface of the body. Ki also flows in defined currents outside the body. Yang energy or Yang Ki flows through downward directed channels found on the outside of the limbs. Yin energy, or Yin Ki, flows through rising, upward directed channels found on the inside of the limbs.

I view Ki primarily as an electro-magnetic phenomenon. If Ki is proven to be fundamentally electro-magnetic, then we are controlling the flow of positive and negative electrical biocurrents.

Feet pointing straight ahead under the shoulders generally results in equal Yin/Yang current flow. Turning your feet inward or outward acts like a valve, increasing the flow of Ki in one direction, while decreasing it in the opposite direction. If you have assumed the correct postural proportionality (correct width and length), feet turned inward, for example, will enhance your arm strength for upward directed technique. Feet turned outward will decrease the current in the Yin Channels but increase Yang Channel strength for downward directed technique.

Prior trauma such as an injury or illness, physical stiffness (muscles held in a chronically contracted state), or mental rigidity from fixed thoughts and prejudices, can block, reduce, reverse, or stop Ki flow altogether.

Few martial artists have a clear idea of how this muscle charge/ discharge system works when selecting a martial posture or technique. Kiko principles are supported by proper body mechanics, but at advanced stages, Kiko can transcend correct biomechanics.

Historically, postures that did not offer viable strength gains were omitted from an art's technical inventory. This is the reason we see so many technical similarities amongst martial systems worldwide. Whether arrived at by intuition or logic, it was understood that certain postures distributed maximum power. Useless postures and patterns were culled in favor of the strongest positions. Selected postures in the traditional arts appear stylized because they were discovered to maximize energy for specific tasks. Some of you may assume I am simply masquerading biomechanical technique as a mystifying Ki-powered skill. As you will see, I will make a case for a clear distinction between these two modalities.

Kiko postures often possess a dual Energy characteristic. They can become either a Yin or Yang posture by slight adjustments in a limb(s). In the Hard Gate system, we want to know at what point the configuration loses its distinction as one or the other. Visually, it may appear a person falls within the correct parameters, but when the Ki flow reverses, that stance or posture loses power for its intended purpose, and must be considered a negative or ne-gating posture. If you need a Yang stance but you mistakenly stand too wide, turning it into a Yin stance, you are in the incorrect position for the task. It's not even necessary to move the feet from their correct placement in width or length from one another, but only to shift the weight front, back or sides, to flip Ki flow from a positive to a negative flow. This is why the detail is taken to heart.

The strength of traditional martial postures and the purposes they were designed for can be confirmed by testing. Martial bunkai, the application of a solo fighting set in a live or partnered assault scenario, was a major part of the old-world testing of both a technique's biomechanical and Kiko principles.

Testing Ki

I owe the advances my organization has made in understanding the internal mechanisms of the Fighting Arts to the extensive testing we have done since 1993. This approach to learning is what the ancient Greeks termed a heuristic method. At one time the Buddha stated that people should not believe anything simply because he had said it, or because it was given by an "authority," or taught because of an ancient tradition or custom. Everything must be tested by the light of one's considered and personal experience and accepted only then. Our testing has provided us with a practical method to continually refine and understand our own experiences.

Testing things by means of direct experience is a method used in scientific fields, along with one other important proviso; namely, that anyone else with the necessary facilities can repeat the experiments and be satisfied that the results claimed can be substantiated. It is precisely in this spirit that I present Kiko. However, it is incumbent on every martial artist to experience Kiko for themselves. The essential point to grasp is that Kiko is not something you believe in, it is something you do.

I never assume anyone's Ki is flowing properly in any martial pattern. I test frequently and assess every new hypothesis with as many subjects available. With extensive testing through a range of physical tasks it is easy to determine if a subject's strength has increased or decreased.

However, we only use subjective measurements of observed and or felt outcomes mutually agreed upon. We do not use any external testing instrumentation except human bodies and occasionally, common objects. I have conducted thousands of these tests with young/old, men/women, left/right handers, beginners, lay persons and advanced martial artists, all with consistent results. Occasionally, we will use a kinesiological Priority Test to determine the optimal action when encountering multiple formulas.

To bring Kiko's potency home to new students, I ask them to push another out of a fighting stance and to keep in mind the degree of resistance they feel when pushing. I then ask them to relax into a *wuji* (empty standing) posture for a few seconds and try the test again. Most participants find the results unbelievable. Not only are they unable to hold their stance against the push, in some cases, they are tossed three to four feet backward where before they barely budged. It's okay if subjects don't believe what happened or think their partner went along with the push. When their friend goes unexpectedly flying—their limited notion of personal power flies out the window as well.

Our strength tests are designed to have a person demonstrate Kiko either by resisting a specific action against them or by using Kiko to overcome a resistive partner. Either way, the results have been statistically jaw dropping, well into the 90% success range. It doesn't matter if the participant is a karate seventh dan, a middle-aged, over-weight, white belt beginner, or a skinny high school student. When you are internally aligned you become significantly stronger than your pre-Kiko, natural capabilities. Our subjects ranged in age from 10 to 90.

Curiously, I have never demonstrated Kiko to anyone who initially thought what they experienced was real. Everyone was convinced I was accommodating them by going along with the test or fooling them by means of trickery. This was exactly how the Frogman and I had felt during my effortless wrist escape. Breaking Stone's grip had felt so easy it couldn't possibly be real. It went against the grain of my too-good-to-be true thinking. It was this very ingrained and limiting conventional ideology that blinded me to the power of Kiko in the first place.

Records exist of Ki-testing *(kitae)* amongst the Asian masters. A somewhat weaker carry over of testing is the grounding of solo formwork with realistic, partnered exchanges. When it comes to martial technique the best course is always 'trust but verify'.

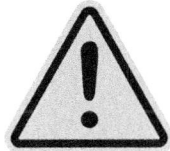

Kiko practice is no more dangerous than external training. However, two precautions should be mentioned when doing Ki work with a partner. Those at the receiving end of Hard or Soft Gate actions can be injured if the moves performed are done too intensely, with too much force. The sudden surge of Ki into the musculature can quickly overpower a subject's resistance and damage their joints. On a more subtle plane, subjecting oneself to repeated surges or dispersals of Ki can throw both the tester and the tested off center as their Biofield's must rebalance.

Single Blind, Double Blind, Blind

A quick look at the ever-shifting tides regarding the contesting of martial theories sheds light on an on-going debate about Ki.

I knew going into this study that I would never coax every-one aboard the Kiko vessel. Is there any novel idea that doesn't attract its critics? As the Chinese philosophers insist, every Yin has its Yang. It's naive to think that there won't be opposition to new ideas or perspectives. One person suggested that if a Dou-ble-Blind study hadn't been conducted on my Kiko work, he could not accept the results or my theory behind the outcomes. He waved away over a quarter century of observations with a snap judgement. I considered his attitude a form of mental blindness.

Absence of evidence is not evidence of absence.
Martin Rees, Carl Sagan

Evidence of absence..., as quoted in the above aphorism, has been a centuries-long subject of debate between scientists and philosophers. Engaging someone who sees something you don't see can often lead to contestation or contention. Fair enough. But for those in denial, a fact isn't really a fact, until it's believed. Odd-ly, belief can trump fact. If someone doesn't want to believe that the earth is round, the earth remains other-shaped in their mind. Facts need belief to pollinate them, to give them traction. Believ-ers of facts pollinate facts. Non-believers of facts pollinate falsities and perpetuate illusion. If blind persons were to steadfastly in-sist that colors don't exist and there were more blind people than seers, the general consensus would be that colors don't exist and laws might be passed to keep their false belief spreading to the destruction of the seers.

There were many individuals who faced criticism for their inno-vative ideas or discoveries, whose work was later proven accurate or had a significant impact on their respective fields. Galileo Gali-lei, the Italian astronomer was harshly criticized for his support of the heliocentric model of the solar system. Alfred Wegener, a Ger-man geophysicist, faced significant lifetime criticism for his theory of continental drift. He was later vindicated with the development of plate tectonics. The work of Barbara McClintock, the Ameri-can geneticist who conducted groundbreaking research on the genetics of corn, was largely ignored by the scientific community until several decades later, when her discoveries were recognized as highly significant. Ignaz Semmelweis, the Hungarian physician who discovered that handwashing could prevent the spread of in-fectious diseases endured a lifetime of resistance and ridicule. His ideas are now recognized as a foundational principle of modern medicine. Closer to the subject of this book is the work of Robert O. Becker who was ridiculed for his belief that the human body possessed any internal electrical system.

Arthur Schopenhauer, the German philosopher, stated that all important advances will go through three stages. First, the proponents are ridiculed, their ideas shunned. Second, their ideas meet with heated argument against them. Lastly, the observations are accepted as self-evident.

Single blind is a term used in science to imply that testing is done with a fair amount of intelligent subjectivity. Fair and intelligent subjectivity begins with acute observation, the foundation of all science. Science is a discipline that tests hypothesis. The Karate master who realized that with the palm of his hand he could knock anyone over and did so with everyone is his class, doesn't need a scientist to prove or say to him he can or cannot do it. His doing it is proof enough. Where it gets dicey, is what caused the knockout.

A Double-Blind study implies that subjectivity is removed enough to warrant that any statistically significant bias is absent in the results—in principle. But here is where Quantum physicists throw a titanium monkey wrench into the works. They say you can't remove the monkey wrench of subjectivity in *any* experiment. There can never be an experiment absolutely free of bias.

How then do you remove the subjectivity from two people interacting to test whether Ki is real, or outside of self-suggestion? You can't. It's the wrong way to test Ki in the first place. Mind is inseparably linked to body. Body is inseparability linked to mind. An event in one dimension will have an immediate effect upon the other. A splinter in your big toe will affect your state of mind. An irritating conversation with your neighbor will affect your mood and might lead to indigestion. We are not machines made of easily definable parts and functions. The whole premise behind Ki is that we are all intertwining, intercommunicating, interpenetrating energy fields, quantumly entangled, influencing one another on obvious and unobvious levels. You are already entangled with me via my ideas reading this book. Is there any instrument that can prove this?

One yudansha, after being introduced to Kiko, was surprised there were not more schools assessing the efficacy of their techniques using a Kiko template. I explained that most martial systems are held in check by the gatekeepers of parochial beliefs preventing their students from looking further into the technicalities of their systems outside where their teachers have told them to look. To progress beyond established dogma, one must challenge the common beliefs and test the theories supporting the challenge. Before you can question outside your martial box you must muster the courage to assail any authoritarian stronghold boxing your thinking about technique into a rigid format. The context of training has to segue from doing what has always been done to doing what has never been done.

Even if you don't think it will work, do what's right.
Thomas Merton

For example, stepping with a left foot will affect the Ki flow in your next limb action differently than stepping with a right foot. I am not speaking of right or left-handedness. When you execute a traditional block, you affect the power of the strike that follows. If you place a lock or have a lock placed upon you, your success in applying or escaping from the grip will be affected by the stance you are in at the moment of the lock, whether you inhaled or exhaled, what your free arm is doing at that moment. Such actions are considered irrelevant by mainstream standards. Kiko challenges this training narrative by introducing an upgraded set of quantum principles.

Kiko's Hard Gate system does not require you to know anything about Ki. Kiko is not a dogma you must believe in for it to work. All you need is to be shown the proper way to organize your body for the task at hand, and relax. This may sound simple but the average martial artist is internally disorganized. It doesn't matter how big you are, how large or sculpted your musculature, how willful or badass you believe yourself to be, if you are internally disorganized you will not be able to derive the optimal power from your physical structure.

Martial technique, with its Kiko principles intact, was preserved and passed along precisely because it revealed, through the detailed arrangement of its fighting sequences, how Biofield currents reinforce and amplify movement. Slight deviations between the Energy Body and the physical body can easily produce a lesser charge and lead to an undesirable outcome.

Before you commend yourself on having joined a school to profit from this immeasurable knowledge, know that Kiko cannot be a taken for granted inclusion in any modern martial curriculum. Where it once may have held prominence in a select few lineages, it has been mostly lost or barely maintained even within the most basic of technique. We can add to this problem the scarcity of teachers and the lack of today's student's interest to expend any time or energy to understand its workings. The union of mind, body and spirit has been degrading in the martial arts for nearly a century. It could also take a lifetime of trial and error to learn this by yourself.

The Five Element Theory & Martial Technique

According to some Chinese martial philosophers, there are five elemental orientations that can be used to characterize any martial technique. Every stance, block, strike or lock, can be classified as possessing the metaphorical characteristics of either Fire, Earth, Metal, Water or Wood. I find this Taoist classification of the elements a more relevant grouping when referring to martial technique than the Buddhist system, where Air replaces Wood and Space replaces Metal. The Five Element labelling is to be understood as a technique's *energy* signature. For each element describes one of five primary Biofield behaviors. For example, every stance generates a frequency unique to its postural configuration. If you make a stance higher, lower, wider, narrower, change your hip angle, the bend in your knees, your respiration, even your mindset, you change the Biofield messaging to both your own and your opponent's body. The manner in which you choose to strike, block and lock engages your adversary's energy field either helping or hindering you. Best to peak under the covers and see what's happening in the quantum arena if you want to up your game.

The *Five Element Phases* or *Five Element Cycles* speak directly to the quantum nature of physical movement. The Elemental Phases link stance to posture, to power, to likely shifts on the subatomic level.

Let's look now at how Kiko's Hard Gating system functions in four technical categories: Stances, Blocks, Strikes and Locks. Hard Gating or Hard Gates refers to the arrangement of the limbs and torso in both static and mobile modes for distributing a greater (or lesser) charge to the musculature. Kiko can be activated when performing any technique or sequence of techniques.

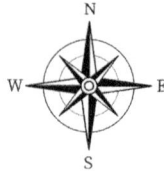

Set Your Bearings

---

*All tests, technical actions, and combative applications presented from here forward are to be understood as being performed North-facing unless otherwise indicated.

Kiko Technique

All limb motions act as electro-chemical pumps. Every martial stance, strike, lock, block, takedown or escape, will have a precise technical arrangement from head to foot to maximize its effectiveness. From the Kiko perspective, strikes are not just brute force limb projections. And stances are not just foot placements. Holding a particular stance or transitioning from one stance to another will follow a specific formula to maintain optimum Ki flow. For example, one of the most common stances in the martial arts, the Horse or Straddle stance (*Kiba dachi*), is not just any parallel, wide-based foot position. Dojos that make little to no distinction between a Horse versus a Seuichin (*Shiko dachi*) miss the opportunity to truly power up their postures. I've encountered sensei who cannot explain the reason why these two stances vary, or the purpose for which they are used. Telling students that outward turned feet in a Seiuchin/Shiko dachi are for those who cannot align their feet straight may be true for anatomically compromised students, but this answer overlooks a larger story.

It cannot be determined from outward appearance alone that there are Kiko and non-Kiko techniques. Kiko should be viewed as an advanced stage of technical execution. A Kiko technique will not only factor in the entire body alignment which includes foot placement, weight distribution on the feet, placement of the knees, hip, arms, neck and head, upper limbs and respiratory pattern but how it's being used. For example, if you had to choose from three right lead stances: Horse, Seiuchin, or T-Stance to bisect an opponent's stance, i.e., cut in between their legs, you would find the T-Stance superior in drawing the optimal charge over the other two. This is all coupled with a simultaneous mental posture, because slight repositioning of the mind will also alter Ki flow.

6* Each traditional stance activates one of five Elemental Phases in the Energy Body.

Kiko Stances

The instant any posture is assumed, a dual action is initiated as each posture is comprised of relaxed and contracted muscles used to sustain the posture. Even static postures pump Ki through the system. Therefore, no two stances create the same charge/discharge formula.

During any kumite, it is rare to find fighters standing still. A moving target is harder to hit. Stances becomes a blur of footwork as the body structure transitions from posture to posture in short, frenetic bursts, often within fractions of second intervals. This is a far more dynamic state of Ki distribution, which is why some schools build foundational skills first, for months, before engaging in free style matches. This parallels the Russian tennis coaches who do not let young developing athletes play any matches until the base skills are imprinted in muscle memory and thus have produced world class champions. A kumite requires fighters possess a high degree of internal control.

In the Wu Hsin Tao, we ascribe the following elements to the below-listed five postures. (Japanese names are given). These are primary stances with the greatest impact on their related meridians. Every posture generates a specific energetic effect defined cryptically as Fire, Earth, Metal, Water or Wood. The chart below, originally created in the 1970's by the British Kempo master, Terrence Dukes, only skims the surface of the relevancy of the Five elements to martial postures.

Earth	Horse Stance	Kiba, Shiko
Water	Rear Leg Stance	Kokutsu
Fire	Front Leg Stance	Zenkutsu
Wood/Air	Cat Stance	Tsuruashi, Neko dachi
Metal/Space	Three Battles Stance	Sanchin

On the following pages are some traditional stances from the Kiko Hard Gating perspective along with their Elemental influences where appropriate.

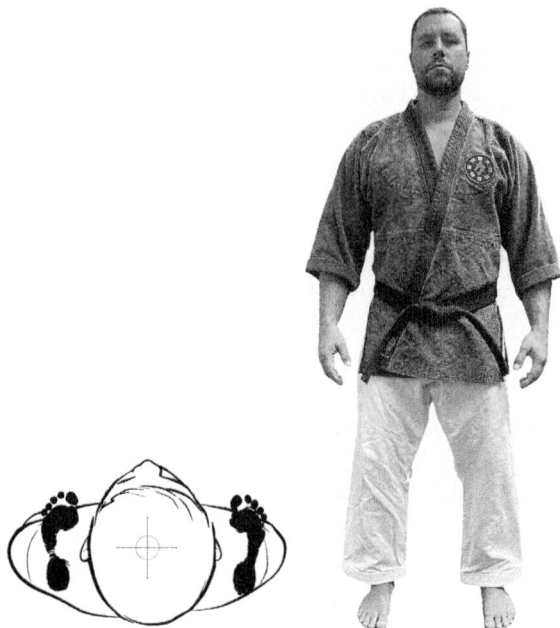

Neutral or Natural stance

Feet straight. Weight centered. Knees relaxed and bent over the toes. The shoulders fall to the outside edge of the feet. The pelvis and chin are gently tucked to mildly straighten the curvature in the lower back and neck. All extraneous bodily tension is released to the best of one's ability. When the attempt is to stand with the least amount of bodily friction to hold oneself upright, this posture is considered a *Wuji* or *Empty Standing* posture.

Purpose: To bring the body into a relaxed, even energy state and to make one aware of extemporaneous tensions. To calm and integrate the nervous and bioenergetic systems by allowing prior actions to find equilibrium.

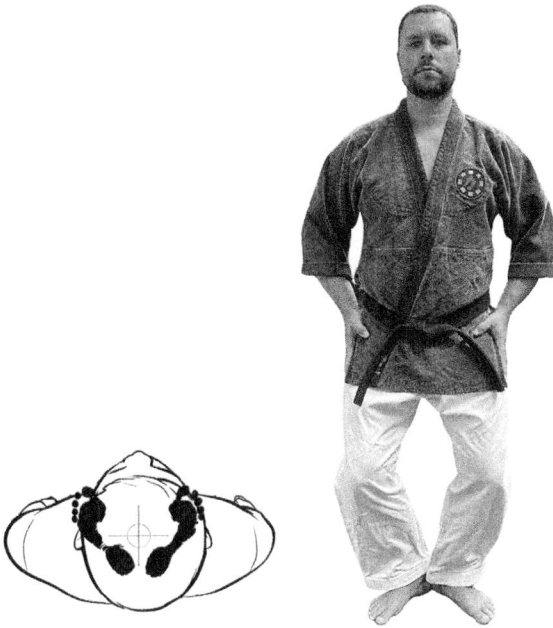

Musubu Stance (v'd feet)

Beginning with the feet together open the stance to 90 degrees pivoting on the heels. Heels can be lightly touching. Knees bent over the toes. Chin and pelvis gently tucked.

Purpose: To protect the nerves and major arteries in the legs from a rear attack. To increase leg endurance when standing for long periods, as in a military sentry. To set up the proper proportionality for other stances like the Neihanchi dachi.

The 90 degree Musubu stance may have been used as a metric for assuming the correct proportionality in the Neihanchi, Tekki (Iron Horse) and Seiuchin dachi. By pivoting from ball to heel to ball in 45-degree arcs all lateral stances can be correctly assumed.

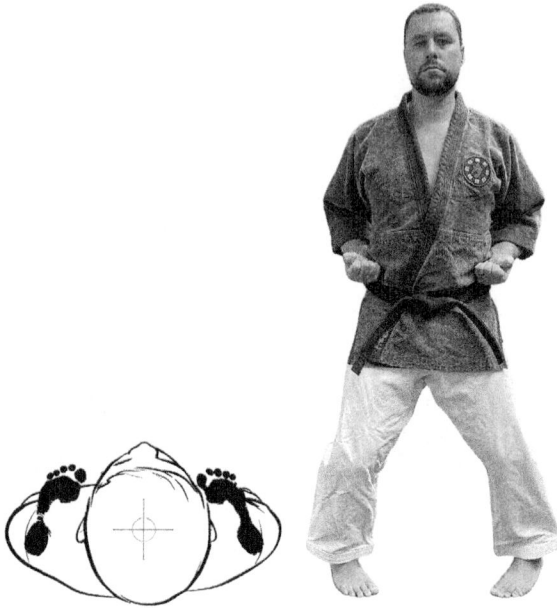

Neihanchi Stance

Neihanchi is an energy rising, Ki-gathering posture. Assume the stance by v'ing your feet on a 90-degree angle with the toes pointing outward. From there, shift the weight to the balls of the feet and move the heels outward until the feet point 45-degrees inward. Place 70% weight on the balls of the feet.

Purpose: To protect the groin. To increase the torque of the hips. To generate rising power in the arms.

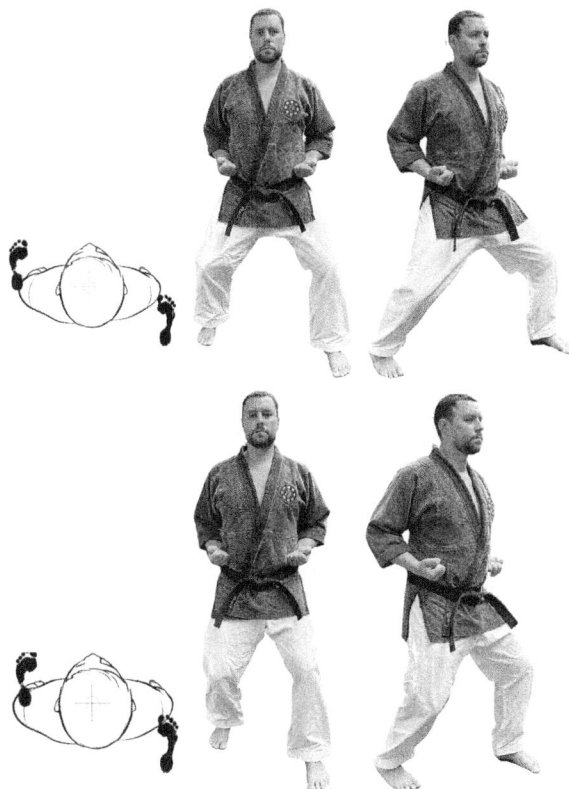

Seisan Stance: wide and narrow variants

The Isshinryu Seisan dachi has the feet point straight, shoulder width, where the outside edge of the feet falls directly under the shoulders. The heel of the lead foot is aligned with the toes of the rear foot. Isshin Kempo's Seisan dachi has the inside of the feet aligned with the shoulders. This foot-width marginal difference between the two systems is enough to shift the upper body posturing as to make IK similar to but not exactly the Isshinryu understanding. When stepping in the Seisan dachi, the foot must stay low to the ground, to absorb the Earth's rising Yin energy. When stepping forward with the left foot, inhale. When stepping forward with the right foot, exhale. This breathing pattern maximizes the Ki flow of each step. In the early stages of energy work, reversing the breath on the step can neutralize or cancel the desired effect.

A Perfect Crescent

Here is one Kiko formula for a perfect, Ki-gathering, Crescent or C-step into the Seisan dachi. Imagine a vertical line down the front of your stationary leg. As you step with your left, brush as close as possible to this line without crossing it. Inhale from your abdomen as you step. (In Shitoryu karate the same benefits are achieved by stepping in a 1/4 arc).

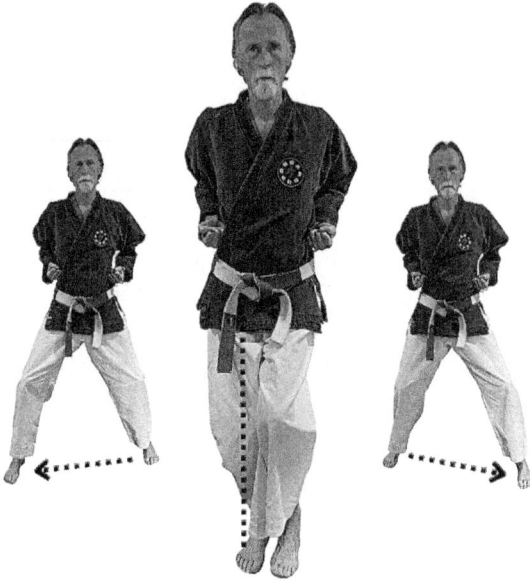

The width of the stepping foot from the supporting leg should spark a debate for some time. The story below explains:

In my early years of training, stances were grossly defined. Teachers were light on detail. As a result, I found myself assuming a wider Seisan dachi than indicated in books claiming the outside of the shoulders should fall to the outside of the feet. Looking back, I favored a wider Seisan stance to better stabilize my 6'4" frame.

Even though students try their best to stay within the guidelines of proper form, technical details frequently drift, much like a car on the highway rarely drives perfectly straight. Since no one corrected my stance, my wide posture stuck.

I later wondered why my upper limb positioning differed from

Tatsuo Shimabuku's kata (note the variations below). I had no idea that grounding myself in a wider Seisan dachi would energetically alter the arm configurations of my kata. It turned out, both positions are correct. To charge the lead arm in Shimabuku's narrow stance, the secondary hand must be placed to the side of the body. By widening the stance, where the outside of the shoulders falls to the inside of the feet, the secondary hand needs to be placed in front of the thigh to maintain the same Ki flow. This slight foot width change, a characteristic that distinguishes Isshin Kempo from Isshinryu, shows how even a minor change in posture alters Ki flow.

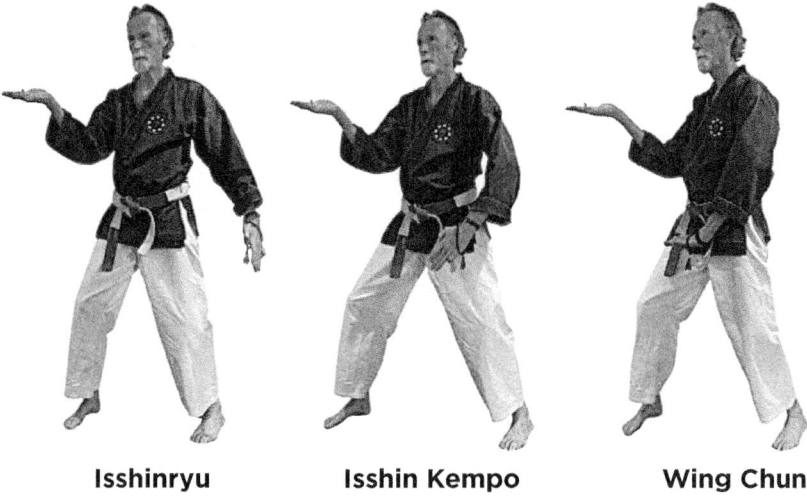

Isshinryu   **Isshin Kempo**   **Wing Chun**

**Marginal differences demonstrated above,
yet all follow correct Kiko formulas**

In Isshinryu karate the outside edge of the stepping foot should land just inside the shoulder. The lead foot should be no more than a foot length forward (one's own foot length). A one-to-two-inch margin of error in either direction is acceptable without experiencing a significant drop in Energy. Exceeding this margin of error reverses Ki polarity, meaning, rather than generating three times the charge, you will discharge three times as much Ki from your arm before you actually push or parry. Energy Body sidedness is far more pervasive in martial arts than most consider.

*Among the subtle energy disciplines, it is acknowledged that the left eye takes in energy. The right eye puts it out. The left hand receives. The right hand sends. Oxygenated blood flows in the arteries on the left side of the body and is carried away on the right through the veins.

When stationary, each foot is roughly 70% forward weighted. This weight shift opens the Bubbling Springs acupoints on the bottoms of the feet to increase Ki flow up the inside of the legs. The Bubbling Springs acupoints act like energy valves. Stretching the ball of the foot opens these valves. Tightening it, closes them. Clenching your toes like gripping sand, similar to making a fist, is a misinterpretation of the stance's proper bioenergetic mechanic. Over-gripping your feet will close the Bubbling Springs and trigger a body weakening due to decreased charge. You want to make broad contact with the bottoms of your feet on the floor. Once this is established, you can apply gripping pressure as long as you avoid bending your toes at the middle knuckles and raising them off the floor.

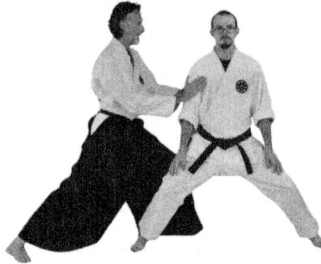

A test: We had subjects resist being uprooted from a Kiba dachi by pushing their torso directly against their rear leg support. When we asked them to clench their toes, they were unable to hold their ground. When they assumed maximum foot contact with the floor and applied a light tension to accentuate the contact, their resistance jumped dramatically.

Some non-kata schools decry the uselessness of traditional crescent stepping. They cite it as cumbersome and ineffective against a highly mobile opponent. These schools miss the purpose of the arcing step. The crescent creates a weaving motion that reduces body target. It can bisect an opponent's stance and disrupt their balanced structure. More importantly, the Crescent step pumps the maximum Ki into the upper limbs for increased arm strength.

Seisan dachi Ki flow when facing North or West:
Forward left crescent step/inhale = energy in =
increased muscular charge
Backward left crescent step/exhale = energy out =
decreased muscular charge
Forward right crescent step/exhale = energy out =
decreased muscular charge
Backward right crescent step/exhale = energy in=
increased muscular charge

Seisan dachi Ki flow when Facing South or East:
Forward left crescent step/exhale = energy out=
decreased muscular charge
Backward left crescent step/inhale = energy in=
increased muscular charge
Forward right crescent step/inhale = energy in=
increased muscular charge
Backward right crescent step/exhale = energy out=
decreased muscular charge

Since Hard Gating is similar to the biomechanics of stacking body weight to add more force behind a technique, the Crescent step must be coupled with the proper respiratory action. A north-facing, left foot forward is coupled with an in-breath. A right foot forward Crescent is coupled with an out-breath.

Purpose: Seisan is an enhanced, yet equal Energy flow posture. In alignment with its external function, Seisan balances mobility and stability without sacrificing either quality. Its exoteric purpose is to initiate an evasive weaving when stepping, and bisect an adversary's stance to unbalance their structure. Its esoteric purpose is to draw Ki when stepping to the outside of an opponent's lead right foot with the left, or to step to the inside of the opponent's lead left foot when stepping with the right. An oblique or angled Seisan stance is also used as a common guard or cover position.

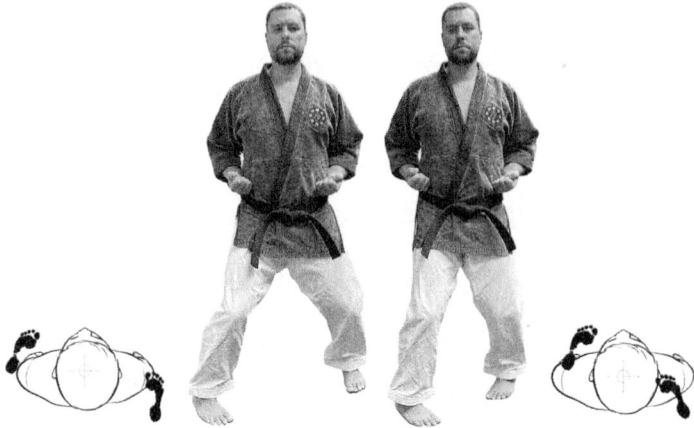

Sanchin Stance wide and narrow variants

There are two Sanchin dachis, the wide and the narrow. The wide only turns the lead foot heel out. The narrow rotates both heels out. Both postures are identical to the details of the Seisan dachi, with the exception of the rotated foot or feet turned no more than 45-degrees.

I believe that the toed-in trait of the Sanchin stance was created, in part, to solve the general problem of how to draw energy up the right leg similar to a North-facing, forward, left leg, C-step into a Seisan dachi. By turning the right foot heel slightly outward, one prevents the usual energy loss, and instead, increases the charge up the right leg. Turning the ball of the foot inward does not maximize the flow but triggers an energy out condition.

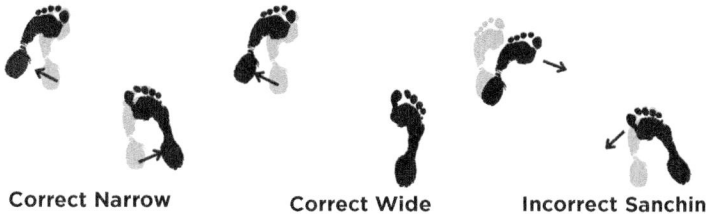

Correct Narrow   **Correct Wide**   **Incorrect Sanchin**

In a static Sanchin dachi weight may be evenly distributed on front and back of the feet. However, this is only a partial understanding of the functioning of this stance and stances in general. While moving in and out of Sanchin, the weight will shift from back to front of the foot while executing upper body limb actions. Weight distribution in stances including forward, backward, inward and outward pressure on the feet represents a dynamic energy phase redirecting Ki currents to different muscle groups, hence, outcomes. Sanchin stance and C-stepping creates an energy-in or condensing (metal) Ki action.

Purpose: To increase the Ki draw when stepping with a right leg. To increase rising Energy in the arms. To protect the groin. To forcefully bisect and unbalance the structure of an adversary who attacks with a lead left leg. From a combative standpoint, it may be necessary to adjust a stance. In the case of Sanchin dachi, if you need to step wider into an opponent, you will need to adjust the upper limb positions to maintain the same power effect. Here you must not turn the rear leg inward but rather, keep it straight.

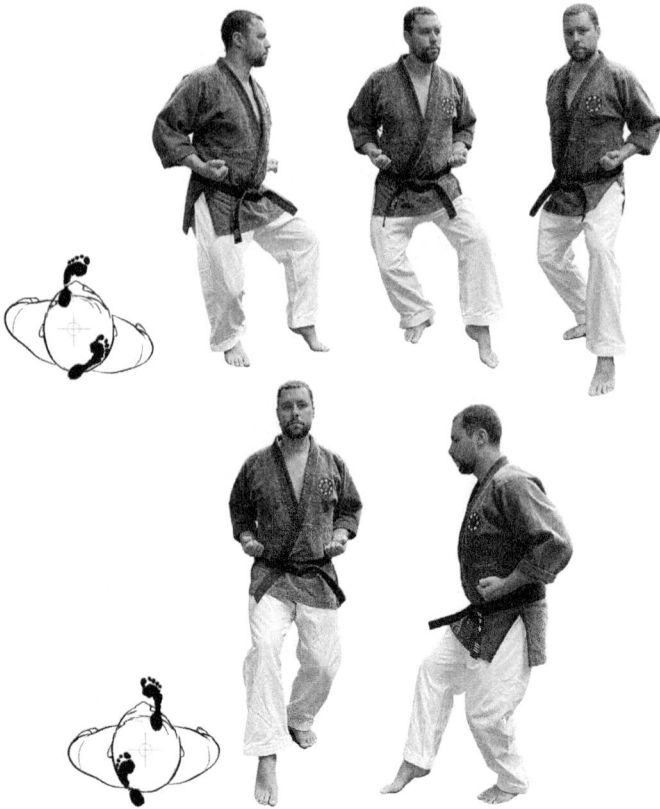

Open And Closed Cat Stance

There are two Cat postures distinguished by the angle of the rear foot and positioning of the hips. In both cases, the heel of the front foot is lifted 45-degrees to open the Bubbling Springs acupoint. When used in conjunction with the proper arm action, the Cat stance becomes a powerful Ki-drawing posture. The Cat is often used in retreat as part of its Ki-drawing function.

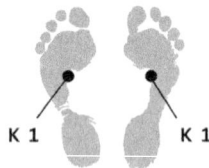

Bubbling Springs or Kidney 1

Approximately 10% of body weight rests on the front foot. The rear foot placed outward 45-degrees is considered an

'Open' Cat. This posture is used primarily when the right foot is the rear leg. A 'Closed' Cat is assumed by placing the rear foot on a 10-15-degree angle and is generally seen when the left foot is placed rearward. In either, case, the feet should be spaced one foot length apart (i.e., your foot length) with a margin of error of no more than two inches. In the Open Cat, the hips are tilted back and angled. In the 'Closed' cat the hips are tucked and face forward.

Purpose: To quickly transition into another stance. To evade without retreat. To draw a strong charge off the opponent in an Open Cat, or energetically overwhelm an adversary by sending a strong charge from a Closed Cat.

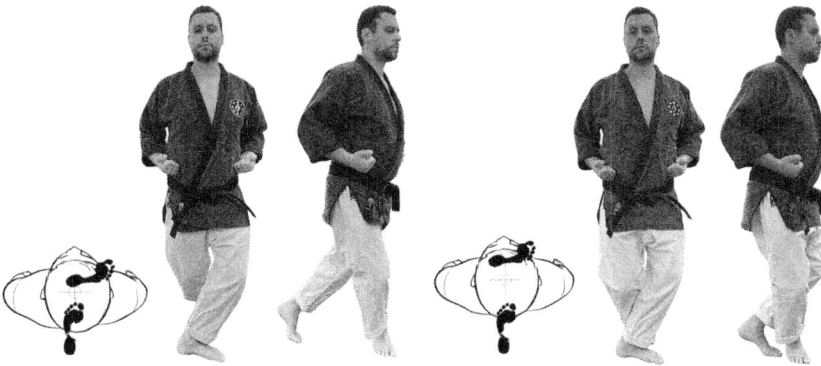

Open And Closed Reverse Cat Stance
(*Kosa dachi, Hook stance*)

The Reverse Cat can be thought of as the opposite posture to a Cat stance as far as the weight distribution on the feet. The front foot is turned outward about 45-degrees and carries up to 90 percent of the body's weight. The back foot has the heel raised while maintaining contact with the toes and ball of the foot. Similar to the Cat, the arching rear leg opens the Bubbling Springs acupoint of the back foot. The toes of the back foot should point toward the heel of the lead foot. The 'open' position refers to the hips inclining toward the rear leg, which is set further back from the front foot. In the 'Closed' Reverse Cat the rear leg hugs close to the front leg with knees nearly parallel and the hips rotated forward. This advanced, transitional, posture, is generally entered into from other stances.

A Reverse cat is entered into by either rotating in place or stepping forward, backward, diagonally, or horizontally into position. The stepping foot should skim close to the ground. The rear foot activates when the heel is lifted.

Let's look at three ways to assume this stance. I call them the Retreating Reverse Cat, the Advancing Reverse Cat (Kosa dachi in Shotokan, Kake or Hook stance) and the Rotating in place Reverse Cat.

The Retreating Reverse Cat is a rearward stepping action coupled with an in-breath. The rear leg extends a foot length backward stopping with one's toes pointing to the heel of the lead foot. The foot must not arc when retreating.

The Forward stepping Reverse Cat is achieved by stepping one foot length ahead of the rear leg and rotating into the posture.

The Rotating-in-place Reverse Cat is achieved by a rotational shift of the body weight forward while pulling the rear leg directly behind the front leg coupled with an out-breath. The affect is cancelled if you leave your back foot a foot length away from the front foot.

Done correctly, all three methods will increase Yin and Yang Ki flow magnifying your strength for upper limb actions. A basic rule in Kiko is not to mix and match the details of one Reverse Cat for another.

Purpose: The Reverse Cat is used for its torquing strength, to extend the range of upper limb deflections or strikes when coming out of other stances, for sinking or dropping weight to take an opponent downward, for deflecting a body coming toward you, for uprooting another's wide base stance and for charging the body overall. The Reverse Cat is an excellent way to draw Ki from an opponent when stepping laterally and diagonally, that is, to one side or another of an opponent. It adds draw power similar to how a retreating Cat stance, done with a straight back, sucks energy from the attacker.

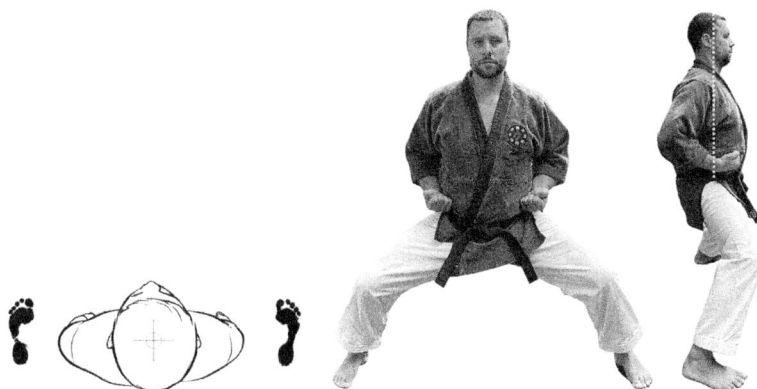

Horse (Straddle Leg) Stance

Feet straight, 1.5 shoulder width apart. Knees bent over the big toes and pushing outward is ideal. Weight falls 70% on balls of the feet. Chin and pelvis tucked inward to gently flatten the curves in the neck and lower back.

Purpose: To strengthen the Biofield's foundational rotational flow. To maintain spinal integrity and open Ki flow when an opponent is being taken toward or to the ground. To resist forceful lateral pushes and pulls.

The Horse stance is an Earth Element posture, not because the spread of the legs and bend in the knees brings you lower to the ground, but because a correct Horse Stance causes Ki to flow with greater volume through the Earth meridians of the body, causing a clockwise or counter clockwise spin of the Biofield extending outside the body. Remember, each meridian charges certain muscle groups. When the Earth meridian is activated by the Horse posture, the Biofield currents outside your body will rotate with more force. The intensity, force and direction of the Ki circulation will also depend upon your respiration cycle and the clarity of your intention in assuming the posture. A Horse stance generates Earth Power or rotational force. The direction of the flow is activated by the breath; clockwise on an exhalation, counter-clockwise on inhalation. An increase in Earth meridian flow will enhance the contractability of all the muscles supported along this bio-circuitry.

Uprooting a Horse

The stability and leg-strengthening attributes of the Kiba dachi has made this posture a staple in martial arts world-wide. When biomechanically correct, it is difficult for someone to be pushed or pulled laterally without leveraging them upward. There are other uses for a Horse stance than resisting pushes or pulls. I will focus on this single purpose to demonstrate Kiko's power.

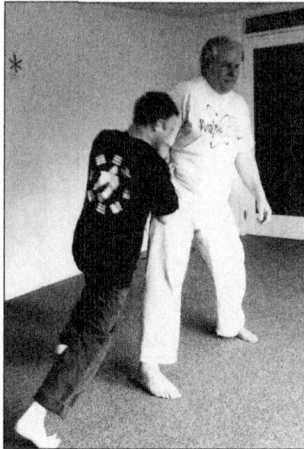

1st attempt pushing   2nd attempt using Kiko

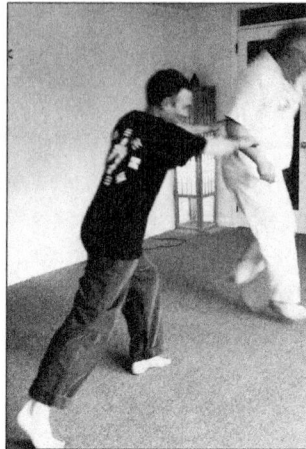

A 160 pound man tries to push a 240 pound man out of his Horse stance (above). In the first image, the pusher barely budges the larger fellow with his best effort. The pusher's handicap was not to push his partner upward. Both men are multi-decade karateka. I then asked the pusher to relax, concentrate on his lower abdomen and hold his Ki back until he pushed. He hurled the man many feet away into the far wall. Observer's reactions; *"It didn't look real."* Reaction by both men, *"It didn't feel real."*

Different body positions signal and prime certain muscle groups for a 30-100% increase in physical output. 100% is the doubling of your physical strength. This posture-to-strength formula is inaccessible to lay persons unfamiliar with martial Kiko except by happenchance. This skill level is also not obvious to most martial artists. Martial Kiko is a subset of strength principles rarely found outside of a small, scattered circles of internally-focused, martial art lineages.

The way blocks are executed in most martial art systems is a case in point. Few students are given in-depth explanations why certain stances have the feet turned out, parallel, or inward while blocking. Reflecting on my early decades of training, neither I, nor any person in our dojo, ever questioned the efficacy of a movement sequence taught to us because it did not feel right.

After fifty-six years of study, I can state with certainty, that most of the Hard style fighting forms carried to Western shores by first-generation pioneers lacked any integral, internal principles. This left later generations lacking this knowledge, creating an ever-widening gap to retrieve or restore these techniques.

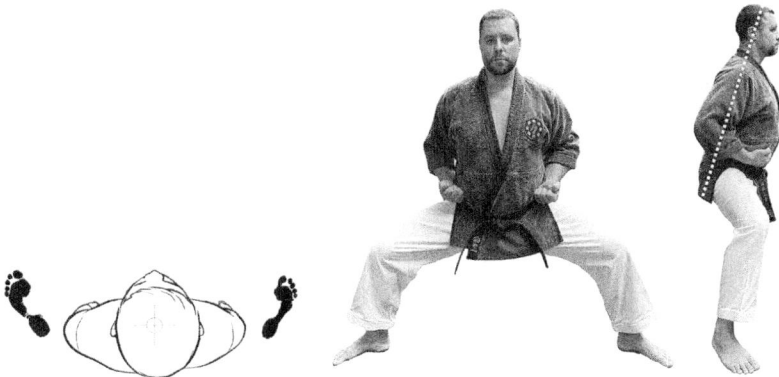

Seiuchin/Shiko Dachi Stance

Feet are splayed outward 45-degrees, 1.5 shoulder widths apart. Knees are bent and press outward over the toes. The pelvis is tilted backward causing a slight forward lean of the torso. The chin and front of the neck are relaxed and gently extended forward.

Purpose: To neutralize someone shooting for your legs. To draw an opponent's arms or body downwards with considerable force. Though appearing similar to the Horse stance, the Seiuchin dachi is a Water Element posture. It increases downward Ki flow. Descending Yang channels on the outside of the legs are activated, directing a strong current towards the floor.

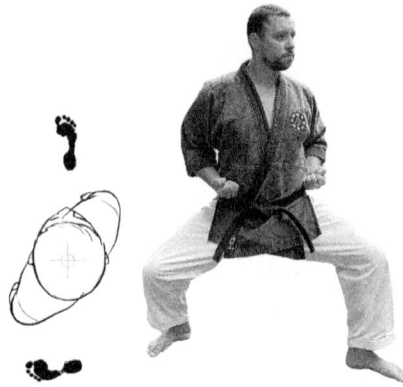

T-Stance (Fudo dachi)

Separate the feet by 1.5 shoulder widths. Point the lead foot straight. Place the rear leg on 90 degree angle. Align the heel of the rear foot with the heel of the front foot. Distribute the weight equally across the feet. Tilt the hips slightly back.

Purpose Similar to a retreating Cat stance, the T-stance draws Ki by stepping forward.

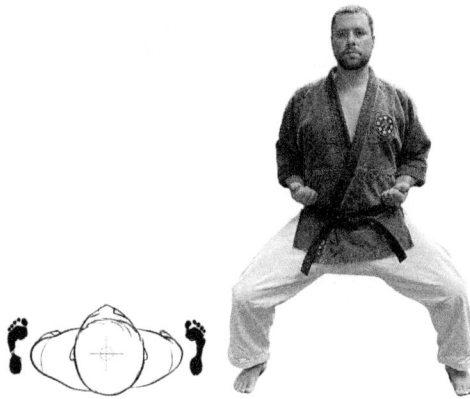

Iron Horse Stance (Tekki)

It is my hypothesis that the Iron Horse is one foot-width narrower than the traditional Kiba dachi. The knees must press outward. Pressure is exerted on the toes/balls of the feet by drawing them inward without moving them. If you want to convert the Kiba dachi into a Neihanchi-activating posture, press the heels outward without moving the feet. Shotokan's Tekki, Iron Horse, can be substituted for the narrower Neihanchi dachi.

Purpose: Same as the Neihanchi stance

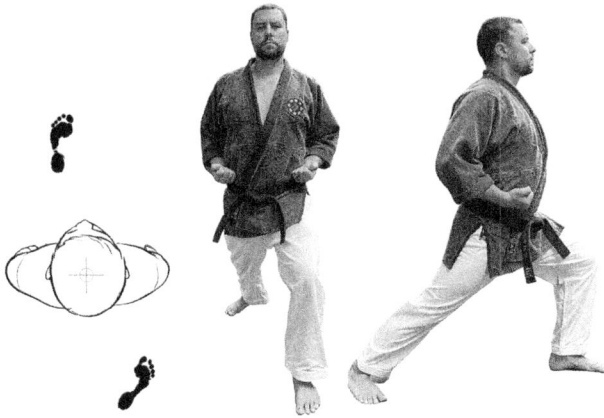

Zenkutsu Dachi

This stance is the hallmark of Shotokan and most Shorinryu and Shaolin lineages. Feet are placed 1.5 shoulder width apart. The rear leg turned out no more than 45-degrees and is either straight or maintained with the slightest bend at the knee. Front foot straight, pelvis tucked forward.

Purpose: To generate maximum forward thrust. To cover a large distance with speed and stability. To generate body weight behind a strike. To initiate a rising action of the Energy Body for potent takedowns. Zenkutsu dachi is a Fire Element Posture.

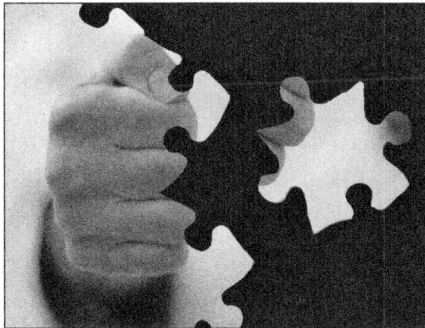

Kiko Strikes

When an action is done
with the whole body,
the whole mind and the whole spirit,
only then, is the result one of true power.

Kiko striking requires the same detailed scrutiny as the other categories of martial technique to unleash its full potential. I will breakdown the internal anatomy of five traditional strikes; a vertical punch, palm strike, elbow, a knifehand (*shuto*), and a front kick

As an expert in the Isshinryu vertical punch, I will start here. You should quickly get the gist of Kiko's influence for clues on how to apply these principles to any martial action.

A unique attribute of Okinawa's Isshinryu karate system is its vertical, thumb on top fist formation. Few are aware of all the reasons why and how the thumb should sit atop this fist formation.

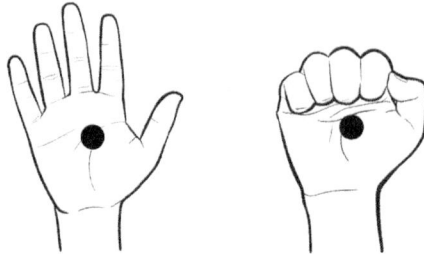

Laogong Accupoint

In Kiko, the fist is made by rolling the fingers into a ball but never pressing them into the center of the palm. Fingertips are placed on the muscle pads of the bottom knuckles, leaving the eye of the palm, called the *Laogong* point (*Labor Palace* or *Palace of Toil*) free of obstruction. The center of the palm and the webbing between the thumb and forefinger are two major martial acupoints. When open, these points allow Ki to flow freely around the hand and arm. Sealing or blocking the Laogong point reduces Ki flow to the deltoid, the central muscle in all forward extending arm actions.

The average person forming a fist will close their fingers and place their thumb over either their pointer or middle finger. Few will instinctively place their thumb on their ring finger, and rightly so. This action shuts off Ki to the deltoid.

There are two critical points on the hand that control the rising and lowering strength of the arm. Usually, one is open while the other is closed. The point called *Hegu*, (*Hand Valley* or *Joining Valley Point*), is situated in the webbing between the thumb and pointer. Stimulating this point helps remove excess heat from your body and can help rid you of stress, migraines, headaches, shoulder tension, toothache, constipation and neck pain. Little known however, is its ability to increase arm strength when used properly.

Thumb as Lever

The thumb in Kiko is used as a Hard Gate to open or close Strength Channels in the arm for different punching heights. The thumb placed atop the fist facilitates a rising arm action. Placed on the pointer finger, it supports a horizontal strike. Placed on the middle finger, a descending strike.

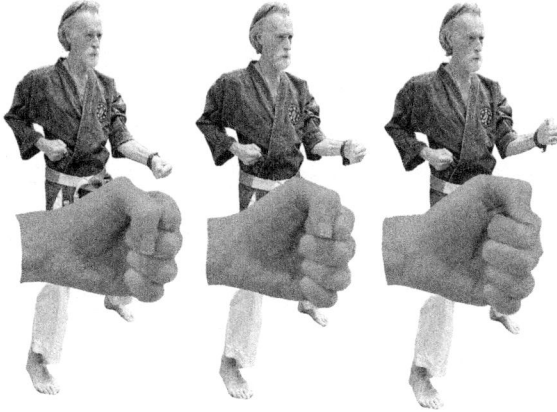

A test: We had subjects stand sideways to a tester and extend their right arm in a vertical fist. They were then asked to place their thumb over their middle finger and resist the tester's slow press down on their forearm, and note the resistance. The test was conducted again with the subject's thumb placed on the pointer finger and finally atop the pointer. Of the three thumb positions, most subjects felt a dramatic strength increase with their thumb atop their fist.

Launched from the side chamber at the waist, a fist strike must rise upward several inches to solar plexus height where a significant body target lies. If you want to punch downward with more force, your thumb will need to cover your middle finger. To punch straight ahead or horizontally, the thumb should be placed over the pointer finger. These thumb positions gate Ki in the arm for ascending, horizontal, or descending motions.

Did you ever hear the Skeleton Song, *Dem Bones*? 'The thigh bone's connected to the hip bone. Hip bone connected to the back bone...' Punching is a whole-body event. The fist is connected to the forearm, connected to the upper arm, shoulder, waist, hip, knee, ankle, foot. The third principle of physics, 'For every action there is an equal and opposite reaction,' holds true for Ki flow.

The fist may be the point of contact, but it represents just one facet of masterful punching.

A Hard Gate thumb position is one of the centerpieces of all punching actions. All joints along the force line of a punch, properly aligned, will supercharge the strike. If you have your thumb in the correct position but your shoulder is raised, the net result will be a decrease in punching power—mere mortal strength. A raised shoulder will negate a correctly gated thumb position. Kiko is a strengthening subsystem functioning alongside proper biomechanics.

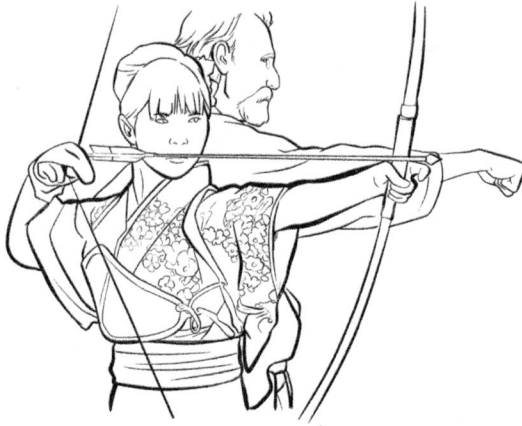

Perfect Form is perfect Ki flow

In Kiko, all joint positions are considered like switches or relays on a circuit board. We want to open or switch on as many relays along the chosen circuit to maximize striking, blocking and locking power.

Priming a punch in a traditional sense builds potential energy in the deltoid. Punching drills often begin with both hands raised at the side above the pelvis in the position commonly referred to as the *chamber*. Chambering primes the deltoid similar to the way an arrow drawn in a bow builds potential force. Stretched muscle draws Ki into its fibers increasing its contractability. If you think of Ki as an electrical current, your goal is to direct the largest possible current into the deltoid. From the Kiko perspective, any change in posture will change the current flow.

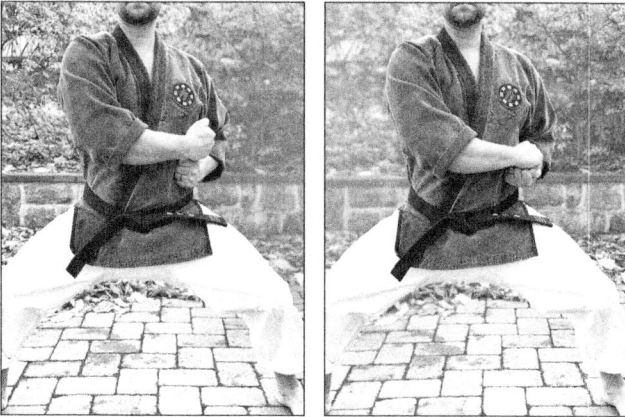

**Different side chambers reveal how an arm is to be grasped
and held and to charge the musculature for a particular action.**

Muscle priming for the upper body begins with the arms drawn above the waist. We are so used to performing simple tasks we never think of this posture as gating Energy. But as soon as your hands rise above your waistline, your upper arms become instantly stronger. This particular observation led me to an unexpected revelation. If you punch with your right, why does your non-punching arm also have to be raised at the chamber height? What difference does it make what your left arm is doing?

In the course of evolution our anatomy has developed a simple method for locomotion. Every muscle that moves a joint in one direction has opposing muscle(s) to move it in the opposite direction. The agonist moves us in the intended direction. The antagonist moves us in reverse. Sometimes these muscle sets fight against each other, hence, the term antagonist. With every muscular action we have a simultaneous charge and discharge cycle. This charge/discharge process is how we locomote.

To bend over and pick up a penny form the floor you have to relax your back and allow it to stretch so you can contract your abdominal muscles to pull your body downward. If there was no charge in your back to rise up, you'd be stuck, permanently bent. Thank God this system is mostly involuntary. The first observation follows Starling's Law; a muscle lightly stretched before contraction will contract with more force. This wasn't the big breakthrough in muscular output. The real breakthrough came when someone must have asked if energy flows from one complimentary muscle group to another. It appears possible to draw a charge from muscles not involved in the immediate action. This is why, when doing a basic punching drill, both hands are drawn upward at the side. The action of the passive hand lifted, drawn back, and held with the palms rotated upward, signals and distributes Ki to the arm about to punch. The result is a much stronger thrust.

A test: We asked subjects to punch with their free arm dangling at their side, then to punch again with both arms at chamber height. Almost every subject experienced a noticeable strength increase with both hands chambered properly.

Kiko in a Vertical Punch

Below is a detailed description of the Hard Gate system for a vertical punch thrown at solar plexus height. When punching, a Ki charge is drawn upward through the legs, concentrated in the belly, then moves through the torso into the punching arm and out the fist. All Kiko striking formulas follow specific rules and use the same underlying principles.

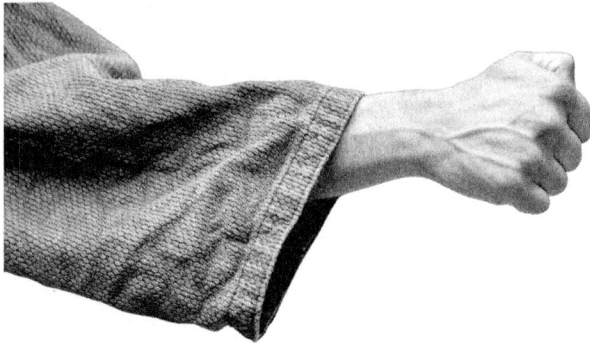

The Hard Gating sequence for a right vertical punch from a Seisan dachi:

Preparation
- Activate the following Hard Gates simultaneously:
- Assume a Seisan stance with left foot forward, weight slightly back on the heels.
- Knees bent over the big toes.
- Hands chambered in fists at the waist crease.
- Palms upward.

- Thumb on top pressing slightly toward the radius bone in the hand. (This seals the channel found in the webbing between thumb and pointer finger).
- Elbows down.
- Pull the shoulders down and slightly back of center.
- Tuck your chin in lightly to increase Yin channel flow up the back of the neck.
- Place your eyes on a 45-degree angle to the floor to better root your mind into your body.
- Inhale into the lower abdomen while slightly tilting the pelvis backward to gather a full charge.
- Keep the belly wall relaxed (relaxed muscle draws charge.)
- Slightly draw the bent knees inward to open Yang channels.
- Close the back by slightly pulling the scapula together to open up and stretch the upper chest.
- Cock the wrist at your side toward the thumb as you squeeze the top three fingers.

Execution: Do these actions simultaneously:
- Exhale through the mouth.
- Maintain the tongue on the roof of the palate.
- Flatten the abdomen upon exhale to distribute the Ki charge to the striking limb.
- Push the knees outward to open the Yin channels on the inside of the legs.
- Tuck the pelvis forward.
- Rock weight forward, placing roughly 70% of your weight over the ball of the foot.
- Aim the punch upward at your solar plexus height and to the centerline of your body.
- Shift the cock of the wrist from the thumb side to the pinky side while squeezing the bottom two fingers as you punch.

This detail behind a single punch is one example of what forms the Kiko art. If you just want a crude smash-and-dash technique, you don't want a traditional martial art. You want a convenient bludgeon.

You might think the reason this punch is stronger is due to proper biomechanics and that I have overdressed the detail. This is the proper biomechanic for a punch. But a strike isn't just about its external mechanics. Punch strength relies upon the distribution of Ki into the striking muscles. Directing Ki flow into the punching musculature is what defines a technique's internal mechanic.

If I ask someone to do all the above posturing and have them imagine a line of energy moving from their fist back toward their chest while they punch, their strike will lose significant power on impact, even though their external positioning and action is perfect. When the mind directs the Ki to flow opposite its intended direction, it deprives the punching muscles of their juice.

If I asked a puncher to clench the toes of their feet while punching, the strike will also lose power because this action seals Ki from charging the lower dantien. If you form a fist incorrectly by pressing your fingers into the center of your palm, the force of your strike will also be reduced because this seals the Laogong point. The more Hard Gates switched off, the weaker the strike.

If it looks like a punch and feels like a punch, it must be a punch, is not true when divining the inscrutable ways of the Asian fight masters. Many fist actions are not punches at all but concealed set up for locks. You have to look at a set or sequence of moves, rather than an individual technique, to make this determination.

Therapeutic vs Combative Technique

Why are there so many different forms of fist striking? Why do the majority of Asian styles punch with a nearly straight arm, palm down, while a minority strike with a stubby, vertical-fisted, short-range burst? If these two punches are so good, why not incorporate both into all fighting systems? Different tactics did not satisfactorily answer this question for me, which led to a radical thought. Has Western martial culture grossly misinterpreted the proper making, purpose, and execution of Asian fist formations? My answer is, "Yes."

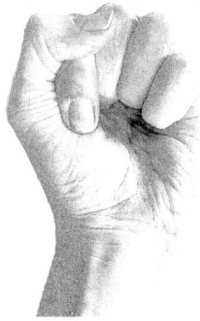

The Motobu Fist

I have read comments from advanced martial artists exclaiming the punching power of this fist formation, when, in fact, it was most likely not designed for striking at all, but rather to increase the grip strength of the ring and little finger and to distribute significant power into the waist for torquing motions. The fist is formed by keeping the pointer finger straight and wrapping the thumb across it. This configuration keeps the webbing between the pointer and thumb (*Hegu*) open. When coupled with the Neihanchi dachi, this fist distributes Ki to the torso.

Not all martial practices and techniques were developed solely for combat. Two other historically valid and influential sides to martial arm extensions were noted; the therapeutic and the meditative, each with further subclassifications. From the therapeutic side, we begin with joint and muscle protection while executing technique. This is followed by Biofield strengthening to increase overall vitality and functioning. On the meditative side, we begin with character, confidence and mind/body anchoring practices. Students are also introduced to rhythmic repetition of specific movement patterns to obtain at-one-ment with one's nature. Consider this a physical parallel of a still meditator counting breaths to transcend the ego mind.

The vertical punch is a combative tool. It is thrown by rotating the fist inward or downward three quarters on a 3/5th arm extension. The more extended full, twist, or lunge punch, commonly practiced worldwide possesses combative, therapeutic and meditative elements. Additional qualities in the way this strike is thrown further distinguishes these methods. To avail yourself of its therapeutic benefits you extend the arm nearly straight while rotating the fist completely down before retracting it. This is done in sync with proper breathing along with a mental visualization; Breathe out on the arm's extension, in on its retraction. During the exhale, imagine a line of energy flowing from the underside of your arm to your fist. On the inhale, imagine Ki moving from the eye of the palm up the back of your hand toward the deltoid.

Both strikes will send a burst of Ki beyond your arm into the opponent microseconds before impact. You might think this is good for the opponent. More energy for them. It isn't. Ki projected quickly at another will momentarily disrupt their Energy Body/Biofield, causing a brief dis-regulation of their Ki flow, which their brain must unscramble to rebalance. By then, they have been hit with the blunt trauma of the physical strike. Shimabuku's odd pop upward at the end of his punches in Seisan Kata, which has mostly disappeared from Isshinryu, stops the back surge of Ki into one's own body after contact—if you interpret this motion as a strike. From the Kiko perspective there are no fist strikes in Shimabuku's Seisan kata. Techniques are not what they appear.

A test: We have a subject stand across from another and punch towards their abdomen with full force and intent to hit, but does not make contact. Immediately after, we test the resistant strength of the target's stance. Most subjects test weak. They are uprooted easily. The test is redone throwing a slow strike at the same target. The target shows significant resistance to the push. Punching slowly allows the target subject to absorb the Ki radiating ahead of the strike, increasing their strength.

During a full, twist, or lunge punch, the small downward twist of the hand at the end of the punch prevents Ki from rebounding back into the striker.

A test: We noted the distinction between subjects executing the two styles of punches, moving them out and back slowly three times from the side chamber, then testing the resistant strength of their stance. The Full Punch maintained Ki in the striker's body far better than the vertical strike. Therapeutic value tends toward the Full punch. When executed correctly, Ki flows down the inside of the arm on extension and up the outside of the arm on retraction, without a loss of energy.

Study of the martial arts is not built upon an either/or choice of its usage value; that is, either you are studying a lethal combat art, or you are studying a healing or meditative discipline. These dimensions are tightly interwoven. Lethality is boosted by being healthy, uninjured, and illness free. Likewise, a clear mind can better rally the motive forces of the body. We want to call forth the appropriate dimension when needed.

Palm Strike

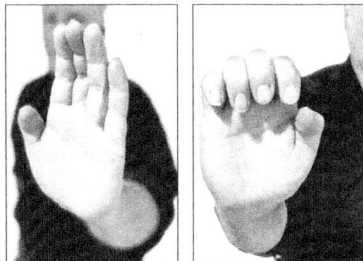

To enhance a right palm strike thrown at an opponent's left side, the fingers are bent at the top knuckles. When using the left hand and directing the strike at the opponent's right side, the fingers remain straight. Both strikes are executed upon an exhale. Done in this manner, and unlike fist strikes, both palms will drain energy from the target. This distinction might resolve some of the confusion I've seen amongst schools that teach the palm strike exclusively one way or another.

Elbow Strike

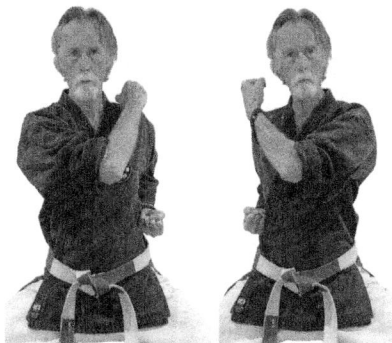

Aside from elbow striking, this action is also used to catch and draw an opponent's elbow for a shoulder lock. In solo practice individual technique needs to follow correct Energy principles to derive maximum strength. One formula to enhance a right elbow is to lay the fist palm's down over the collar bone at neck height. The fist of a left elbow should lay palm's facing the neck on the right side. Solo versus partnered kata practice present subtle differences in performance posturing. These differences allow one to accommodate Energy flow when dealing solely with your own energy field versus another's energy field.

Spear Hand

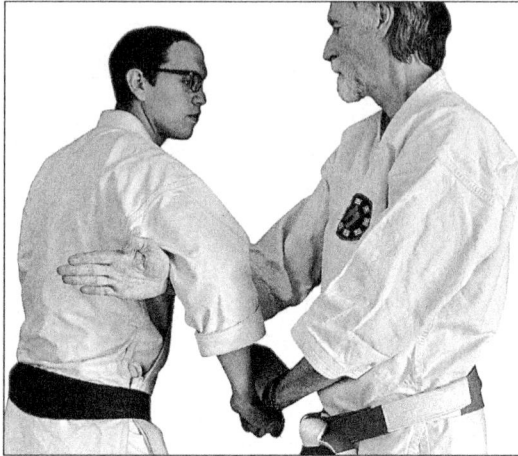

In my opinion, the spear has been misunderstood. Few people possess the finger strength to damage another's torso by jabbing it, even with a fair amount of training. More likely, one will destroy their own weapon. Jabbing to the eyes and throat—fine. Viewed differently, the spear solves a central grappling problem. To gain control of another's arm it is often necessary to wedge your arm between their torso and arm. A fist is a poor fit when an adversary assumes a defensive guard with elbows tucked at their sides. A spear is the perfect shape for slipping into such tight spaces. Furthermore, a 'soft' spear will have the energetic effect of cutting Ki currents in the adversary's torso. A Spear Hand held with rigid fingers is referred to as a *'hard' or 'closed'* spear meaning closed to Ki flow. Fingers held with the barest of tension defines a *'Soft or open'* spear meaning free flowing energy. Sanchin kata's multiple spear thrusts were likely used for controlling an adversary's elbow.

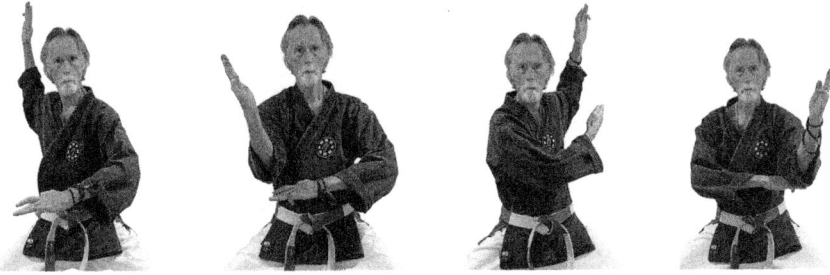

Knife Hand or Shuto w/Defensive Guard

I have no problem with creative technical interpretations if you can make them work. Improvisation has its place in training. I was initially taught to shuto the neck, collarbone, or weakness in the Temporal region of the skull. A basic shuto might include a defensive guard using the non-striking arm. This arm is drawn across the chest to either deliver a mid-body shuto, deflect and/or catch a strike, or simply guard the abdomen.

To maximize this technique's impact, when raising the arm, the thumb should open the eye of the palm by placing a slightly bent thumb over the pointer finger. When striking downward or diagonally across body the thumb must shift to close the eye of the palm. The chopping action should also differ between the left and right hands. A left shuto begins with an inhale while drawing both arms up and away to the left. A right shuto begins with an exhale. A defensive, left hand guard directs a 'soft' attack to the other's dantien as the right arm draws away and upward. It's not necessary for contact to be made as this action alone will disrupt the opponent's energy field.

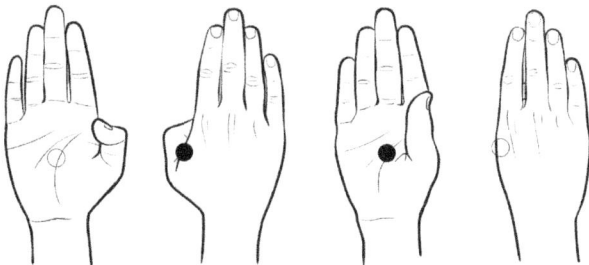

Laogong Open   Hegu closed   Laogong Closed   Hegu Open

Kiko isn't exclusive to martial technique. Kiko can enhance any physical activity or sport. I give examples of Kiko's benefits to a broad variety of physical activities in my book, *Internal Karate: Mind Matters and the Seven Gates of Power*.

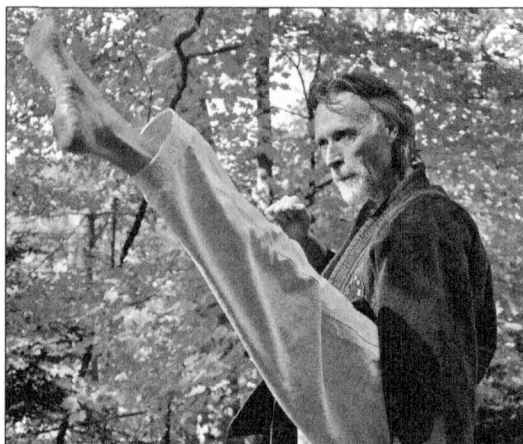

Front Kick

Kicking is one of the hallmarks of the Asian fighting arts setting them apart from Western pugilism. Front or forward kicks can be executed as snaps or thrusts. In the former, a quick lift of the upper thigh snaps out the foreleg with the ankle up, toes up, for striking at angled surfaces, or ankle down, toes up, for striking vertical surfaces. A thrust kick adds penetrating drive through with the hips and torso.

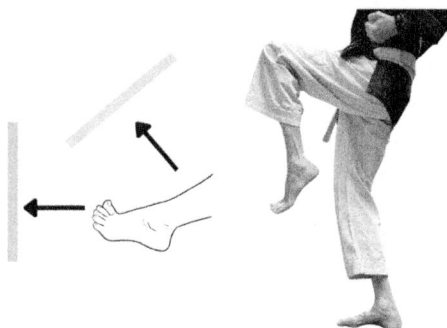

Less emphasized but highly effective is the use of the shin and in particular, the tibia, the largest of the two foreleg bones for striking. Shin kicks spare the toes and delicate bones on the top of the foot from injury and add more diversity to leg techniques. The sharp edge of the tibia considered the cutting edge can be acutely damaging to an opponent's muscle tissue.

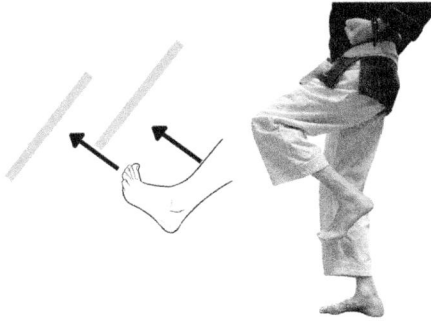

Adding Kiko to kicking technique broadens the use of the legs to improve both acceleration and drive thru and cuts off Ki supply lines to the opponent's musculature as set ups for further technique. Kicks executed above the waistline are done with an exhale. Kicks in which the upper thigh is positioned lower than the waistline are executed with an inhale for maximum results.

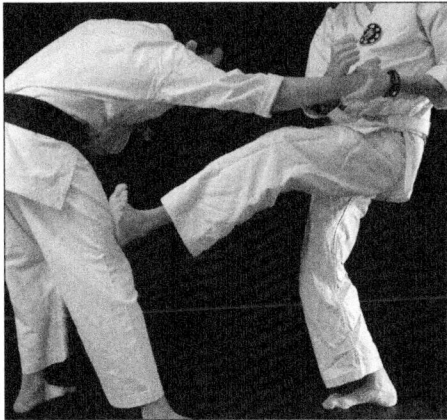

The bottom arch of the foot is highly effective when used to brush, slice or thrust into meridian channels.

Kiko Blocking

During my thirty-five years teaching karate at Drew University in Madison, New Jersey, I met many martial art students from a wide variety of styles. I would marvel at the technical diversity they shared. One young man demonstrated a high block with his wrist cocked toward his pinky. His only explanation for the unique wrist tilt, "That's how I was taught," a common dojo *mantra*.

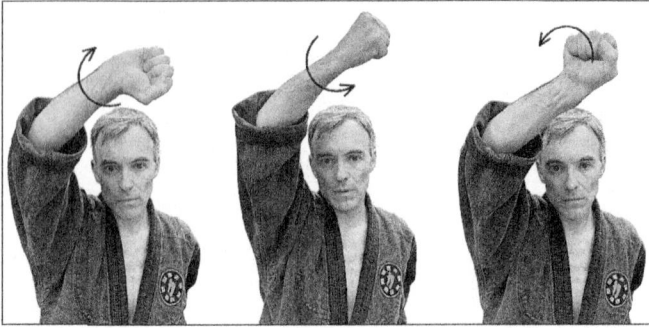

Most blocks found in the Japanese, Okinawan, and Korean martial arts are initially executed from a side chamber or guard position and make contact either with the flat back or the sharper ulnar edge of the forearm. As long as a practitioner's arm reaches its final destination, few schools care how it gets there. With Kiko, origin to finish matters greatly.

Crescent Blocks

The most powerful Kiko parries/deflections move in a semi-circular arc, rarely in a straight or diagonal line. This action is similar to the Crescent step, which is a more potent Ki driver due to the arcing action of the leg. Kiko forearm blocks are essentially C-steps done with your arms.

There are four ways to execute a traditional low, middle, or high forearm parry. Starting from a side chambered hand a block can:

1. Move in a straight diagonal line toward the target.
2. Move with an exaggerated rotation.
3. Crescent close to the chest then away from the torso,
4. Crescent away from the body and arc back toward the torso.

In every case the block will end in the same location.

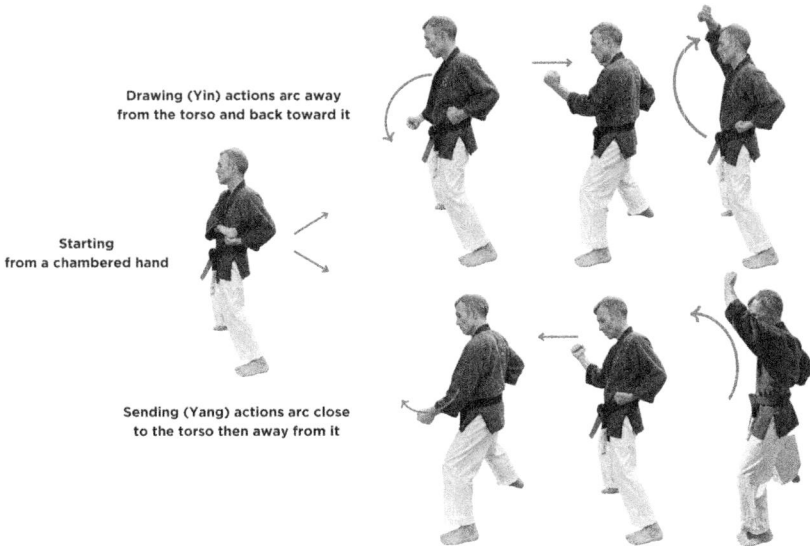

Drawing (Yin) actions arc away
from the torso and back toward it

Starting
from a chambered hand

Sending (Yang) actions arc close
to the torso then away from it

These methods exist because each action exerts a distinctive influence on an opponent's Biofield and subsequently, mechanical structure. Blocks thrown on the opposite side of the body must also be done with slight variations. Fighting systems that execute identical blocks on the right and left sides downgrade their technique. The reason for this became clear when I discovered the concept of sidedness (Observation 36).

The unintended decision to standardize bilateral martial technique, or the misassumption that each side was to be performed identically, removed the arcing nuances from these parries, probably to make them more palatable to a broader clientele. This degrade likely occurred with the Japanization of Okinawan karate in the early 1900's. This decision, or innocent oversight, excoriated Kiko from traditional systems leading to the further decline of the body's natural sensitivity to feel this distinction. The evidence points to the traditional martial art community engaging in subpar blocking/defense. Let me illustrate Kiko's buried wisdom in a forearm Middle block.

The Middle Block

You may have noticed that some schools teach bone edge blocks and others, flat forearm blocks. I originally thought these methods boiled down to tactics. Working with Kiko revealed a different rationale. Bone edge blocks are essentially taught as deterrent strikes against an attacking limb, specifically aimed at pressure points. The two-boned, flat side, forearm blocks downplay the sharp arm hit with a focus on quickly reaching the primary target of the face or torso. Styles that use bone edge blocks are coincidentally coupled with full, lunge or twist punches where the fist ends up palms down at the end of the strike. By contrast, systems that use the flat top of the forearm are coupled with vertical strikes where the fist is thrown with the hand in a vertical, thumb up, pinky down, position.

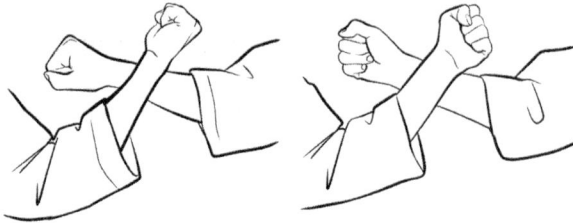

Correct formulas

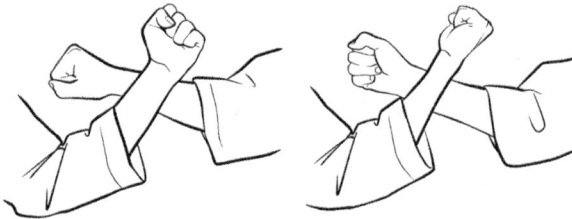

Incorrect formulas

The eye opener came when I tried to block a full punch in slow motion with the flat side of my forearm. It tested markedly weak. Blocking with the bone-edge proved far stronger. The same held true in reverse. Slow parrying a vertical punch with a bone edge block also tested unusually weak. Blocking with the flat of the arm made it unexpectedly strong.

In the heat of an intense exchange, who will ever have enough time to choose which block to use fast enough? How do you know what kind of punch an opponent will throw? The above formulas couldn't be right, otherwise Shotokan was best designed to defeat Shotokan and Goju to defeat Goju, etc. That's when I came across several experts discussing the potency of the three-quarter arm rotation. The fist is neither vertical nor horizontal but rotated at a 3/4 angle. A more complete picture began to fill in, for it turns out that a 3/4 three-quarter forearm position resolves the blocking issues above. A block executed on a 3/4 angle will effectively sweep both a horizontal and vertical punch aside.

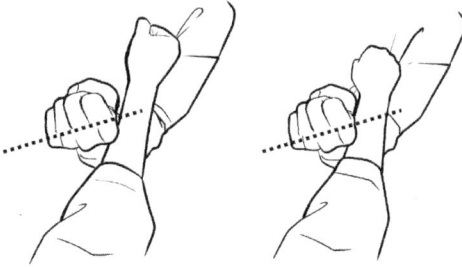

Effective against both vertical and horizontal strikes

Do We Need Big Blocking Motions?

You never see boxers or MMA fighters do anything remotely broad like traditional martial art blocks, yet they don't lose a bit of lethality. Many Asian fight masters use subtle arm parries, sometimes moving only inches in actual fights. So, what's going on? Are these gross blocking actions later shucked in favor of tighter deflections? From a biomechanical viewpoint, mainstream practitioners have been misled about these broad blocking maneuvers. To begin, most traditional blocks consist of a two-hand action. One hand, considered the inside hand, is the actual parrying limb. The other, the outside hand, or what most think of as the formal low, middle, and high block, are mostly follow-up strikes or set up for locks.

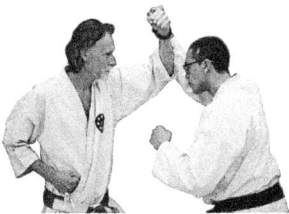

Common use of the Upper block   **Uncommon use of the Upper block**

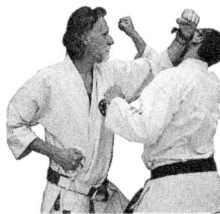

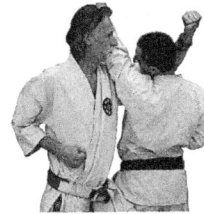

Kiko clears up the mistaken characteristics of these actions. Aside from deflecting strikes, the essence of these blocks lies in their underlying value as receivers and transmitters of Ki. These big deflecting moves suck Ki out of the opponent for more damaging strikes to follow. They also weaken the opponent's stance for a major assault on their structure and reduce the effectiveness of a counter attack. Big blocking motions highlight the Ki exchange making it more tangible, more evident. As your internal skills advance, these moves can be reduced to smaller actions without losing their effectiveness. This skill progression is best exemplified in the Sanchin kata where visually obvious undulations of the torso, like the tuck and tilt of the pelvis, rise and fall of the chest, done at early stages of training, are reduced over time to imperceptible actions without losing their Ki-generative or Ki-dispersive functionality.

Moving Limbs

I've spoken about the Energy Body as the medium by which Biofield signals direct Ki to power specific muscle groups through static and active body postures. Liken a limb motion to a sink faucet; One direction turns the water on. Full blast equals big flow, big charge. The other direction turns the water off, equals no flow, no charge.

To understand Kiko, we must begin where the block originates and how it reaches its endpoint. When executing a traditional block, many students naturally focus on the point of contact; the radius bone of the forearm for a bone-edge middle high block, or the flat side of the arm. Few consider these blocks can be done in one of four methods. A high, middle or low block can follow either a diagonal line, one of two different crescent actions, or a slightly exaggerated rotation.

Circular Blocks

There are three ways to perform a circular block. One type of circle will cause a striker's arm to rotate, making it difficult for them to resist the deflection. This type of block uses a non-Kiko principle I call complex torque, which I discuss in my book, *Internal Karate, Mind Matter & The Seven Gates of Power*. Complex torque is a sophisticated biomechanical technique. Its principle lies in introducing an oblique force against a strike in such a manner that a striker will unconsciously shift the force line of his strike to counter the oblique force, lessening the impact of their strike. Whenever a block causes an adversary's limb to circle, however slightly, it stymies their ability to adjust, for as soon as they mobilize muscles to resist, the circling action cancels that muscle's reaction. Common linear blocking allows an opponent to quickly adjust.

Two other types of parries use a half-circle or crescent action. One method draws KI. The other sends Ki. Just as we have crescent steps, we have crescent blocks.

A typical forearm parry will move diagonally toward its contact point. This is the most energy-neutral action and the way most traditional arts teach blocking. But two other methods exist. The forearm can arc close to the torso and move outward to its finish point at a 90 degree angle of the elbow joint. This block is called a *send*. It transmits charge. The second method is to have the forearm arc away from the torso then drawn back toward a 90 degree elbow joint angle. This type of block is called a *draw*, as in physically drawing the opponent's arm toward you. This action receives charge. These latter two arcs convey different energy signals to the opponent with powerful effect.

A Primer on Hooking Blocks

Over the years, students have asked about the purpose of flexing the wrist when blocking. Let me answer this query with the illustrations below. Imagine a right punch is thrown at you and you chose to parry with a right closed fist, outside, mid-body forearm block. Basic blocking skills can usually deflect the strike, image (1). One thing a defender cannot control however, is the degree of rotation in the puncher's forearm. If a vertical fist is thrown, the parry will be more effective if your wrist is cocked (fingers in a fist) so the first and/or second large knuckles overlap the striker's wrist in image (2). This overlap draws the Ki current moving down the underside of the striker's forearm to the defender's advantage. If the striker's fist is rotated palm's down, the bent wrist will be less effective. It becomes necessary to open the hand to a palm's up position to draw that same current, image (3). Different traditional fist and hand positions were selected to maximize absorbing Ki from the opponent.

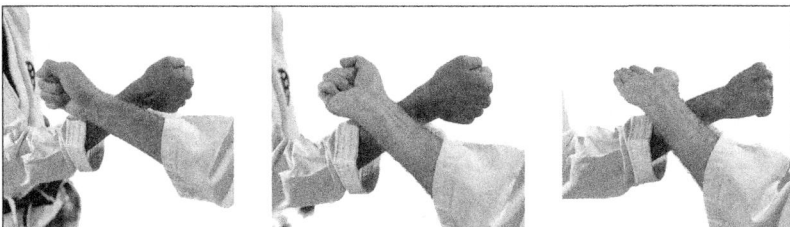

1   2   3

One example of blocking to the inside of an attacking limb below is the different use of the right versus left open hand. To maximize a left arm blocking a right punch requires a drawing, soft (relaxed) palm during an inhale (top image). A right blocking a left punch requires a fast send with a soft palm, wrist cocked outward during an exhale (bottom image).

Draw the arm in the direction of the current

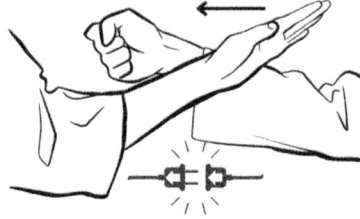

Send the arm in the direction of the current

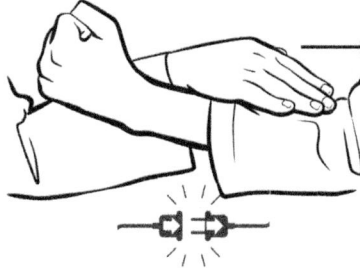

Think of a left block as a socket-in-motion drawing the opponent's right arm (plug) into you. Interesting wording when you consider if someone tries to 'sock' you, your response could be to 'plug' them, in this case, with your block. I could analogize an opponent's action to a *tori*-sending cathode terminal discharging electrons into a *uke*-receiving anode terminal in a charged lead-acid battery. In a combative situation the attacker sends a charge of electrons toward the defender. If properly trained the defender can draw these electrons into his or her system to power up their musculature. Too often however, both parties send a wave of electrons crashing into one another.

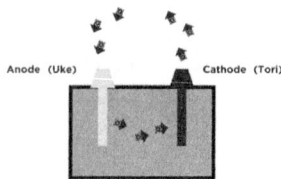

Uke (receiver) —Tori (sender)

Rotating Forearms

Another overlooked characteristic to blocking deals with the rotation of the blocking forearm prior to, or at the instant of, contact with a striking limb. A forearm that rotates toward you will draw energy from a striker. A forearm that rotates away from you will infuse Ki into the striker. Look at the action of a bone-edge versus back of the forearm middle block. The forearms of these two actions circle opposite one another. The bone-edge block rotates the thumb toward the striking limb while the back of forearm block has an ever-so slight reverse action. Each of these rotations result in a different effect upon a striker's Biofield. Proper blocking action will instantly weaken an adversary, a goal over and above a block's external function to deflect the strike.

Blocks, such as closed-hand versus open-hand blocking, or blocks done with various fist, finger or wrist formations is a deep subject, especially considering that some blocks are not solely intended for the purpose of parrying. Suffice it to say, that traditional parries become a unique plug or socket, designed to maximize or minimize their Ki-altering contact.

> **Mental Deflections:** After explaining the energy boost in the middle block to another martial artist, he got testy and wanted to prove whose martial art was better. I told him Kiko would give his technique the ability to pound me more effectively into the ground! He laughed. Situation defused. An appropriate mental parry can prove as advantageous as a physical one.

Kiko Joint Locks and Holds

Martial artists have two objectives in regard to locks and holds; to quickly and effectively subdue an opponent and, if on the receiving end, to escape from such with equal dexterity. Here is an overview of Kiko as it relates to the arm bar, a common elbow-locking action in many schools.

Five considerations for placing an effective joint lock:
- Using the correct line of force
- Maximizing weight behind the force line
- Destroying the opponent's structure/stability for resisting the lock
- Maximizing pain
- Correct Ki manipulation

Arm bars

An effective arm bar will hyperextend an opponent's arm rendering it impossible to bend the elbow joint and create enough pain to cause most persons to submit to further action. What's often missing is how a left or right arm bar must be executed differently for maximum effectiveness. Using Kiko we draw Ki when barring the right arm and send Ki when barring the left arm.

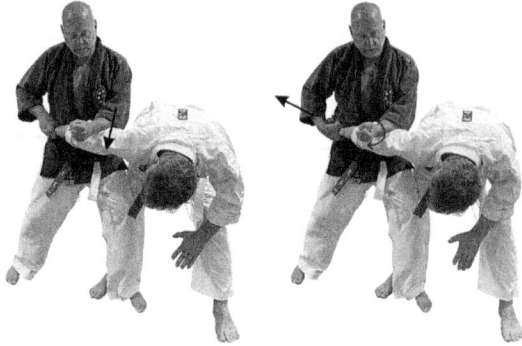

Applying a right arm bar facing North:
Draw the arm toward your right chamber while inhaling. Apply downward pressure in the groove just above the elbow joint (see diagram below) rotating the cutting edge of your ulnar bone in a counter-clockwise motion.

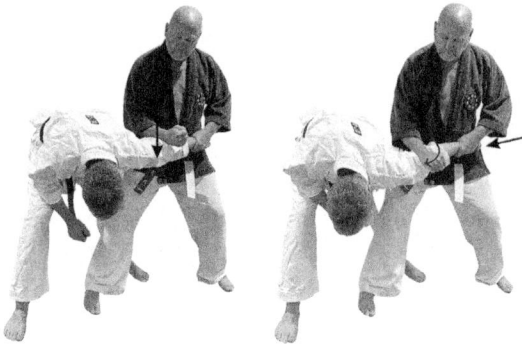

Applying a left arm bar facing North:
Press the arm toward their shoulder while exhaling. Apply downward pressure in the groove just above the elbow joint rotating the cutting edge of your ulnar bone in a clockwise motion.

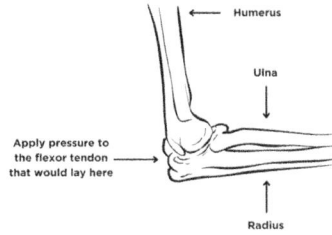

A Front Choke release:

Let's look at a simple front choke (or lapel grab) release.

To draw Ki: Grip the right wrist around the joint with both of your thumbs on the inside. Inhale and squeeze the joint as you pull your right shoulder back a few inches. Twist the wrist clockwise until their pinky faces upward. Throw your left arm over their wrist and apply an arm bar.

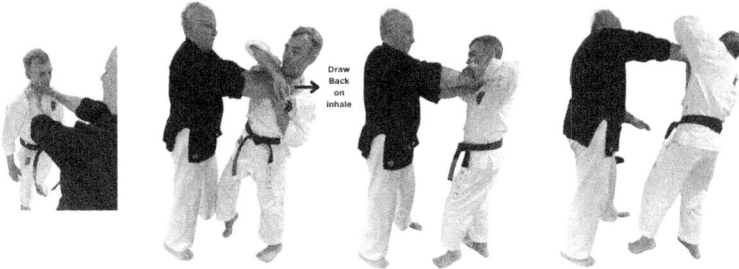

To send Ki: Grip the left wrist around the joint with both thumbs on the inside. Relax, exhale quickly while pressing your shoulder slightly toward their left arm while rotating their wrist counter-clockwise. Lift your elbow over their arm and finish with an arm bar. Complimenting this action with the appropriate stance will increase the drawing or sending force.

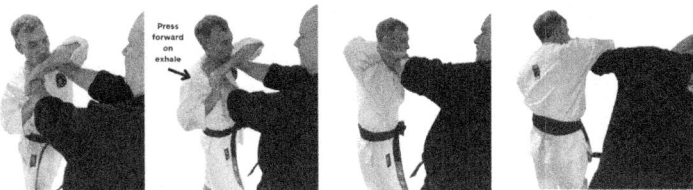

Medicus Emptor! (Practitioner Beware)

Many martial actions today have decoupled from their bio-energetic mechanics. Commercialization continues to strip Kiko nuances even from a system's *kihon* (basics). It remains unclear whether this was an accidental or intentional omission. Certainly, the breath's role in generating martial power has been considerably downplayed in modern fighting systems. Kata pacing generally fixates on fast only. Where there are pauses or stops in traditional forms, a clear rationale is often absent. The kiai also appears to have lost its broader tonal dimensionality and purpose. These downgrades line up with Western societies falling out of touch with their Energy Body's signaling mechanisms.

When Kiko Doesn't Work

Make it simple but significant
Anonymous

In the end, Kiko boils down to simple adjustments in a fighting form to unleash extraordinary force. When it works, it is highly impressive. No one doubts the efficacy of pressure points when you watch a Kyusho expert render a subject unconscious. Likewise, a direct experience of Kiko's thunderbolt power, the foundation of pressure point work, is equally astounding.

However, in the early stages of Kiko training, much can go wrong. I view this no differently from external training challenges. Nobody picks up a roundhouse or side thrust kick in a few days. It takes the average student months, even years, to develop lethality in some strikes. Kiko presents no differently as a new skill set. Patience must become a consistent virtue in all training modes.

Internal training does not need to be wrapped in vagueness or ambiguity. Its principles can be stated clearly and understood by any lay person. More importantly, the strength results are often strikingly dramatic. Like any technique, though, there may be counter forces at work that give a person the idea that internal techniques don't work. This would be a mistake, because the essence of martial art lies within this hidden dimension. It's only hidden because minds are looking elsewhere. The Hard style community cranes its neck toward a Hard style event horizon.

I would not have pursued the study of Kiko if the results had been spotty or marginal. It would not be worth years of painstaking investigation just to gain an extra percent increase in strength. But when I saw and felt the exceptional and effortless power, often exceeding a 50% increase, it was impossible to walk away from this power surge.

Kiko study is currently so far afield from the mainstream martial mindset that an experienced guide becomes a necessity. You will also need a partner. In the three decades my organization has been testing Kiko principles, we have gone through an enormous range of meticulous trial and error experiments with other open-minded seekers to arrive at our conclusions and theories.

The main reason I see a failure to achieve significant results is a lack of understanding about all of Kiko's moving parts. There are enough facets to the Kiko story to easily overwhelm someone unfamiliar with the subject. Our energies are in constant flux and entangled with the energies of our partners, opponents, surrounding objects, the clothing we are wearing, time of the day, direction we face, etc. Even deep relaxation, an important element in Ki cultivation, is not an easy state to assume given how much tension is carried in the average body and mind.

Many times, during my investigations into Kiko's technical behavior, a hypothesis based upon the outcomes of a previous test failed to produce the desired result with certain people. Seeking the cause for the anomaly almost always led to a breakthrough understanding behind the outcome and just how personalized Kiko study must be.

7* Because respiration is a mechanical as well as an electro-chemical action, its musculoskeletal dynamics form part of Kiko's Hard Gating system.

In my opinion, there is no physical, spiritual or healing practice in the world that does not address the intimate link between breath to strength, health, mental wellbeing, or spiritual insight. Martial arts are no exception. Because breathing is a physical as well as an electro-chemical action, the muscular nature of respiration forms part of Kiko's Hard Gating system. Breath work is integral to Kiko training.

To learn a martial art without instruction in the proper way to breathe is to miss one of the most critical elements in executing correct technique. Current explanations for breath work run the entire gamut from the ridiculous to the sublime. One instructor told a student he had to learn to breathe in and out simultaneously, leaving the young Phd. completely baffled. It was a nonsensical instruction.

Kiko practice is not illogical, ambiguous or mystical. If you end up baffled by someone's explanation for a breathing technique, ask for a better explanation. If you do not understand something, it's possible it was not meant to be understood but rather to cast a spell upon you to keep you entranced in another's martial drama. No matter how complex a rationale might be, if it's a worthy explanation, there should be a logical pathway to understanding it. Feeling it might be more difficult.

To understand the breath's connection to physical strength, shift your attention away from the intake of air to oxygenate the body, and look instead at the muscular mechanisms that draw and expel air from the lungs. Breathing can require movement of the diaphragm, the intercostals, (muscles in between the ribs) for chest expansion, and the scalines (neck muscles) to lift the ribcage to allow for additional lung space. All these muscular actions make up what I call our *respiratory jacket*. The actions of this jacket become a prime distributor of Ki.

Although we all breath in and out daily, if you were to look carefully you would see that throughout the course of any single day you will utilize your respiratory jacket differently depending upon your mood, activities engaged, state of mind, time and quality of the day, level of health, and other, more esoteric variables. In monastic martial study we note three distinct levels of breath.

Chinese boxing masters engaged in an exercise called *Tai Si*, which included the *'Lore of the Three Depths Breathing'*.

Mune kokyu – Upper chest breathing integration.

Suigetsu kokyu – Middle stomach breathing integration.

Fukushiki kokyu – Lower diaphragmatic breathing integration.

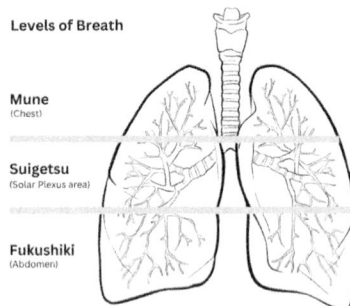

Levels of Breath

Mune
(Chest)

Suigetsu
(Solar Plexus area)

Fukushiki
(Abdomen)

These three levels of breath encompass all manner of psycho-emotional expression. That is, every psychic and emotional state has a corresponding breathing pattern associated with it. These breathing levels are not only related to the physical art of *kokyu* (breath practice) but are symbols for three types of insight and wisdom engendered by their practice. To firmly control these levels requires insight into the depth psychology which they represent.

Upper breathing is chest or shallow breathing. In chest breathing your lungs get the least stretch, the least volume of air. Middle breathing is observed in the motion of the lower ribs expanding with minimal chest rise or abdominal protrusion. Lower breathing is commonly referred to as belly or abdominal breathing. It is most noticeable in the expansion of the lower abdomen as you force the diaphragm to press downward into the belly cavity causing the bottom portion of the lungs to fill. This level of breathing brings the greatest amount of stretch and volume of air into the lungs. What does breathing have to do with Kiko? Most cultures have been conditioned to think of breathing mainly as a means to oxygenate the body and dispel CO_2. This is far from the full story. When you breathe in, your Biofield concentrates, densifies. Deep abdominal breathing primes the entire muscular system. Conversely, when you exhale, your Ki diffuses as it discharges from the body.

A test: We asked subjects to push one another from a rooted stance at the beginning of their inhale, then repeat the test pushing after the peak of their inhale (i.e., the beginning of the exhale on the push). A noticeable strength difference was observed. Weak on the first test, strong on the second. This test alone is significant enough to establish that martial moves must be done with the proper breath cycle; in versus out. A general rule is to exhale with pushing actions, inhale with pulling actions. However, certain high-level fighting Forms teach a reverse breathing pattern from this general rule demonstrating that one can decouple the bioenergetic from the biomechanical.

The ideal time to strike someone is at the end of their exhale, when their Energy Body is at its most dispersed and weakest juncture. Damage from a timed strike like this will be far more devastating as the opponent's Ki-shielding capacity is significantly reduced.

Belly Breathing: A Big Pot O'Breath

Belly breathing coupled with the attention held on the lower portion of the torso fills the lower abdomen with Ki. Stretched abdominal muscle draws energy. Contracted muscle discharges energy. Belly breathing is a principal method of Kiko to build an impressive physical body charge.

The lower abdomen serves as an Energy reservoir. This reservoir fills with Ki that rises up the inside of the legs on every inhale. During exhalation, the Ki is distributed away from the belly and through the limbs at a particular pace where it passes out and/or around your fingers. Think of Ki like a wave rolling atop the ocean's surface. Your Ki is always present, but you can cause waves on its surface either by body posturing (Hard Gating) or mental projection (Soft Gating).

Choosing to breathe in the upper, middle or lower abdomen is part of the Hard Gating system. Each level distributes charge to various parts of the organism. Deep abdominal breathing generates a strong, multi-limb charge. The other two breath levels offer a slightly different distribution of this energy. Many martial arts activate an explosive Ki discharge by means of reverse breathing where the belly wall is drawn inward on the inhale and expanded outward on the exhale. Taken as a whole, the three breath levels and their variety of respiratory activations express the entire range of Ki distributions throughout the body.

Contrary to common thinking, your ability to concentrate is controlled by your breath rate and depth, not by your mind. Next time you find yourself in a deep state of concentration notice the depth and rate of your breathing.

Abdominal breathing firmly anchors your mind to your body. It draws the head, so to speak, into the belly. This action re-establishes the psycho-physiological center of gravity in the lower belly where real physical power is generated. Upper breathing routes energy to your head for thinking. Notice what happens to your thoughts when you hold your attention on your lower belly while breathing deeply into the bottom of your lungs. Thinking and your awareness of thinking shifts. You will become much more aware of your physical self. You won't stop thinking, but the quality and pacing of your thoughts will change. A pervasive whole person awareness is established. Because of the heady fixation of modern societies, many people divide their energy between rooting their senses in their body versus pushing a train of thought in their heads. This phenomenon has to do with the West's fixation on cognition. Western societies are so habituated to dwelling in their heads that when they shift their awareness to their belly, they find it buoyantly rising back into their head. With consistent practice however, you can maintain a root in your belly which leads to a more quiescent mind.

From the Soft Gate perspective, meditation does for your mind what rooting the mind into the belly does for your body. Both actions lead to a refreshing stillness. What meditation does from the top down, belly breathing accomplishes from the bottom up by grounding the Biofield.

In a fight, you want to be a unified, one-piece unit. You are not just a body fighting another body while you mind observes securely from its ivory-like, cranial tower. We want mind and Biofield backing our body's efforts.

Breathing Spectrum: Hard, Hard/Soft, Soft

Breathing patterns and breath controls will change naturally as your awareness evolves. A hypothetical story illustrates this evolution:

A young man, fearing for his safety, seeks out a martial art school to learn self-defense. By happenchance, he chooses a traditional martial system. He tells his teacher that he feels a personal assault is imminent in his crime ridden neighborhood. He is introduced to various self-protective techniques and concepts. At some point 'breathwork' enters his training equation. His teacher tells him, "If you are attacked, you will likely over tighten as an instinctive re-action to the fear of injury and the shock of the adrenaline dump. I am going to introduce you to some respiratory methods to overcome this handicap."

The student is encouraged to kumite/spar. As expected, his body over-tightens from the intensity and fear of getting struck. He finds himself holding his breath then gulping large quantities of air to make up for shortchanging his system. His breathing is disorganized. His erratic breathing pattern, brought on by the stress of the kumite, distracts and prevents him from executing solid technique.

The master continues, "To avoid inhibiting your own Energy flow I am going to teach you a form of breathing called *ibuki*. He is instructed to coordinate his inhale with an imaginary line descending down the front of his body into his lower abdomen, then exhaling by the reverse route. "This will keep your Energy from stalling in your over-stiff form." Later, he is introduced to the Sanchin kata to teach him what it feels like to be tense and relaxed under stress. Sanchin's self-imposed stress occurs by way of contracting the musculature on the exhale, then relaxing it on the inhale.

During this solo practice the student begins to identify and repattern his body's reaction to stress.

As this student moves between kumite and kata, he finds pockets of relaxation amidst the intensity of the fight and his own self-imposed tensions in his Sanchin kata. At this point he is instructed to change from ibuki to *Microcosmic Orbit* breathing. In this new breathing pattern, he must still visualize his breath descending down the front of his body, but instead of returning it by the same path, he is taught to imagine his breath returning by passing under his perineum and rising up his back and over the top of his head. As his body sheds the tensions that arose from his previous agitated mental state and adrenaline dump, and as long as he maintains a state of semi-relaxation, the microcosmic breath supplies his muscles with the necessary Ki.

Over years, in the forge of kata and kumite, the student is able to maintain a near constant state of relaxation. He learns to regulate his breath to be deep, slow and rhythmic. His Sanchin kata performance has moved him through three stages; unable to relax (Hard), able to find pockets of relaxation (Hard/Soft), and finally, able to completely relax (Soft). At this latter stage, it is no longer necessary for him to practice his kata with antagonistic tension for he will have removed the majority of physical barriers preventing his free flow of Ki. He has also calmed his restless mind which led to his tense state and has learned how to flow with his bodily instinct and hormonal energy system.

The Breath Mind

Our physical center of gravity resides in the lower abdominal region, the center of body mass. But our body's psycho-physical center of gravity, the point where mind and body intersect, generally lies north of the solar plexus. In Western cultures this intersection is usually situated in the upper chest. The higher this center is located, the less physically rooted and the less potent one's martial technique. There is a distinct and improved qualitative feeling practicing a martial art holding your attention in your lower belly rather than in your head.

Our Mental Cups Overfloweth

The Mindfulness trend in the West has misled some to develop an overflowing, over-engaged mind. Western culture is already spending far too much time in their heads, leading to top-headiness and less grounding. Instead of calling this trend Mindfulness, we ought to re-brand it as the Breath-fullness movement. In this way we can remedy two problems at the same time; over-dwelling in the mind and fixed, shallow, or upper chest breathing.

Abdominal breathing draws the awareness down into the lower torso where gathered power can be distributed to the limbs. The torso is undervalued in Hard style training. Ballistic martial systems frequently and mistakenly over focus on limb actions. Different martial theories exist about power development and expression. Ballistic, Hard arts like Karate and Tae Kwon Do build power in the extremities first. Practical effectiveness is almost instantaneous. Shortly after learning to throw a punch, one is good to go with some measure of force. With consistent effort and time, limb power eventually links up with the body core so you can hit with more weight behind your strike. Conversely, Soft arts, like Tai Chi, generate strength from the core outward to the limbs. Thus, the Soft arts take longer to connect core torsion to the limb actions. Eventually, the Soft stylist catches up in effectiveness.

Whether you train in a Hard, Soft or hybrid system, your own sensitivity for how to move will also engage your art. Everyone possesses some measure of innate guidance. But some of us have better gut teachers than others. My father was a very physical man. He played sports, sailed, swam, liked to build things. He had excellent coordination, a trait all his offspring share. Today, however, many people find themselves in a physically pacifying era. Modern life has become more mentally active. This doesn't bode well for the future coordination of our youth, who more often exert themselves running or slinging picks in Minecraft.

To counter balance modern society's habit of shallow or upper chest breathing you must establish a firm root in your physical nature. You can do this by holding your attention in and on your physical self. More specifically, you must work consciously with all three breath levels. This can be as simple as spending time aware of and feeling your breath. To hold your attention in front of a computer screen you must shift your Ki to the upper dantien to keep energy flowing into your brain. This results in tranquilizing the body, denying its normal allotment of Ki. The more time you spend shallow breathing, the more you reinforce the behavior of directing Energy into the upper body.

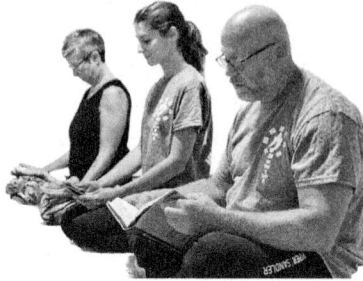

Lft to rgt: Notice the similar neck positions. Yogic Throat lock, woman looking at her cell phone and man reading a book

A Society Atilt

The slight downward tilt of the neck, common during cell phone use, computing, reading and writing, reduces the central flow of Ki in the elliptical pattern called the Microcosmic Orbit. Instead of freely running the length of the spine, continuously filling your belly, Ki pools in the skull, concentrating it like a yogic *bandha* (interior throat lock) in the head. When your Ki gets dammed, energy meant for the whole body is diverted to the brain. This condition was less prominent before the digital revolution. To break this habitual pattern, it is essential to maintain an upright head and neck.

One obvious and intuitive allure to sports, body disciplines and physical activities in general is spending more time with and inside your body, invested in your body. Attending to your body increases vitality. I can't say enough about this fundamental remedy for many of the health issues plaguing society. Practicing martial moves with proper breathing will also increase the force of your technique.

Martial breath control isn't about how long you can hold your breath, how fast you can expel it, or how loud you can shout, but rather, how changes in the respiratory jacket during various breathing patterns jockey power throughout the Biofield system.

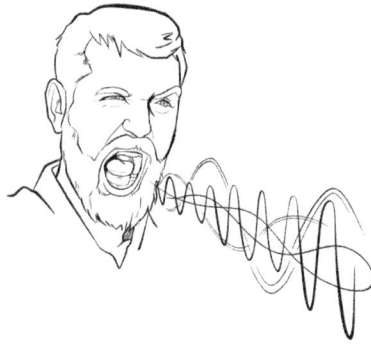

The Kiai

The martial kiai or *spirit shout*, deserves special attention. The kiai is not a simple vocal explosion. *'Kiai'* means spirit harmony or energy harmony. A proper kiai is an energy-moving vocalization in harmony with your intentions. A lot of Ki is moved when we shout. When Ki moves, it carries an informational signal to all within earshot. Yes, a shout startles at a basic level, but this is the kiai's lower function. The pitch and duration of the shout can be modulated to decrease or increase your energy potential.

High tones are used for striking high targets, low tones for attacking low targets. Different vocalizations are used for pulling versus pushing actions, for clockwise versus counter clockwise motions, for rising versus lowering maneuvers. Each note in an octave will affect your body and those of others in proximity in specific ways.

If we were to go back in time, we would find that kiai's made at junctures in various kata would have been of a particular tone, not just a blanket bark.

Avital Hedva in his research on Chinese Military history argues that, rather than mere ornamental "military music," drums and bells were perceived by early Chinese strategists as indispensable sonic communication devices, which played a crucial role in victory or defeat in battles. He notes that sound activates a certain form of qi in humans: negative sounds trigger negative qi. Positive sounds activate positive qi. This process is based on a natural mechanism of stimulus (*gan* 感) and response (*ying* 應).

Look at how powerful sound is when speaking to another. The intention behind a voice can elicit tears, laughter, anger, fear. A voice can lift one to incredible heights of motivation or sink a person into despair. A voice can break glass, cause you to cover your ears, draw you closer, hypnotize you, con you, psych you up, or out.

Imagine the sound you might make shooting a basketball. Now think high block. Let your instincts guide you. What sound might you make if you were driving a shovel into a pile of gravel. Now, think downward heel thrust. Your body has a primal awareness for coupling sound(s) to certain actions. It knows what sounds will maximize certain physical efforts. Based on the activity, sound signals your Energy Body to juice the needed muscles.

Evidence of the power of sound is all around us, but we rarely reflect on how to use our voice to enhance our physical power. Although we see plenty of evidence in the grunts, groans, huffs and puffs we make doing certain tasks around the house; lifting, twisting, pushing, shoving, reaching, bending, all these sounds distribute energy to the precise muscles being challenged in each and every activity. The sound you release to pull an object will differ from the sound you use to push it. We sigh to release anxiety. We bellow to let loose the charge of a joyous, funny, or buoyant moment. We inhale with wonder. We burst with emotion when something great or horrible happens to us. Animals use sound to terrify and paralyze their prey, to lure mates, to locate other members of their species—all expressions of the dynamic interplay between sound and power.

Each of us possess a unique range of vocal tones, that can evoke strength and courage, or echo weakness and fear.

The Rishis of India discovered the universal master sound *Aum* or *Om* thousands of years ago. Repeating this simple mantra consistently, even silently, will draw energy into your body and open blocked Ki channels.

External Sounds

In Kiko, we work initially with three basic sounds; *Who, Ha, He.*

External sound is air sent through the vocal cords to project sound waves thru and away from the body where they are picked up by other's ears and Energy Bodies. Our Energy Body will translate detected sound as either foreign, friend or foe. But our auditory perceptions do not stop at this simple recognition. When a sound is perceived as unfriendly, our body goes on muscular alert and gears up for a level of Fight or Flight.

In kumite and kata performance distinct sound modulations can be detected in a student's breathing. These sound shifts may be barely perceptible, but are there if you listen carefully. Because people have fixed sound patterns and distinct voices, we want to break vocal fixations and expand the tonal range for better body control. An observation will explain:

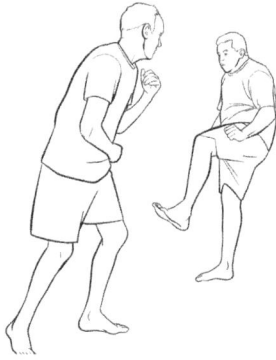

Bob weighs 240 pounds and stands over six feet tall. Whenever he strikes during kumite, he blows air from his pursed cheeks. He centers high in his upper body, evidenced by his high stances and straighter legs which puts his balance at risk. I point out his vulnerability. I provide him with a particular vocal tone, the sound 'who' as a remedy to drop his attention into his lower abdomen. It is impossible not to feel your lower body when you breath abdominally. Exhaling with a 'who' sound accomplishes the goal. Bob adjusts his breathing but quickly gets consumed in the heat of the kumite and again reverts back to his instinctively fixed higher center. The evidence can be heard in his breathing as he exhales with a higher pitched "ha".

A proper kiai is the perfect tonal quality of the breath supporting the move being executed. There is no one sound that fits all technique and every person save for the universal sound, *Om* or *Aum*. Specific vocalizations are uttered to activate the necessary muscles.

Internal Sounds

Internal sound is consciously imagined sound, released silently in your mind with the same intention as an audible utterance—in stealth mode. By using an internal sound, you can prevent others from picking up a direct vocal intent through their ears. Although their Biofield will detect the sound, most listeners lack the sensitivity to decode the message. The effectiveness of silent sound can cause changes in another's Biofield under their awareness.

145

Imagine at your work environment your boss, a bully, wants to talk with you. You can't stand the man. You hear yourself wishing he would leave the room. On the surface, however, you are all smiles and praise. Which 'sound' speaks your truth? The words uttered out of your mouth or the words spoken silently to yourself? Did your boss pick up on your distaste for him?

Japanese Samurai wore long skirts called *hakama*. Hakama were initially designed to protect warriors against thickets and brambles and to conceal footwork. I used to think, how much could a hakama hide of one's footwork? I could easily tell if you had lowered down or not, even if your feet were hidden under your skirt. It wasn't until I studied Kiko that it became apparent that even if I could tell someone had lowered or risen, this wouldn't tell me what muscle groups were primed by the specific foot placement hidden under the hakama, thus giving away the type of sword cut possibly intended. Internal sound functions like the hakama. It hides energetic intent.

Sound As Antidote: An Inbuilt Natural Defense

A senior black belt once applied a shoulder lock on me that elicited a grunt. Somehow, I knew instinctively if I uttered this sound prior to the lock being fully secured it would counter his move. It did.

Have you noticed how a body collapses, gestures, or aurally expresses a painful event? Why, for example, does someone let out a moan, sharp exhalation, or flail their free arm in a peculiar manner when placed in an arm bar? How did their body learn to gesture this way? You might reason when the body is thrown off center it instinctively reacts with a counter balancing action. When we looked at these reactions from a different perspective, we saw something extraordinary.

Many after-the-fact, reflexive actions appear to be energetic remedies or protections for the strikes and locks applied against us. This reminds me of how herbologists will tell you that Poison Ivy often has its remedy in Jewelweed, growing nearby. When we looked carefully at our gestures, sounds, and posturing during the application of certain locks, we found these actions to be strong unconscious counter measures if activated prior to the finalization of the lock.

This places a different light on the use of the Kiai (spirit shout). A Kiai is not a random yell. It is a vestigial, reactionary defense. Even if you are just trying to startle someone, the Kiai is powerful, preemptive verbal counter measure against a physical assault.

Without this tonal neutralizer, a lock or strike placed upon you could be more damaging. It appears to be our Biofield's last-ditch attempt to send a surge of sonic energy to protect a stressed joint and musculature.

This raises a similar question to the age-old dilemma of which came first, the chicken or the egg? Was there a time when primitive peoples reacted with this kinetic antidote simultaneous to the moment of attack? Or, was this defensive mechanism observed thousands of years ago, just as I have observed it with my students, and someone got the idea to replay the sound back prior to a lock being placed, for instance? These defensive sounds appear to possess a specific frequency or tonal quality unique to each person. What works for me will not necessarily work for you. It was uncanny that my body knew exactly what sound to make to counter the lock. It was not a sound I would have consciously considered. This sound also revealed to me the specific respiratory tensions used to shuttle Ki.

One clue why sound might strengthen or weaken us is given in the study of Cymatics. Cymatics demonstrates that water molecules take a particular shape when exposed to different sound frequencies. If different sound frequencies are known to produce different shapes in bodies of water it's possible that upon hearing certain tones these restructured water shapes within our bodies convey information resulting in instant increases or decreases in our physical strength. Science has proven that ultrasound heals but doesn't know why it heals? Why can't sound affect our strength?

Primitive Reactions

When I duplicated the sound originally evoked from the pressure of the lock, my arm became so resistant that my partner was unable to conclude the technique. The kiai doesn't function so much to startle, as to suppress another's Strength channels, similar to the way sound waves can cancel one another out.

The art of the Kiai likely evolved from hostile situations like the above. Perhaps, in conditions of dire stress, sound does, in fact, elicit before the terminal point of a technique. We just don't have enough instances to observe this phenomenon outside the dojo. Prior to my own experience, I would not have considered such actions noteworthy. I now acknowledge that our primal, unconscious utterances provide an aural antidote, an acoustic counter, for resisting joint locks and absorbing the shock wave of blunt force traumas. Acoustical counters applied to locks have made us more impervious to pain. At the very least, they have increased our pain threshold enough to give us precious seconds to escape locks placed on us.

Spontaneous Concealed Counters

Sound is not the only antidote in our primal arsenal. Our body possesses other built-in Biofield fail-safes. I was testing a senior black belt named P5W (Prince Five Weapons) who was doing multiple crescent steps toward me to test his body's overall charge. My body must have sensed that I was going to get uprooted. The moment his hands touched me, my right arm, farthest from him, spontaneously sprung upward. I was pushed over in the test. But following my hunch about sound, we repeated the test. This time, I lifted my arm prior to his contact. He couldn't budge me. Nor, could I move him when we reversed the test and P5W repeated his own gut response.

Subtle gestures like grunts, groans, huffs and puffs are visceral premonitions indicating that our bodies hold an instinctive wisdom for negating energetic attacks, even if these actions come post event. Watch how martial students make distinctive utterances and/or odd physical gestures when they are struck or have joint locks placed on them. Observe your own reactions carefully. By mimicking sound(s) or gestures made prior to a lock being applied, your partner or opponent may suddenly find it difficult, even impossible, to conclude their maneuver.

8* Aggressive movement toward you by another will generally send a Ki wave ahead of their action.

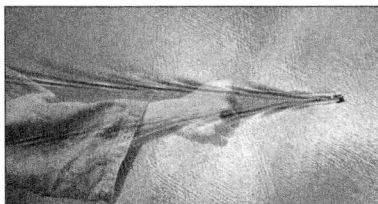

A boat leaves a trail called a wake.
What is the wave pushed forward by the bow called?

It's called a *Way*. As in, 'Get out of my way.' 'You are in my way', or 'Make Way!' A boat's action upon the water is a perfect example of how Ki precedes all forward directed technique. Tai Chi and Ai-kido practitioners lead their opponent's Way. They accelerate the attack by pulling their adversary off center into a tactical trap. This same action exists in Hard style fighting arts, but it is less apparent because the limbs are moving too fast for most to notice the Ki affect. When you parry in a manner that draws your adversary in, you are leading their Way, manipulating their Ki. Kiko takes this tactic one step further. It has you energetically pull the opponent before actual physical contact is made. We want our Ki to lead their Ki. Kenji Ushiro in his book, *Karate And Ki*, notes that Hard style combatants prefer to project strong Ki at one another hoping to cut through the other's assaultive Ki wave, but in doing so, miss a vital strategy of leading the other's Ki to their advantage.

9* Kiko integrates our non-physical nature with our physical structure.

Every bodily structure has its physical/material and non-physical/immaterial dimension. Like a magnet's invisible field, we too exist with both a material and non-material nature with our own unseen Biofield. One dimension presents a see and touch world, a realm that can be easily sensed, like our physical form. The other dimension can neither be visually seen nor physically touched. Here we encounter the amorphous realities of mind, thought, emotion, electromagnetic fields, photonic emissions—unseen, unconscious sub-drivers of behavior.

We have material organs like our heart, liver, spleen, etc. and their immaterial counterparts, like our heart's electromagnetic field emanations. If you do not believe you have an immaterial heart, how do you explain that a blow to the heart meridians on the inside of both arms can cause the heart to cease beating. We literally wear our (immaterial) hearts on our sleeves. Deprive the heart of its electrical field, it dies.

The official definition of death used to be the absence of blood circulation. Today, 'death' is defined as the cessation of all vital functions of the body including breathing, the heartbeat and brain activity, which stops within 20-40 seconds. The immaterial side of human life was referred to by ancient peoples as 'spirit,' the untouchable world. You might sense it, but you could not touch it.

The so-called Death Touch masters understood one's life could be taken away by stealing this spirit. They knew this spirit, aka Biofield, in an empirical sense, could be damaged. Overloading or underloading another's Electrical system were the two primary internal killing methods that emerged in the Eastern internal fighting arts.

10* Your kinetic pattern defines your Energy personality.

If we could drop out the visual background of our lives and video record our physical motions at high speed suspended in space, I believe that we would appear as an atomic structure with movement patterns as individual as our thumbprint.

I mentioned earlier that any martial technique can be defined as one of the five elements. Your Energy Body will also exhibit prime behaviors that fall into one of these five elemental categories. These signature behaviors are a co-creation of heredity and environmental factors. For example, I possess a Wood Element Energy Body with a strong Fire element nature. A Chinese astrologer might say that I inherited a certain energy persona being born in the early Spring when Earth energy was rising strongly from the ground. Put another way, I was in the path of rising Yin energy at birth, orienting my Energy Body around this immaterial parenting. My liver/wood meridian was flowing strongly.

One author on the subject of the Five Elements pointed out that Wood natured persons need expansive environments to allow release of Liver energy. I never realized the significance of this characteristic until I began to work with the Five Elemental energy flows for, prior to this knowledge, I had always sought wide-open spaces. I find them rejuvenating. When teaching, I always made sure I arrived at the various dojo sites early to sit or stand quietly in their large open and empty areas. Apparently, Wood Element people make good teachers and innovators. Coincidentally, I not only chose to become a teacher but I am also head master of a school. Being in my head a lot aligns with my Western astrological sign, Aries. My mind is always active. I can easily relate my thoughts to a fast-growing wood. Coincidentally, I was given the spiritual name *Hayashi*. The monk who chose my name, told me it meant *Forest*—woods! I instinctively added a graphic touch to the Bagua trigram for my business logo by placing a flourish to the *Sun* or wind gua just to the right of the Greater Heavenly north gua sequence. Each of the Bagua's eight trigrams is related to an element. I wondered which element wind (*Ch. sun)* represented. It turned out to be number 4 wood! There are two wood elements represented in the Bagua; number 3 and 4 wood. Number 4 wood represents a tree's trunk and canopy. The 3 Wood, its roots. Was this just a series of uncanny coincidences? Simple formulas for determining your own elemental natures can be found on the Internet.

11* Large quantities of energy drawn into the body can cause an effect known as Induced Ki Flow. Large energy outflows can cause its opposite effect, reduced Ki Flow.

It is not uncommon for meditators, yoga practitioners, and internal martial artists to encounter involuntary physical movements during certain practices. These spontaneous, reflexive movements can manifest as sudden jerks, spasms, tingling, tics, or more typically, a gentle swaying. Regardless of the reaction, an instinct is triggered to move differently than what one has consciously planned.

I never encountered this phenomenon during my early training years. That changed when I began seated and standing meditation, even more so with specific energy-cultivating martial patterns.

I have explored many movement avenues outside of traditional martial arts; I've engaged in various forms of meditation, Chinese yoga, Tibetan exercises, free style dance and induced Ki flow activity. In my own private space, I do not feel any inhibition about the way I move. I often set aside time for free form movement where I let my body move spontaneously. In essence, I invite my unconscious to direct my body.

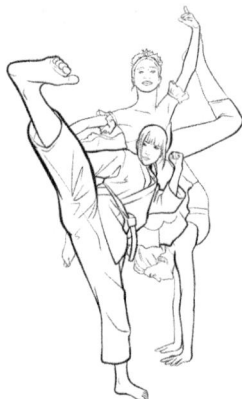

The Trance Dance

In 1995 Dr. Valerie Hunt, who holds advanced degrees in psychology and physiological science, published *Infinite Mind: The Science of Human Vibrations*. Hunt was the first to discover vibrational patterns during pain, disease, illness, and in emotional and spiritual states. Hunt found scientific evidence of subtle Biofield happenings between people and within groups. What caught my attention was her experience with a dancer named Emilie Conrad who claimed she danced in an altered state and wanted to know what was happening to her. Hunt's research team set out to answer her question. The woman was hooked up to various bio-recorders and began her dance, which gave typical readings. Five minutes into her dance however, Emilie began defying all scientific understanding. As she danced vigorously, even acrobatically, all recordings fell to near zero despite the intensity of her movements. Her heart rate did not elevate. There was little to no galvanic skin response as her muscles stretched and contracted. When asked how she did it, Emilie apparently said, "*I create a field of energy and ride it.*"

Allowing our bodies to move involuntarily and uninhibited can offer great insight into the healing powers of motion and the workings of Ki. Conversely, disallowing involuntary motions will too often suppress Ki flow.

Many martial students are not comfortable moving outside of prescribed training routines unless they are engaged in free-style kumite with another. Sanctioned movements are fine but unsanctioned moves can reveal physical inhibitions. These inhibitory states are precisely what prevent one from riding their own self-created energy waves.

Five States of Ki Flow.

1. Super-charged: Yin and Yang channels are flooded with Ki giving us peak strength for any kind of activity. It this state, our body may feel like it has a mind of its own and move involuntarily.

2. Charged Yang state. Strength is formidable but one-sided. Forward directed for certain actions like pushing, punching, lifting. (Observation 65)

3. Neutral flow: Yin and Yang meridians carry an equal but neutral charge. This state represents our body's average, everyday charge-carrying capacity.

4. Charged Yin state. Receiving strength is at its peak but only Yin directed for certain actions like pulling or pressing.

5. Super-discharged: Yin and Yang channels discharge a large amount of Ki. This condition can lead to lethargy, including a loss of will and drive, leaving one weak and vulnerable to injury and illness.

Exhibition Vs. Inhibition

Not everyone wants to step out on the dance floor, belt out a karaoke song in front of strangers, or enter a martial art tournament. Others can't wait to strut their stuff. When Ki is given free reign, it can have a mind of its own. But its current all too often yields to the moorings of the ego.

One day I was doing a *Wuji* (empty-standing) meditation, when I felt an urge to shake my shoulder. It's common when standing for a long length of time for the body to micro-adjust to avoid feeling uncomfortable. I didn't realize that my body was speaking to me via sensation about my own Ki blockages. That jerky shoulder turned into a repetitive bounce, which gave way to a tic-like neck twitch. I wasn't worried about my mini-spasms. They felt somehow beneficial, if not a bit strange. Instead of suppressing the twitches, I relaxed more deeply into them, which only exacerbated the swaying, rocking and jerking of my back, shoulder and neck. My right shoulder would bounce up and down dozens of times, then my left shoulder would catch the beat and do the same. My body began to sway, shake and shimmy wildly. Suddenly, I felt a pop in my upper back and all the strain that I had felt for days subsided. It was then I realized that what had just occurred. Induced Ki flow is an innate healing mechanism addressing imbalances in one's musculoskeletal structure. I felt as if a higher intelligence, or intrinsic body wisdom, was working on my behalf. The tightness I had felt in my upper back had been completely relieved by these strange gyrations.

I could not have consciously activated these motions with the same intensity or specificity to remedy my back tightness. Mesmerized by this emergent force, I chose to simply observe myself as if overtaken by an alien force.

The Chinese internal masters noticed that certain people would have specific types of wiggling, jiggling, jerking and swaying, later cataloged as indicators of certain blocked Ki channels attempting to self-clear. Historically, these observations came to be called the *Five Animal Frolics*, as the spasms reminded the observers of certain types of animal motions. These Frolics further evolved into Asia's Five Animal Kung fu systems.

My meditation practices occasionally placed me into a deep enough state of relaxation to cause a physical release of previously bound muscle energy. I had experienced induced Ki flow. This release sent a wave of energy to flow along its prescribed meridian course until it hit a blockage where it then pressed, pressured, and pounded until the impediment was removed.

I could have stopped this involuntary action at any time with the slightest intention. I liken this to the control of holding our breath at any instant. Had I been inhibited or over-controlling, had I determined the jerkiness to be superfluous, useless noise in my system, had I felt self-conscious and shut these instinctive motions down, I would have missed a truly insightful event.

Induced Ki flow is one of the most overlooked outcomes of doing martial formwork, particularly in the Hard styles, and from my inquiries, even with many Soft-style practitioners.

The current insensitivity I see in martial artists underlies how we all have been conditioned into a collective myopia in regard to physical disciplines in general. We are given a set of moves to practice and, once done, we are told to move on to the next task. Western athletic training only pauses long enough to catch one's breath or build up motivation for the next drill. Few ever pause to watch and feel how their body is handling these exercises. Little to no value is attached to passive Yin states in Western athletic practices. This absence of Yin awareness, and Yin practice, has led to an imbalance of Yang-based over-practice.

The reason for this overlook has to do with how Western cultures objectify physical training. We are taught to think of training in terms of discrete, quantifiable units; numbers of repetitions, time frames, limits. We rarely train by feel. But everywhere we look in the animal kingdom we see a contradiction to this type of training. Animals move entirely by feel and their power-to-weight skills are across the board impressive.

In Okinawan karate, the most popularized, premiere, energy-cultivating kata is the *Sanchin*, or *Three Conflicts Form*. Students will sometimes rehearse this form to near exhaustion then move to another exercise. The missing value to all Energy work is standing still and relaxed at the end of the practice to watch, feel and allow any unbound currents to pass through the body. More importantly, one must not allow inhibitions to stop any tic, sway, spasm or novel mental experience that occurs. The moment you pause to relax, you are summoning and releasing a healing genie inside your body bottle. Once the energy genie is let out it will attempt to push through blockages inside you.

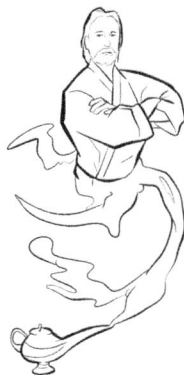

I have since had many induced Ki flow moments, some lasting up to twenty minutes. Others, seconds. With all of them, I finished feeling far better than when I started. I have never injured myself in any way, never passed out, never threw my back, neck, or any joint out, no matter how violent my shaking became. I once mentioned this phenomenon to my chiropractor who seriously inquired if I had had a seizure. I told him I was having an *un-seizure*. I was unwinding, unbinding myself.

Initially, I could only trigger the phenomenon through standing meditation. For reasons unknown to me, seated meditation rarely let my energy flow as freely.

My first experience with induced Ki flow occurred after doing an unusual Sanchin variant taught by a former Isshinryu adept, Aston Hugh. This Sanchin form was three times longer than Okinawa's traditional long form. (The shortest Sanchin is three steps forward, two steps back). One day, after performing Hugh's set multiple times, I followed up with a standing Wuji meditation. As soon as I relaxed, my body started powerfully jerking me about like a puppet on a string. Now, after any Ki work, I make it a habit to stand quietly for several minutes.

No Shake No Gain?

Induced Ki flow isn't something you must strive for, or feel bad if it doesn't happen to you. A free, open body with an unblocked energy field may not sway or shake at all.

After experiencing Hugh's esoteric Sanchin, I experimented with Isshinryu's Sanchin kata. If Sanchin was a Ki-cultivating form, why hadn't I experienced Induced Ki flow? I wondered if I was performing it incorrectly or simply had never considered standing still after doing it.

After numerous trials to elicit an induced Ki flow event, I concluded that I had probably been given the correct external sequence but not its internal map. I had been taught to tighten my whole body upon exhale, which turned out to be a gross misassumption of the proper tensing sequence. I intuitively began to reconstruct Sanchin with the principles I had previously discovered hoping to restore the kata as a more potent energy cultivator.

Another remarkable event emerged during this pursuit. Whenever Ki strongly surges through someone's body that person will appear visibly larger. It's a true perceptual illusion. The Ki-filled subjects are not actually or measurably taller or wider, but there is a distinct shift of awareness creating a sense of their expansion.

I eventually understood what lay behind this phenomenon. As Ki fills and flows through the body, charging the muscular system, the Biofield balloons, densifies. To the observer this creates a mirage of sorts. Though their body does not appear distorted in any visual way, their more concentrated Ki field creates a felt impression of expansion, for one has become electrified!

We are electrical beings having a physical experience
not chemical beings having a physical experience.
Dr. Robert Young

Many of you have already experienced this magnification process and its opposite state; shrinking, condensing, withdrawing, albeit more than once. Recall any time in your life when you felt really connected, where your mood was giddily elated. At that moment you might have felt larger than life; buoyant, elevated, explosive, overjoyed, lit up. These are common terms used to capture this emotionally charged, Biofield-expanding, state.

I used to have a young, energetically active, highly engaged assistant who stood five foot four. I rarely thought of him as short, even though I towered over him by a foot—until he got sick. That's when I noticed his small stature. Illness diminishes us. When we are ill, injured or traumatized our energy field collapses inward. We look and feel shrunken, spent, hollowed out, gutted of energy.

Larger Than Life
After a student has been working on Sanchin's energy mechanics for several months, I test them to see how effectively they can draw Ki into their system. Both of us square off, standing about six to eight feet away. I ask the student to assess our height differences. Most note I am taller. I stand 6'4". I then have them perform Sanchin. When finished, we stand across from one another again to reassess our height differences. I don't put any words into their mouths. Many can't believe how much taller they seem. I can usually notice the difference and confirm their observation. Sometime a student will seem unchanged or produce the opposite effect, appear shorter or diminished. This tells me the student either has not drawn a charge into their body or has lost charge and needs more work on their Form.

An amusing example of Biofield distortion is how often people misjudge my weight. People consistently overestimate my body weight by up to thirty pounds. A dense Biofield makes people appear heavier.

When Student Becomes Teacher

Some people find solutions to problems during their nighttime reveries and dreams, others from hitting the books, some from raw trial-and-error, or by surrendering the problem to their unconscious. I sometimes draw major insights by listening to students remark about their training.

Eric, is an athletic, middle-aged student who possesses unusual body sensitivity. He heals quicker than the average person. He needs twice the anesthesia for any surgery. He told me his great grandfather could bend iron and steel tools in his bare hands. Eric had been training with me for over twenty years when one day he admitted that doing Sanchin kata caused his eyes to bug out of his head. He would get so physically juiced it took him hours to calm down. I realized in that moment the Sanchin kata might not be solely teaching one about charging up but also how to release or discharge excess Ki. Eric could easily build a huge charge in his body doing Sanchin, but he had trouble letting the energy out. If a kata like Sanchin had been designed solely to draw in energy it would cause men like Eric to explode, figuratively speaking.

Carrying too much energy in the body is no better than holding too little. The tension and relaxation cycle typically seen in many variations of Sanchin gives us a strong clue about its purpose. I am convinced that Sanchin teaches one how to draw and release energy, a logic I've ascribed to this Form for decades. The tension/relaxation cycle was introduced to help students discern these two states from one another for greater control over their Ki flow.

Most people studying a martial art are likely practicing one primary style. Even within styles, it is not a one-size-fits-all practice. An astute sensei will tailor their art to meet each student's strengths and fill in their weaknesses. In terms of Kiko, if you habitually take in too much energy you will need to familiarize and work with opening your Yang Gates, the channels that let energy out. If you are someone chronically tired, physically weak, you will need to focus on opening your Yin Gates to bring in a greater charge to get your work done.

Traditional Chinese Medical theory can be helpful here. Any acupuncturist will tell you that an excess in one area generally implies a deficiency in another. The excess of holding too much energy belies the deficiency of not being able to let it out. And vice versa. The excess of letting too much out implies the deficiency of not being able to hold it in. The repetitive practice of Sanchin offers a tool to both scrutinize and remedy imbalances in our Energy system.

The Four Dimensionality of Kiko-induced Strength

Physical strength is not a one-dimensional phenomenon, as in solely a body reality. Everyone displays some degree of strength, but likely far from optimal when certain conditions are absent. Healthy body tissue holds a better charge. A hydrated body holds a better charge. Nourishing foods helps the body hold a greater charge. Proper respiration is a more efficient distributor of the charge. A mind free of mental clutter and stress holds a better charge. An outer structure that aligns with inner channel flow holds a better charge. All these dimensions aid in clearing the human circuits, removing impediments to your power.

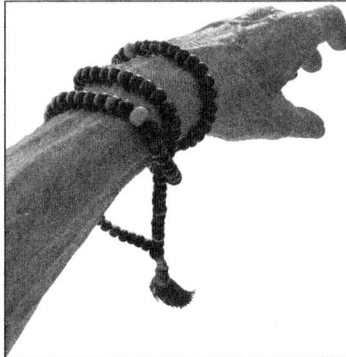

The Mala and the Sanmitsu

I wear a meditation bracelet called a *mala* on my left wrist. The mala represents the Buddhist concept *Sanmitsu*, the *Three Mysteries*. These are the mysteries of mind, body and speech, the latter which we could broaden to sound/*mantra*. Though the mala might first appear as three separate bracelets, it is one strand wrapped three times. The ancient sages understood that although we project three separate appearances to the world; mind, body and spirit. We are one living, united strand.

12* Your Energy Body can move independently of your physical body.

Your Energy Body can move independently of your physical actions. It can leap ahead, lag behind, or run opposite any bodily movement. Initially, we want our Energy Body to move in sync with our physical form. Feeling the movement of your Ki, Energy Body or Biofield indicates a major stride in internal martial development.

In your most relaxed state, when internally at rest, your Energy Body will move in sync with your mental and physical actions. But any degree of conflict or stress can easily throw the Biofield out of kilter, causing it to shift signals and resources toward rebalance. When you feel out of sorts; anxious, fearful, restless, agitated, too hot, too cold, hungry, unfulfilled, your Energy Body is the first to respond to the disequilibrium.

Consider that martial artists may train for years to get used to the intensity of kumite (free fighting). Likewise, it will take most students years to fully comprehend the dynamism of their Biofield.

The most common observation of a student out of sync with their Energy Body is physical awkwardness; too stiff, too loose, or mis-paced. Less obvious disconnections might be a wrong mind-set, or a reversed electro-magnetic polarity in the limbs.

Tai Chi practitioners move slowly precisely to align their actions to the speed at which Ki naturally moves in and around it. Liken Ki flow to an even-paced breathing rate, the lapping of waves, the heartbeat. Ki flows in a constant, steady, rhythmic pulsing motion.

Moving suddenly can cause one's Ki to move out of sync and thus difficult to feel. This is why most Hard style ballistic practitioners miss internal factors. Energy moving ahead or behind a physical maneuver will affect a partner, an opponent, a competitor, or a bystander differently. Advanced Kiko students can feel this lag and will adjust quickly.

Five ways limb actions and Energy Body move:
1. Limb and Ki flow run parallel, in sync, simultaneous, and even.
2. Energy flows ahead of the limb action becoming projected energy.
3. Energy lags behind a limb action, resulting in a disconnected technique.

4. Energy flows counter to the limb direction, either resulting in a weak technique or acting as a Ki draw.

5. Energy does not move into the limb. This results in a 'dead' arm or leg. Dead means, void of energy, absent of charge. This method can be employed in advance of being hit in a pressure point or to seal against a direct internal attack against the Biofield. A strike directed to an acupoint on a dead arm will not be as acute or even activated.

Projecting or withholding Ki can be either an unconscious or conscious action. The mind can control the Ki flow or simply allow it to move at its instinctive, preset rate. What does Ki feel like? Sensing Ki might be as simple as the following exercise:

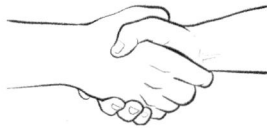

The Hand Shake

Imagine a scenario in which you are going to shake hands with two different people. The first person is a dear friend of yours whom you have not seen in years. The second person is an abusive, condescending bully. If you feel different sensations shaking with these two imagined persons, you have just felt your own Ki moving. Beyond noting your psychological state of liking or not liking a person, Ki will flow unimpeded down your arm when shaking hands with your long-lost friend. By contrast, you may feel your Ki recede, or not flow in your arm at all, no matter how vigorously you shake hands with the bully. To an observer your hand shake will look identical in either case, but one hand shake will be ki-filled, the other, devoid of Ki.

Where the mind goes, your Ki flows. Where your feelings flow, your Ki flows. My own *Ah ha!* moment came when I tried to resist a wrist takedown by Stone, who pointed out, "If you're going to put all your attention into your hand, I'll take you down easily." At that instant, I understood exactly what my Ki felt like. I needed to place Ki in the resistant musculature of my forearm, not in my fingers.

Epigenetics is the study of how our behaviors and environmental factors can cause changes affecting the way our genes function. The word 'epigenetic' means 'above the genes,' implying changes in gene activity that do not involve changes in DNA sequence. This emerging science is finding that we don't just inherit our genes. We inherit, through nature and nurture, our emotional patterns, constitutional health, personality traits, etc.

If your parents were athletes and your grandparents were athletes, they may have produced high-functioning offspring both as a genetic trait and due to the exposure to people with athletic ability in a fitness environment. If optimal or suboptimal biological systems can be genetically and environmentally passed to us, why not our Biofield patterns? A sub-functioning Energy Body could be the result of an epigenetic degrade reflected in disorganized Ki flow.

Gaining awareness of the workings of your Energy Body is the first step in controlling its movement. I have many students who can manipulate their Ki to disrupt their partner's strength or avoid the same happening to them.

13* The average martial artist is unaware of the complex interactions of their Energy Body during training. Most Biofield effects are registered below awareness.

During thousands of tests conducted on the functions of the Energy Body with a broad range of people, I rarely encountered individuals who had a firm and conscious control over their Biofield. It did not matter if they were a lay person or a karate eighth dan with fifty years' experience. If they had not done prior Ki work, they demonstrated no better method for resisting a push, a pull, or a lock then their biomechanical strength, skill, and coordination afforded them. I guesstimate around 1% of the population is able to solidly connect with their body's full ability to generate power.

Modern societies do not teach their youth about their Ki or Biofield, nor is there any particular emphasis or care to develop intuition. The West has instead focused heavily on and promoted cognition, mind over body, and relentlessly touts technology as superior to feeling. If you are consistently taught that your feelings are subordinate to your mind, at some point you will begin to suppress, deny, or disassociate from your feelings altogether. Conversely, connecting to physical sensations is your strongest link for understanding Ki flow.

Due to false beliefs and physical blockages, many high-end

martial art concepts remain invisible, thus out of reach to most practitioners. This ignorance is not bliss. The consequence is the suffering of being left out of the bigger game of life. The Energy Body functions by degrees on all three levels of our being; conscious, sub-conscious and unconscious. Kiko will usher you into a backroom of self where a bigger game is played and larger life gains can be achieved.

Heart Felt

One way in which our bodies interact without touch is through the heart. Any person within close proximity to you will immediately experience a heartfelt communication, but not the touchy-feely kind.

We know from scientific studies that electrical heart entrainment, or cardiac synchronization, is the phenomenon where the heartbeats of two individuals become synchronized when in close proximity. The exact distance required for this phenomenon to occur varies on a number of factors. One factor is the strength of the electrical fields produced by the hearts of the individuals involved. These fields are generated by the electrical activity of the heart muscle. Science has yet to determine what these interactions mean. However, I believe the transmission and reception of such signals cause a shuffling of inner resources leading to up or down surges in physical strength. Who is to say our muscles don't shift their charge when feeling friend or foe nearby?

The closer two people are to each other, the stronger the interaction between their electro-magnetic fields. Factors such as the angle and orientation of the bodies, as well as any physical barriers between them, can affect the strength of the interaction. The American neuroscientist, Joe Dispenza, has registered the body's magnetic field at distances of up to 9 meters (29.5 feet), depending on the circumstances. From a martial standpoint, I was most interested in interactions taking place within a three-foot range. Overall, it seems that the exact distance required for electrical heart entrainment to occur is highly dependent on the specific situation.

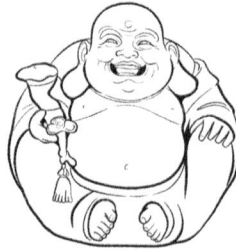

Haragei: Gut Art

There was a time in Japanese culture where it was common for the average person to engage in a social practice called *Haragei*, literally, *Stomach Art*, a form of interpersonal communication.

In Haragei a person attempts to link, or measure, their gut connectivity to another for a sense of their mutual compatibility or intentions. Haragei is silent communication, an exchange of thoughts and feelings through nonverbal means, the essence of a refined Kiko sensitivity.

In martial circles, Haragei extends to the practice of perceiving threats and anticipating an adversary's movements. This sense can be so finely tuned that it is possible for one to perceive a specific attack before any physical movement, no matter how slight, has occurred. This form of silent exchange picks up intention and meaning through alterations in the other's Biofield.

We assess our environment through our head, heart and gut. These systems are not identical mediums though they share information with one another. Which carries the greater truth for you, your heart, your gut, or your head? This question needs to be investigated to get at the bottom of situations you find yourself in or you may get confused by the information you pick up.

In his book, *Gift of Fear*, author, Gavin DeBecker, tells victims of near-death assaults that they instinctively sensed things were wrong at the outset but neglected to act until nearly too late. DeBecker points out to the victims that their gut felt the danger but their head canceled their impulse to react. These victims admitted something felt wrong but justified their actions because, as some victims described, their predators "said or did all the right things," tamping down their fears. Stories like this tell me we are losing our ability to accurately read or discern the messages coming from other's Energy fields.

The closer you get to another, the more intense the Biofield exchange becomes, and the more you will discover about them. Standing inches from anyone often elicits very strong sensations. This is the physical essence of intimacy. Most people are uncomfortable in such close proximity because of the intense sensations aroused. If you feel uncomfortable when someone stands too close for comfort, imagine how you might feel if someone began pummeling your face. Partnered training is meant to break down and declaw the fear-inducing part of the proximity threat intensity. It's meant to acclimatize you to playing with the fire, so you can more accurately read or feel other's intentions.

14* Your Biofield is affected by proximity to the radiating fields of animate and inanimate objects.

Kiko and the Proximity Formulas

In my private studio, I began to note where students stood in relation to the room's layout. Most naturally selected the center of the studio. Others choose off-centered spots. I wondered if theirs was a purely random selection, for I believed their Energy Body knew precisely the best spot for them to stand. I devised a test to prove my hypothesis. I asked each student about their preferred placement in the room. Most admitted that certain areas of the studio called to them despite their lack of logic why they felt this way. I divided the room into quadrants and tested students standing in the center of each quadrant. Sure enough, when tested, their strength varied significantly from one quadrant to another. Often, their intuited position proved strongest. It became clear that the center of the studio, free of any obstructions, was also the one spot least influenced by the radiant Energy fields of the walls, wall hangings, and objects placed alongside them. This was the spot chosen by the greatest number of subjects.

I discovered another Biofield behavior when two people stood in casual closeness. What seemed like a benign action, standing one to three feet away from another, altered their strength as their positions changed. Subjects were asked to simply stand across from one another with no particular intention other than to chat. I noted whether they chose chest-facing, or askew, left, right, or center, arms crossed or at their sides, etc. In almost every case, we found significant strength shifts when testing various resistances shortly after, for the Ki field is constantly adjusting to the exchange of the other's posture and mindset.

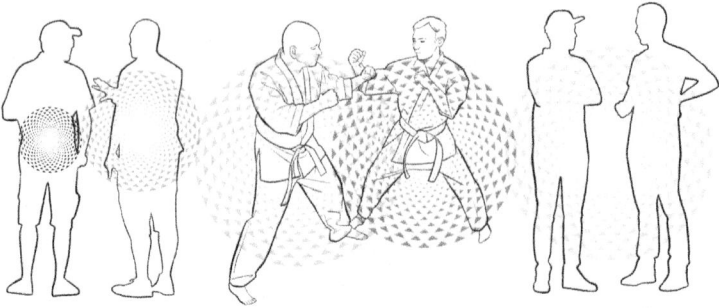

Our biofields can react radically different depending upon the nature of the interaction

My thoughts jumped to the choreography of kata. If a casual, social context had this effect upon another's Ki, it was highly probable that kata was constructed to continuously strengthen the performer and weaken the opponent. I am not talking about strength gains from doing a kata consistently over time to build muscle tone. I am talking about an instant, easily testable affect. Years of analysis determined this is exactly the case in most kata. It makes a significant difference which side of the opponent you orient toward, or align your legs and torso to, depending on the Kiko formula selected and whether you want to send or receive Ki. As further confirmation, I tested every opening move of Isshinryu's entire kata syllabi to find they all, remarkably, increased the strength of the performer and diminished the opponent.

ISSHINRYU KATA

The initial step in each of the eight Isshinryu Forms
charges the performer and weakens the opponent

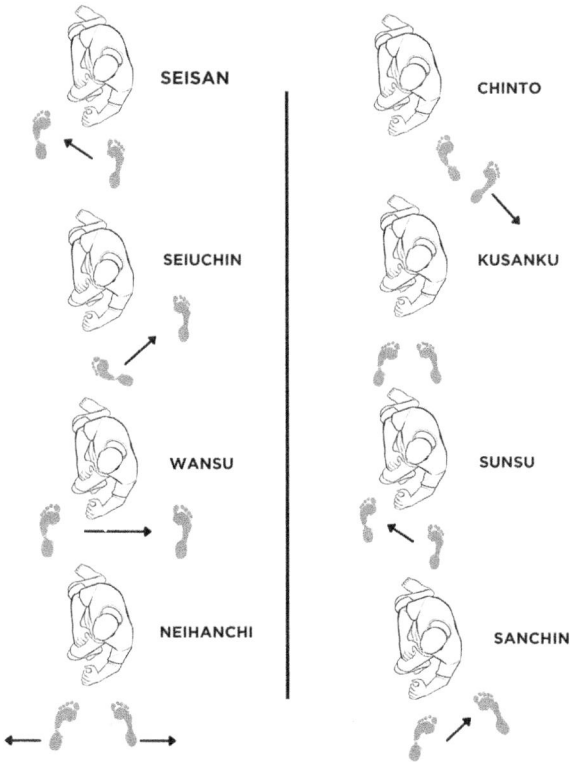

SEISAN

CHINTO

SEIUCHIN

KUSANKU

WANSU

SUNSU

NEIHANCHI

SANCHIN

**The only direction not indicated in the isshinryu kata syllabi
is to move on a retreating left diagonal.**

**15* Persons in proximity will exchange energy
and information on seven distinct levels.**

You are in continuous communication with all aspects of your world at every moment whether you are conscious of these exchanges or not. I call these exchanges the *Seven Conversations*. Each conversation can be correlated to one of the body's seven energy centers denoted in the Hindu chakric system. These conversations, in total, represent a private, complex, multi-level, sensorial dialog. Your Biofield weighs the stimulus of each chakra against a personal standard of feels good, not so good, bad. Then it reacts, like a hand withdrawing from a flame, adjusting the chakric spin before your mind ever realizes what is happening. Sometimes the signal is strong enough that we become cognitively aware of the need to act. As the therapist and author Stanley Kellerman wisely noted in his book, *Your Body Speaks Its Mind*, our body has an innate mechanism through posture and gesticulation that displays complex feelings, which he and others possess the ability to accurately decode. I did not fully understand the import of this seven-layer communication cake until I researched the Hindu chakra system and anchored each conversation to one of the body's seven energy centers. I have since adopted this heptagonal template as a means to evaluate students, competitors or opponents.

The next time you stand across from someone, see if you can disentangle the seven conversations in your own mind by asking yourself the following questions from the template below. Each question relates to one Energy center in your body, beginning with the crown chakra at the top of the head down to the root chakra at the base of the spine:

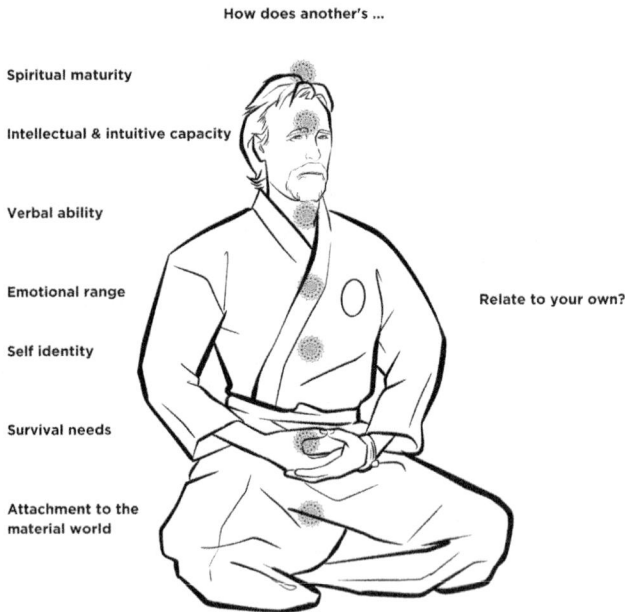

How does another's ...

Spiritual maturity

Intellectual & intuitive capacity

Verbal ability

Emotional range

Self identity

Survival needs

Attachment to the material world

Relate to your own?

Don't worry if this inquiry feels daunting at first. Once you get the hang of this self-inquiry checklist, you should find it helpful for guiding or determining your actions with others.

MIND MATTERS

16* The Energy Body can be manipulated mentally through intention and visualization in a method I call Soft Gating.

The most powerful weapon in the world is the human mind.

My decision to formally enter Buddhist martial practice was motivated by the single statement; 'If you do not understand the nature of your own mind, you will never understand authentic power.' I found this comment hugely compelling. Its truth became more apparent with every passing decade. Outside of physical limitations, the biggest obstacle I observed confronting martial students wasn't their bodies, it was their mindset. Their concepts of power were often limited, leaving them on the one extreme, either lacking confidence and fearful, thus leading them to overestimate adversaries, or on the other extreme, leaving them over-confident and self-absorbed, leading them to underestimate their opponents.

Soft Gating: The Hard, Hard/Soft, Soft Continuum

Ki is gathered and stored in the body just as a battery holds a charge. We can't move Ki without our body just as the charge does not exist without the substance of the battery. Our energy field conducts Ki by way of continuous signals received from our internal and external terrains.

However, Ki can be pushed through and around the body purely by the mind through clear intention in a process I call *Soft Gating*. But this is not an action derived solely by thinking. Thought is the production of ideas in one's head. Intention is the engine of thought. Intention is the producer, the prime actor, that leads Ki around the body. Until you sense what Ki is you will not be able to consciously transmit or receive it as you will be confined to the involuntary presets of your Biofield system. In the Soft Gating process, it is your willing that sets your Ki in motion along with the assistance of your imagination.

Exchanging ideas is a form of psychic manipulation, something we in the West are quite skilled at. Though an energy transaction takes place, it initially moves each other's mental fields or upper dantien.

Limited awareness bound by limiting beliefs leads to restrained expression. Take the concept of physical power. As youths, many of you probably witnessed situations where a larger, stronger person prevailed in contests of strength. This may have impressed upon you that unless you are bigger or stronger than your competition you can't be victorious. Size has relevance. But size alone does not determine the victor. One's level of organization does. A larger, disorganized competitor can lose to a smaller, highly organized person. A perfect example can be found in Rickson Gracie's reign as an undefeated jiu jitsu champion for two decades where he proved time and again that a smaller person can defeat a larger opponent. Sometimes brain defeats brain or brawn defeats brawn through better organization. Let's look at how Kiko relates to the brain-versus-brawn equation and draw a finer line between physical and mental posturing.

Six Mental Pillars of Kiko

How do we tap the power in our minds as martial artists? We obviously need an affirming, can-do attitude. Such a mindset comes from being confident, psyched up, sure of oneself. Such an attitude, if not inherited from our parents, is generally built brick by brick through positive, reinforcing experience. In an ideal state, these experiences are crafted by the sensei in the forge of the dojo whose crucible is the fire of intensity through calculated intra and inter-psychic practices and bodily challenges. From these trials students come to identify and apply their mental tools.

Six primary mental tools make up Kiko's Soft Gate system. Refining and using these tools correctly will allow you to direct extraordinary strength into all manner of martial technique.

Interoception: developing your perception of internal sensations which includes emotional, imagistic and somatic experience. This is a critical platform for a firm grasp on directing your Ki. It requires spending time looking and feeling inward.

Memory: recalling and installing past Biofield templates of successful behaviors or outcomes. Memory allows us to call forth previous winning strategies and avoid faulty ones.

Willpower: the raw, psychic fuel that powers our concentration and intentions.

Intention: the projection of a clear desire powered by our will that activates Biofield signaling to bring one's goals about. Intentions are formed through the twin faculties of logic and intuition. Intention is the seed of our behavior and more importantly, can create unique energetic fields.

Concentration: The gathering and condensing of the Biofield, strengthened by mental work and consistent repetition of physical technique along with integrative movement sets.

Attention: The steady projection of Ki into and onto the object(s) of focus.

Mental Breakdown

Is Ki manipulation all in the mind? No. But the mind is involved. All bodily actions have some level of brain engagement or management. Mind and body, as vibrational structures, occur simultaneously though function at different frequencies. No layer of one's self is completely partitioned from another, although such effects might be too refined to be felt consciously. This is why they get overlooked or presumed non-existent.

What is the mind's role in Energy work? What are the psychic factors involved in Ki transmissions? Let's look at some Biofield mechanics.

All we have in the universe at its core is the flow and interaction of energy vibrating at different frequencies. Energy is never static. Terms like mind, body, emotion describe various states of energy phenomenon. These labels do not do justice to these intricate interacting fields. Energy flow in the body impacts energy flow in the mind, and vice versa. A tidal motion of Ki coursing through the whole system generates currents within currents and cycles within cycles. This system is always adjusting toward a homeostasis specific to each of us.

Awareness gives some of us greater degrees of mental and physical control over previously involuntary processes. For example, we can control our breath, our diet, our emotions, our thoughts, what martial techniques we want to use, all to varying degrees. It's unlikely that lower creatures possess these same controls with the same predetermined effect as humans. I don't see a chimpanzee practicing breath control to see how it might improve its Biofield functioning, or a squirrel thinking it could improve its jumping skills by hopping an extra fifteen minutes each morning on alternating legs.

How do you think the average martial artist introduced to Kiko would receive the idea that it is possible to weaken someone without touching them? I've seen a wide range of reactions; surprise, doubt, skepticism, blind faith, enthusiasm, awe, or a wait-and-see approach.

I believe that every attitude correlates to a shift in energetic structure on the molecular level. In other words, if we could look at our mental functions on the quantum level, we would probably see subatomic distinctions amongst all the above-mentioned states. Even accepting or rejecting a belief in Kiko would reveal a different quantum pattern. But no such looking glass exists, except for highly sensitive minds. I doubt if every scientist would disagree that something shifts in the quantum field.

If the above attitudes are indicators of shifting energy currents, we can look for their effects on the physical body's musculoskeletal system. It's here I see a remarkable expression of physical change coupled with our mental postures. I have observed the outcome of a physical strength test vary between a doubtful subject compared to a confident, receptive subject. A shift in attitude not only reveals degrees of muscular strength or weakness, but implies that the mind has the ability to override our involuntary control of the meridian flows in the body. With a strong enough mental directive, postures that would normally distribute energy to bring about one outcome can be overridden to produce its opposite. How does this occur?

The function of memory might help us to understand the answer. Most people think of memory as a personal data retrieval system. Say you need to recall a former classmate's name. You search your mental databank and up pops the name 'Bill'. A more complex retrieval might recall a mathematical formula and how to apply it. But this does not describe the entire memory mechanism. The mind also imprints/activates precise energetic formulas for every one of our successes and failures into our Biofield. If you are shown a method of making your wrist twice as strong, your mind will recall the exact Ki flow and postural pattern your body needs to duplicate that feat. It will open or close the necessary Energy Gates and channel Ki to the needed area. It will remember this template even if you consciously cannot. Where the process goes bad is when the ego insists upon validating its powers of recall by trying to access the correct formula, when this is not the actual function that does the retrieving. For example, a senior student having been introduced to Kiko principles, boldly states, he feels very strong in a posture, but when tested he actually turns out weak. His ego had convinced him, by an erroneous internal cue, he must be strong. His was a case of wrong state of mind.

There are several methods to call forth a success formula. One method is through memorization and rehearsal (such as performing a kata sequence). Another method is to activate it by way of practices designed to bypass the conventional (ego) mind as the above example illustrated. One can invoke a success formula by means of a connection to a higher power; God, a deity, trust in Nature, etc. thus allowing an intuitive, unconscious manipulation to take place.

The Electrical Component Behind a Takedown

In the Wansu kata of Isshinryu there is a step backward into a Horse stance that concludes a leg takedown. The Horse stance activates the Earth Element rotation of the Biofield. Proper rotation of the Biofield makes this takedown far more potent. Those who deny any internal electrical system involvement are baffled when 1. They attempt the throw from another stance with far less affect, 2. Are told to imagine they are stepping back into a Horse stance and find the throw easier or 3. Are told to imagine the appropriate direction for the Biofield rotation (clockwise vs. counterclockwise) and notice how much easier this maneuver becomes.

Success has energetic shape. Successful people project an aura of confidence, an 'air' of accomplishment around them. Thoughts of success or victory is not just an airy ideal spun in your head that dissolves into nothingness when you stop thinking about it. Success is a formulaic, recallable, projectible energetic field. The British Scientist, Rupert Sheldrake suggests such may be part of a morphogenic field, which, in part, I call a 'success field'. It can be summoned and activated. We limit ourselves when we think of memory solely as a type of robotic, binary inner hand that either grasps the correct classmate's name, or fails to remember it. This is only the tip of our Biofield's genie powers.

A fundamental problem however, arises in this discussion. We cannot presume that anyone's internal systems is working without obstruction or impediment. The human energy system for many is essentially corrupt (as well as corruptible). Amongst the general populace, it is inefficient. Our mental software is frequently marred by glitches. The vast majority are simply not attuned. The main problem is twofold; a lack of knowledge for how to tune ourselves up and the lack of follow through when this knowledge is in our hands. I could analogize this issue to the wielder of a martial staff. A small circle made with the hands at one end of the *bo* results in a much larger orbit at the other end. Similarly, a small motion in our psyche can lead to a much larger and pervasive bio-current. This is why the mind can wreck a good Ki experiment. Shifts in mental focus result in simultaneous shifts in the Biofield. Martial Buddhists were onto this observation. Single pointedness achieved by meditation held the monk's mind to a razor level of acuity. Their inner practices paid attention to the subjective qualities of their experiences to halt mental aberrations and illusions.

The development of inner experience often begins by calming and balancing the physical dimension first. Achieving inner stillness immunizes one from external distraction or disturbance. Our minds need training to project clear, pure intentionality. The more refined the intention, the more dramatic the energy flow, the faster the outcome. There can be no doubt, no hesitation, no second guessing, no tension, no fear, no holding back. Buddhist Qigong recognizes four necessary steps to develop miraculous abilities; The intention to do so. Gradual progress. One pointedness. Intense visualization.

You need more than hope or pretense to be victorious in the ring, on the street, or in life in general. Victory must be felt in your bones. You must want it so badly you taste success in your mouth. Do not let outside thoughts dissuade you from your goal. Once your mind is clear about its objectives, the next step is to transform your desire into action. You must become like the samurai who prided themselves on their single-mindedness, their ability to prevent distracting thoughts from intruding and diluting focus from their ultimate goals.

17* Intention drives Ki

Thus, humans have the latent ability to utilize their own specific intentions to alter various properties of their own body's tissues, muscles and organs in beneficial ways if they will only believe that they can do so and make the personal effort to train themselves to do so.

William A. Tiller, Phd

The strength of any intention is determined by the force of your will. Will power fuels intention. The stronger the will, the greater the intention. The greater the intention, the greater the Ki charge generated. Coupling a strong emotion with a clear intention infuses the system with more motive power. Emotion turbocharges the frequency of your Ki wave.

Think of intention as a signaling mechanism, a thought projection converted into an electro-chemical stimulant leading to the manifestation of that which you desire. I contend that one who initiates a clear intention will control all the other surrounding weaker fields, if only for an instant—enough time in a confrontation to be decisive.

18* Mental *chi nate*, (throwing energy) is supported by imagination and visualization.

Visualization is the ability to craft a clear picture or a desired outcome in your mind. Visualization was the primary mental tool used by the esoteric Asian masters to cultivate and direct their Ki. We can divide visualization into static and moving images.

Static images can be simple shapes; a triangle, square, circle, cross, etc. These images will cause Ki to move in unique ways. Even a static image will cause Ki to move. This is why still images can be potent activators. For example, visualizing a triangle, will cause your Ki to move upwards. Inverting the triangle (point down) will cause your Ki to flow downwards. A clear intention felt in your body will direct the Biofield to project itself (Ki) outward, the basis of *Chi Nate*, or throwing energy. Moving imagery can be divided into: Pictorial images; a waterfall, flame, spinning top, etc. and Conceptual images; holding desired ideas, concepts or outcomes in your mind's eye.

Active imagination isn't child's folly. It is an interfacing perceptual system that gives us access to our inner world. Ancient Asian, internal martial masters took visualization to a high level of detail. The power of visualization is rarely discussed in martial training. Visualization is a non-language intermediary between the conscious and unconscious mind that can be used as a potent Ki activator. We consider it a tool in what one psychologist calls, *'inner physics'*. Visualization brings into reality that which it conjures. It is part of the mechanism of manifestation to get what you desire. A strong visualization stirs the Energy Body and activates our primal nature signaling to the outside world this is what I want and I am coming for it. I am not talking about fantasy, or escapist thought, though visualization can serve this purpose if one's mind is out of balance.

The noted Japanese Ninjitsu master, Masaaki Hatsumi, speaks about the importance of focusing 'only on the outcome.' Morihei Uyeshiba, of Aikido fame, stressed holding the mind on one's center. These statements suggest that if your concentration is strong enough, your goal can be achieved with less effort. The power of concentration focused on a task can direct your unconscious to redistribute and restructure your Biofield to bring about the desired result.

True imagination is the activation of imagery on an unconscious level as a gating mechanism causing Ki to flow as intended. Visualization is an archetypal tool dating back to human's earliest relationship to the world. Before we had verbal language, the world spoke to us through images.

Kime: Focus

I often asked university students early in their self-defense course, "Do you think your physical strength is affected where you hold your attention in your body? They are not sure. So, I pair them up and designate one group the pushers. The others assume a strong Horse posture. I inform the resistors they will be pushed three times, each with a different focus of attention; the top of their head, the bottoms of their feet, their belly. What do you think resulted when they were pushed?

Focusing on the top of their heads and bottoms of their feet, most were pushed over easily. Focusing on their lower belly they found themselves strongly rooted in their stance.

A correct visualization, or bodily locus for the mind to attend, does not mean there aren't blockages preventing a desired outcome. Some students focusing on their dantien still get uprooted. If you have a great piece of music for the guitar but you've never played guitar, your musical score will remain trapped in your head. Therefore, it is important to feel what you think. To effectively move Ki, you must feel the visualization in your body. Do not confine images to conceptual snapshots in your mind.

Feel what you think.

I conducted the above experiments year after year in each new semester's class. As the years passed, a shift occurred. Even though maintaining their focus on their lower abdomens, fewer and fewer university students were able to hold their ground. I concluded that the reason more of them got uprooted was due to their inability to get out of their heads into their bodies. This presents a foreboding future. Today's sensei's have a steepening, uphill battle ahead.

Clear Mind to Empty Mind (*Mushin*)

In the same way you might declutter your abode of unneeded, useless things to make room for the new, a similar process is used to declutter the mind. Achieving *Mushin* (empty mind) is not a static event. You must actively clear your mind. It is a misunderstanding that meditation is solely a passive activity. It's true, the body is quieted. But the mind must remain alert and actively detach from the sway of thoughts and desires that clammer and clog it for attention, otherwise it is continually absorbed in muddling itself with unnecessary worries and concerns. Mind clearing is the first step toward mushin or mind-emptying, the alignment with the ever-present, universal 'I'.

Three Mind Paths for Generating Power.

1. Let the Hard Gates dominate your Ki flow by relaxing into the moves. Focus solely on the physical organization and actions of your limbs and what you want them to do.

2. Visualize your Ki moving along the meridian pathways (or musculature) you want to activate.
3. Activate the appropriate static or conceptual imagery. This can be the visualization of a specific shape, symbol, or thought stream. You can also hold a picture of the desired outcome in your mind and let your unconscious fill in the rest.

For Ki to flow freely you must avoid, reduce, or resolve any discord between your mind and body. Disharmony can happen for a multitude of reasons; remaining in your head while working on technical preparation during execution will split your Ki flow between your mind and body. If you pick an incorrect visualization, an incorrect thought stream, wrong Ki flow direction, or you lack confidence in your process, you will reduce or cancel the effect of your Hard Gates. Always take a moment to transition from one desire to another. Form a clear image of what you want to accomplish. Then set to it.

Discord and Ego: Which Way To *Wu Wei*?

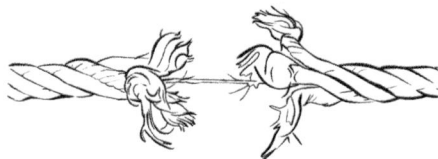

"The man who has no tincture of philosophy goes through life imprisoned in the prejudices derived from common sense, from the habitual beliefs of his age or his nation, and from convictions which have grown up in his mind without the co-operation or consent of his deliberate reason. To such a man the world tends to become definite, finite, obvious; common objects rouse no questions, and unfamiliar possibilities are contemptuously rejected..."
Bertrand Russell, From The Problems of Philosophy

A person's martial behaviors can reveal a great deal about their life philosophy. Having taught thousands of individuals the means to defend themselves, I've observed that rare is the student who uses their art to step out of the need for a defensive or offensive mindset altogether. This is a seldom achieved, middle state, mental ground. The mere suggestion of such a possibility would raise eyebrows as martial hypocrisy in most dojos. Nevertheless, the question, 'Is it possible to train in the arts of self-defense to transcend the need for any defensive or offensive mindset?' drew my curiosity.

Personal protection is one of the central reasons people seek out martial disciplines. Some individuals are dogged by constant friction; smack-down struggles, chaos, ill health, and/or repeated failures in their lives. The idea of acquiring skills that might end or prevent current or future struggles; slay the enemy, defeat the bully, avoid the pain, stand up to criticism, feel worthy, is very appealing to them. In their minds, if they could just clinch the black belt, gain the stamp of expert, defeat the competition, all their ongoing and future problems might resolve. But seldom are life issues starkly black and white. And it's rare that material skills alone will provide anyone an absolute remedy. That Universal Energy works at all upon our anatomical energy is primarily to realign our spiritual and material natures that have fallen out of sync with one another.

Within the Asian contemplative disciplines there emerged the concern that an acute need for personal defense might create a slippery slope. For a defense implies an offensive. This notion marches in line with the concept of Yin/Yang but where opposites generally viewed as interdependent forces are skewed as antagonistic forces. That is, daytime becomes dependent upon the reality of a night time. Hot has no relevance without cold. A defender or victim decries the existence of an adversary, imagined or real. The competitor needs the competition of a challenger/opposer, else what is there to defend or champion against? This notion must have presented a philosophical enigma to some early martial philosophers. For does one who carries a knife, a gun, or trained limbs in any way manifest an opponent to validate their choice as defender?

For the average person, no, not really. But there do exist persons for whom the acquisition of martial talent does little to stop a vicious cycle of violence and abuse in their lives. These are students convinced the world is out to get them and who in turn, must righteously assert. In return, their world provides confirmation by hurling at them all manner of provocation. These are the students quick to get into a heated kumite, quick to ignite with the slightest goading, quick to justify their cheap shot after the match is called, quick to aggressively assert their point of view and who lack the sensitivity to see the damage they inflict. These students do, in fact, unknowingly invite violence into their lives to justify their quashing it with their acquired power. This is the cyclical drama of the wounded, disorganized psyche that can lead one into a downward spiral that gradually distorts their reality to keep them dancing on a hot plate of personal transgressions.

I believe we are an inherently positive species by nature. But if you insist the world is out to get you, it will offer you offensive proof to reinforce your self-projecting, defensive or offensive mindset. Such a person has severed from their own positive nature.

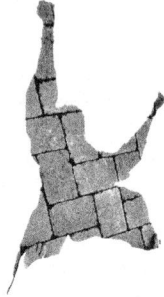

Shadow boxing with the ego attempts to dispel mental illusions

Imagine trying to defeat your shadow in a fight. You swing, your shadow swings. You jump, your shadow jumps. When you step into the sunlight, your shadow hides under your soles. When you cleverly get a flashlight and shine it under your feet your shadow clings ninja-like to the ceiling above. Every move you make will be futile. You are neutralized at every turn. It matters not that you are an eighth dan or a combative champion. This type of shadow boxing explains how some people's egos, in an attempt to resolve the source of their discord, only extend the drama. The ego's strategy is fraught with challenge because ego is but a small part of our Pure Mind and often the very root of the problem.

Allow me to wax philosophical. Think of discord like the severed end of a cord seeking reattachment. People speak of being on the mend, picking up the pieces, pulling themselves together—reconnecting. What are they reconnecting to? I suggest their reattachment is to the once Unbroken Thread of their own positive nature.

What could break this Unbroken Thread of positive existence? Did an evil, mysterious force pull it apart? Was life always this way? Is the idea of one's severance an illusion, a mental illness? Are people trying to mend something that only seems broken?

To sever a cord requires an oppositional force or friction, a tension strong enough to snap it—an opponent.

If you were to honestly look at all the counter forces that exist in your life, you will see that many are generated from a world view consisting of oppositional forces. How many people blame the source of their bad luck or suffering on something outside themselves; God's will, Nature's will, a Divine plan, other people's stupidity or aggressions, enemies, maligning events? The ego is first to decry that something else, something beyond themselves, must be responsible for severing their thread. We never think we might be the source of our own upsets.

Whenever our intentions are complicit in separating us from our positive nature, a mirror is instantly created in its reflecting shards. All the oppositions that plague mankind could be seen as divides of our own separated parts.

All manner of discord can be cured by bringing into accord, alignment, attunement, the disagreeable, the maligned, the separated, the out-of-onement experience. Harmony and discord can move with the same intensity. The main difference is that harmony is movement of the parts seeking union with the whole, while discord is movement in reverse, a dis-integrating, destabilizing division of the whole, fragmenting into further pieces.

It has been my experience that the Dō side of the Martial arts offers a platform to observe our inner dramas in the hopes of resolving the bigger universal puzzle of human suffering. It presents a method for reattaching severed pieces of self toward a more unifying picture. This transformation, this reconnection, or reconciliation, occurs through keen observation of cause and effect. Students who enter combative disciplines with an open mind may come to realize that the Martial Ways present a mini-world, a microcosm, of the larger interplay of everyday life. The dojo distills the world into a more manageable grasp of fundamental cycles giving one the chance to see Life in its naked state. As each year of hard training passed, I realized that I was being given an opportunity to observe my own aggressive tendencies, my own core beliefs, the nature of my conflicts, the natural cycles and actions of men and woman as they charge and discharge their desires, power struggles, dramas, and their ego's sly role in perpetuating aggression. I realized that authentic power only comes from wholesomeness, from being whole. And I could not be whole unless I had a clear picture of what it meant to be and to feel whole and connected. The world at large is too big, too complex, with too many moving parts. The dojo brings it down to size, presents its layers systematically. The Dō of the do-jo points to a uniquely personal inner way in calculated, manageable steps.

You've heard the adage, 'Be careful what you wish for.' Intention can be a curse or a cure. The wrong intention curses us by generating more friction in our lives. The moment you act as a separate, severed strand of the Unbroken Thread, the cycle of discord revolves. This is a tricky matter because all movement presumes some level of opposition. Movement cannot exist without the resistance of something to push against. But, do I move this way or that way? To stop discord, to stop severing, you must stop opposing, stop negating, stop blaming, and simply start being. When you embrace a philosophy of duality, of oppositions, you inevitably invite discord.

This brings me to the principle of *wu-wei*, the action of inaction, moving without exertion—nondoing. Wu-wei is a unique mindset that reinstates positive Universal spirit, restoring one to a spontaneous state of harmony, a state of non-opposition. In a balanced state, people will act appropriately without fearful or aggressive intent, without self-criticism, without self-justification. There is no opposed or opposer, no need to filter one's actions through an inner critic.

An animal attacked by another animal simply reacts. It does not reflect, 'This is my enemy, I am justified in fighting back.' The animal behaves in accordance to its nature without self-identifying, or self-analyzing. Likewise, when you take root in your own unsevered nature, your actions will flow naturally with conviction. Do you think if a river possessed consciousness, it would say to itself, 'Am I going at the right speed? Do I have enough power? Am I heading in the right direction?'

The sages recognized that no mind (ego) equals no opponent. No intention equals no friction. No friction brings one to the time before any severance. What you send out, what you radiate, what you transmit, reflects back like a mirror image.

How does the universe mirror our intentions? M was an angry student. One day he released his anger on a junior classmate during a round robin kumite. Needing to feel superior, he struck his partner. M felt justified to release the internal pressure of his anger on his victims. I pointed out to him that his partners lacked his skill, to take it easy. But M had broken his positive thread in the past. He hurt another student, then another. M had splintered into unwholesomeness and his splinters began to damage others working with him.

Spirit is not mind, yet it permeates mind. Spirit is not body, yet it permeates body. It's an illusion of the ego that our mind, body and spirit are separate threads. When we sever our connection to spirit, to life, we fragment. A fragmented self sets a de-evolutionary course into density, darkness and inertia. When spirit coheres, it generates light and lightness of being. The Unbroken Thread is a positive weave of the spiritual, mental and material worlds.

Movement consumes space by filling it. This 'filling' stirs both destructive and creative transformative energies. The destructive sires the creative which births the destructive in a circular manner. How you determine which cycle is active depends upon your perception and definition of what is creative and what is destructive.

Negativity creates reality X. Positivity creates reality Y. Do you seek more friction or the absence of friction in your life? Are you successful in this venture? No matter what reason brings you into martial arts there will always be an underlying positive or negative current regarding your personal protection and assertive rights. And this will determine whether you attract light or darkness into your life.

There is no soil for you to manifest an opponent unless you distinguish yourself as separate. The moment you acknowledge your separateness, you invite the friction of opposition. You've cut the cord. And ego is quick to sever. It has had generations of practice. For it assumes that our self-identity and self-identifying actions are necessary to survive in this world.

Concepts of *God* and *Ego* represent polarized end points on the spectrum of universal intentionality between the sacred and the mundane. Ego acknowledges opponents by making distinctions based upon life's perceived dualistic reality of a good guy requiring a bad guy, a 'this' requiring a 'that' to exist. A personal God or impersonal Dō opposes nothing. The concept of God or Dō unconditionally allows everything to occur because they represent the world as a single unifying field. The cosmic intentionality of God's or the Dō's vibrations create a grand game board, the pieces, and the rules. You and I, as pieces, create a subgame with smaller pieces and narrower rules. For the majority, their micro view of the whole consists of disparate pieces in a constant fight for reconfiguration that often leads to disfigurement instead of wholesome reconstruction.

The Buddhist *Middle Way* offers a still point between the self-split worlds of heaven and hell, good and bad, love and hate, war and peace. Walking the Middle Path dissolves all the inner and outer battles by choosing to hang in that rarified space where nothing ever separated in the first place.

19* Your Biofield patterns are reflected in your foundational beliefs, forming the platform upon which your physical and psychological behaviors spring.

To expand your skills, you must challenge your foundational beliefs about primary concepts; power/force/strength/enemies/justice/morality/destiny, etc. Think of your beliefs as active psycho-ingredients in all your day-to-day decisions. Their programming runs constantly, shaping your life philosophy, which in turn activates your behavior and life choices. If you believe that fighting is good for you, you will fight. If you believe that fighting is toxic, you will avoid fighting. You become what you believe. If what you believe is what you receive, but what you want is not what you get, then you either have not waited long enough for the results to occur from impatience, doubt, ignorance, or misinformation (you are not believing something correctly), you don't really want it, or karmic forces greater than your conscious actions are blocking your beliefs/desires from manifesting. I call these foundational beliefs our *Platform*.

Martial greats like Aikido's Uyeshiba, Judo's Kano or Mifune, Karate's Funakoshi, or Jujitsu's Gracies, all transcended their basic platforms allowing them to ascend to superior technical functioning defying even above average martial artist's comprehensions.

20* Examining your beliefs can unleash your full powers by revealing limited or obstructed Ki flow.

Karma is a root energy that carries your past actions into your current and future patterns of being. Karma refers to 'action,' more than a predetermined fate. People who accept karma as fate often struggle with the term because they entangle fate with inevitability, which offers no wiggle room around life decisions. If it is your lot that you will never earn your black belt or defeat the bully, why struggle to succeed? This is not the right way to think about karma. Simply put, all our actions have consequences. This has been scientifically and psychologically established. What you do about these consequences defines your karma. If you go around hurting others, beware. You may experience a rude comeuppance, not because it is fated that you will get payback, but a strong probability exists that you might.

A single karmic action could be likened to the expanding ripple from a pebble dropped into a pond. Karma is merely an empirical cause and effect. Once this wave hits the shoreline (a resistant structure) it will return to the center of the initiating action (you). On a metaphysical level, karma holds us accountable for our actions. If you want positive outcomes, engage in positive efforts.

Conceptual *Kumite*: A Cognitive Duel

Martial art teachers are not trained psychologists, though they get to witness a great deal of psychic energy at play in daily dojo dramas. And there is no scarcity of dojo drama. There are the occasional pep talks to elevate the downtrodden student or calm a bruised ego after a heated kumite. But overall, the mind is given little credence as a major part of the learning spectrum compared to the attention given to the body. This is unfortunate, because we need to train our mind as diligently as we train our body to develop real power.

The Buddhist monastic approach to martial arts differs from mainstream goals by its broad focus on quelling hidden enemies both within and without. Here, the goal shifts to removing our ignorance about the nature of reality, unearthing past traumas and faulty beliefs that hold us back from progressing.

In Isshin Kempo we create a psychic arena to engage in a Conceptual Kumite. This partnered didactic has been crafted to advance martial concepts. It is part of the Dialogic Movement that aims, in our case, to refine the art of conversation into a vehicle for martial transformation via intellectual discovery. This practice has proven just as valuable a means for overcoming our ignorance about the nature of mind as physical bouts for sharpening one's fighting skills to overcome a flesh and blood adversary.

Rules of Conceptual Kumite: Two students pair up. Rank and age are inconsequential to the coupling. A novice can be paired with a seasoned black belt. Both individuals then share what they know of a mutually selected concept through personal stories or academic acumen. The goal is to cooperatively elevate one's understandings of the concept through discussion and compassionate debate. It is unacceptable for a partner to condescend to the other for any lack or level of understanding. Several significant results can be expected; at least one party is elevated, context is built between the partners, and a mentoring relationship enables any wisdom to be imparted.

Meditation

The mainspring of all Buddhist training is meditation. Meditation is a method which enables us to truly see just where we are in the present moment. From this vantage we can best see what we need to improve. The most effective way to discover more about our nature is to watch it in action. This is what happens when we practice meditation. Think of meditation as a mediation between discordant parts of yourself toward a psychic settling. Meditation is the practice of candid, non-judgmental, honest observation of oneself. If you don't know who you are, or how you function, you cannot expect effective change for the better.

From the Kiko standpoint, meditation is also a direct portal to energy sensitivity. For every person in proximity to you is engaged in an on-going multi-modal, Energy dialog. Your ego is either participating in or oblivious to these conversations. The more you understand what is taking place within your own Energy field, the more power you have available for making decisions to get what you want.

A Disturbing Trend

I have observed a growing and disturbing trend regarding modern youth entering the martial arts. Many have trouble holding their full attention on their moves and exhibit less coordination than previous generations. These young minds too easily stray. Some mistakenly believe that as long as they are outwardly doing their motions, it is okay to let their minds wander. This bifurcation only causes their Ki to disperse further. Rather than concentrating or packing Ki in their muscles, a divisive, counter-signaling misdirects their energy, often into their heads.

This trend portends the coming of a great mental reset in Western culture. For we are shunting Ki away from the lower dantien, the body's true physical power center to the upper dantien, the soon-to-be new and illusory center of power. I say 'illusory' because the head cannot become the center of power without sacrificing our humanness, unless we give birth to a completely new human species. For the mind currently get its mojo from the lower dantien.

Each year more studies come out that children are growing weaker, that, for example, 75% of our adolescents are not getting enough exercise. This suggests we are producing a generation of weaklings; less fit, less active, more sedentary and, in many cases, heavier, with more fat and less muscle mass. Arm strength and grip strength are on the decline. These weakening youth will challenge future sensei and reshape the future martial landscape.

Tasks that premodern generations could easily do, today's youths are finding more difficult. The preference for passive activity replacing vigorous physical pursuits is only part of the story. I see four trends changing our youth's physical landscape:

1. The increase in electronic screen time requiring more physical passivity.
2. The increasing number of children in proximity to synthetics and electronics, nudging their organic world into the background. Children today are literally less grounded to the earth.
3. The increasing number of distractions in young minds due to the constant bombardment of information tailored to lull them into an addictive consumer complacency.
4. The steep rise of anxiety and other mental issues.

21* Skepticism is Soft Gating.

Attitudes have a kind of inertia. Once set in motion, they will keep going, even in the face of the evidence.
M. Scott Peck

There are two ways to be fooled.
One is to believe what isn't true;
the other is to refuse to believe what is true.

Søren Kierkegaard

Peck's statement is particularly apropos to the current attitude about the existence and function of Ki. In my pursuit for the rationale behind the effortless power I felt with Stone in 1992, I paid little attention to a scattered community of skeptics who do not believe that any hidden, secret, ki-charged techniques exist, nor how narrow or belligerent their positions could be.

I've encountered advanced martial artists who readily dismissed Ki's existence or value. What I find disturbing is their reluctance to take a deep look at the subject. Few in the Hard arts understand Ki or how it functions in their own disciplines. Having spent years absorbed in their arts and not seeing it, some arrive at the false assumption that Ki is a fantasy power, a dog chasing its tail.

I do not fault anyone for feeling skeptical when reading about my accounts of dramatic strength surges from Kiko. I would have been right there with these skeptics with a raised brow. I didn't see this side of the art because I wasn't looking for it. Our prevailing cultural context and ideologies do not support this vision, and may even lead to a conditioned mental myopia. Several scientific studies prove however, that we can be completely blind to otherwise obvious events.

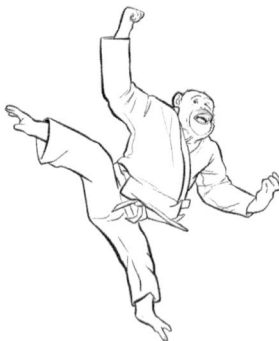

Monkey Mind

A dumbfounding study called the 'Invisible Gorilla' test conducted in 1999 by cognitive psychologists Daniel Simons and Christopher Chabris asked subjects to watch a video of basketball players and record how many times players dressed in white passed the ball. During the game a life size, gorilla-costumed subject walks across the floor. Amazingly, the majority of test subjects failed to notice the gorilla, though staring right at it. We are far less aware of our world than we think. The testers call this effect 'inattentional awareness'. They concluded that it is easy to miss details you are not looking for. Ki is a costumed gorilla in many dojos.

I saw a Ki gorilla in my practice. I experienced marked strength shifts week after week, year after year, now running over three decades playing with this beast. What set me on my quest after my initial reaction with the Frogman, was to prove that what I had experienced was real. I wasn't content to wave away the results as a freakish, one-off event. I was willing to expend the time and effort to find out what lay behind the phenomenon.

I fully understand the skeptic's mistrust. I studied Okinawan karate for twenty-five years and never encountered any such power—until the day I did. I've since spent three more decades following its intriguing clues in kata, painstakingly assembling an amazing puzzle of Ki's essential principles and behaviors in many of our universal martial practices. Ki is astonishing, inspiring, elevating and has given me and others a deep appreciation for the essential martial disciplines originating in Asia. Each one of them contains rare gems of insight in their advanced practices and principles.

How Kiko Gets Discounted

Someone reading about Kiko to enhance their physical strength might discount its existence if they try a Kiko experiment and it does not work. The reason for the failure however, might not be because Ki doesn't exist, but rather the inability to see the variables that shut their Ki flow down. This is not much different from the student who cannot pull off a joint lock maneuver because of a faulty understanding of its biomechanics, then claims the technique is useless.

I've conducted many tests where something that worked well previously, suddenly failed to work at all. With persistence, however, I often discovered the reason for its failure was a factor previously not considered.

It is difficult to let go of well-entrenched, parochial views, especially, if you are successful working with what you've got. There is a long history of such in every known field of endeavor. For decades the medical establishment believed that blood serum was a useless substance with the sole purpose of conveying blood platelets through the body. Years later, it was discovered the serum itself was an important source of electrolytes and transport for fatty acids and thyroid hormones which act on most of the cells in the body.

We can also take the once historical fact that the world was thought to be flat. Of course, this paradigm proved flat out incorrect. But it wasn't false science. It was science not stretched far enough. If the world had better instrumentation to look over the edge of the supposed flat earth to see its curvature, everyone would have agreed the once blasphemous round world view was spot on. It takes time for new paradigms to root into mass consciousness. Kiko presents us with another paradigm challenge.

I don't fault rigid thinking built on previously sound observation. There is always a prevailing notion until its reign ends. Flat earth explanation was the best that science could offer civilization at the time. It's the complacency or refusal to consider or debate new ideas that prevents one from taking the next evolutionary step. Times change only when beliefs change. Civilization may go up or down, but it rarely remains still on evolution's ladder.

On the other hand, we need the challenge of critics to help us separate the chaff from the wheat, otherwise the charlatans get to run wild. Even Einstein showed us that the most long-standing theories may be open to improvement, even radical change. Open criticism is the lifeblood of progress both in science and culture at large. You may have noticed however, that open criticism, even intelligent debate is being censored across many fields today.

From a different angle, skepticism, or doubt as to the truth of something, should be addressed as a form of Soft Gating. The skeptic who rejects a new idea simply on the grounds it is not what he or she has seen or believes, activates a Soft Gate manipulation of their Biofield preventing access to any validation of the information being denied.

I have experienced two types of martial skeptics; healthy and unhealthy ones. The unhealthy skeptic chooses to believe the martial world remains ki-less and will do everything to assert this belief. The healthy skeptic challenges the existence of Ki pushing its believers to find stronger arguments for its existence and value. I assert the existence of Ki. I also remain open for it to be proven otherwise.

If someone told me fifty years ago a man could poke the bottom of my foot using one finger and make me pass out, I would not have believed him. But I would have been curious to observe the feat. Do I believe everything I'm told? No. Do I believe what I see with my own eyes? No. I've encountered posers capable of tricking my mind. I do tend to believe what I directly experience, particularly, if I can duplicate the feat and attach a sound rationale to the outcome.

22* False gatekeepers may block your martial advance through misdirection due to their limited knowledge and/ or restrictive convictions.

The world is filled with charlatans and con artists who operate at every stratum of society. These are the false gatekeepers claiming to possess various truths about the martial arts, which they do not possess. Trust your instincts, question deeply. Experience for yourselves the real from the illusory. I've encountered individuals with lengthy martial credentials who were quick to discount the knowledge I am sharing in this book because they hadn't witnessed it for themselves. It is neither my path nor my purpose to change the fixed mind, particularly minds that mistakenly view my presentation as a challenge to their supremacy. In truth, our realities are challenged at every turn. Kiko's behavior upturned my beliefs on a life-changing scale.

The biggest critics of internal work seem to fall into three categories; those who live viscerally only for the fight and thus reject any conceptualizations, those who do not want to change, and those who want to control information. These attitudes measure the value of their martial way through a narrow lens. One supposed, half-century expert vented to me that, "There is no chi. There is no hidden technique, and kata is for beginners." Anyone can take a magic mental wand and erase the 3,000 year Asian history of the evolution of Ki in their mind if they choose. Mental power doesn't imply intelligence-based.

Every sensei and shifu, every disciple, contributes their experiential threads to a grand, ever-weaving martial loom, whose total creation in any given moment represents the collective reality of the Martial Ways. No single person holds all the answers. No one possess the omniscience to know what is meaningful to others. There are plenty of pitfalls without adding an arrogant, cock-sure teacher, a delusional skeptic, or the student who does not or cannot listen. Don't let your shepherds lead you into wolf country. Many dead and wounded casualties lay strewn across the martial field.

23* All manner of negativity causes suppression, drag or friction on your Ki flow.

Negativity is the result of any physical or mental activity, or lack of such, that resists or moves counter to your intentions, hence, your Ki flow. Your body communicates positivity and negativity through sensation; too hot, too cold, too tight, too loose, not right, etc. The mind reveals positivity and negativity through feelings states; love, joy, peace or anxiety, irritation, anger, hate, fear. Our brains register and remember positivity and negativity by outcomes; I failed the test. I beat the game. I earned the trophy. I lost the match.

It's important not to erroneously entangle the concept of effort or work to negativity. When effort is applied to your betterment, resistance will be encountered, but the resulting friction is called growing pains. These pains are recognized as a means of progress to a better state of being. One becomes like the seed pushing through the weight of the soil above it. All attempts to move beyond a limitation will generate positive friction. Once the resistance is overcome, the result is higher functioning. An elevated state of being frees up Ki flow, resulting in less friction, more positivity, better health and, in regard to your martial pursuit, greater physical strength with better outcomes. A generative cycle is brought about by positive training.

Do not confuse negativity with well-focused effort. Exerting to better yourself will shed layers of negativity, like a snake sloughing dead skin.

24* Mind and body co-depend on correct energy and information to function optimally.

There is no separation between the mind, body and Biofield. When optimal, a fluid interpenetration of information and energy occurs among these mediums. Correct information provides us proper action, and gives our Energy Body the means to carry the action to its conclusion. The greater the corruption of this three-tiered system, the greater the increase in life frictions and the more incoherent the information received. We only separate these mediums in an academic sense to bring clarity to certain levels of information and functioning. Our potential is a seamless communication between brain, body and Biofield. Consider the mind like a stream and the body, the streambed, with Ki acting as the underlying motive power. Or, think of your mind as your body in Hard form and your body as mind in Soft form. Without your head, your body cannot function. Without your body, your mind loses relevancy.

KI Flow

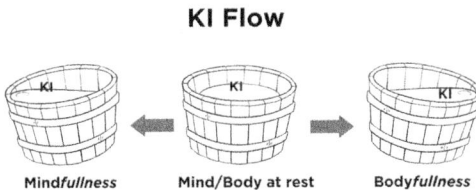

Mind*fullness*   Mind/Body at rest   Body*fullness*

Imagine a large tub (body) filled with water (Ki) representing a human. The left half of the tub represents Mind. The right half, body. Any mental or physical action sets the water in motion, as if the tub was tilted toward one end or the other. The water will slosh from side to side until everything calms and reaches equilibrium in stillness. Mind spills into body. Body spills into mind. Each biological system: mental, circulatory, musculoskeletal, neural, endocrinal, depends upon the other systems for energy and information. The human entity always functions as a one-piece unit.

Before you even throw a strike, you need confidence that you will be successful, followed by the intention to strike. You need neurons to carry the impulse of your intention to propel your limb forward. You need primed and conditioned muscles. You need an idea of proper striking technique. You need the breath to sync with the muscles to help push more Ki into them.

Striking always generates a dual shock wave. For every action there is an equal and opposite reaction. One wave will move into your target. A simultaneous counter wave will travel back through your body. When the striking form is incorrect, the return wave can damage you. If you don't understand the significance of this principle, imagine striking a block of cement as hard as you can. You will be injured. The greater resistance of the cement block will send the full force of your strike back through your striking limb. To generate maximum power, you must train to properly ground every returning shock wave.

Likewise, for every action in the mind there is an equal and opposite reaction in the body and Biofield. A mind trying to overturn an unwilling body will meet resistance. A body trying to direct an unwilling mind will also encounter resistance.

25* Mind and Body govern your Energy Body via conscious and unconscious intent.

I believe what we call Mind or consciousness is our subtle human Energy Body. The part we label ego is just a small piece of this larger mind which the ego claims. Our ego's primary purpose is to preserve and to protect its identity (you) as a separate self. Ego however, lacks awareness of its own Biofield capacity. This is why people can find their unconscious intentions antagonistic to their conscious desires. When one part of us wants to go left and the other, to go right, we've gotten in our own way. The ego, ordinary mind, the small self, gets into frequent skirmishes with our Higher Self, or Pure Mind. This puts an odd spin on the idea of self-defense. For how do you defend against your own maligned ego?

26* You can instantly install Biofield templates of past successes or failures.

Success starts by feeling desired outcomes in your body.

Science has not fully determined exactly where our memories are stored. The British scientist, Rupert Sheldrake, holds that memories might actually be held in, what he terms, a *Morphogenic* field, an energy field existing outside of our bodies. Is this field our Energy Body or part of it? Wherever memories are contained, I've noted our mind is acutely aware of our successes and failures and is quick to recall and/or install them.

I have conducted hundreds of simple tests demonstrating how just recalling a past, positive or negative event has an immediate influence on our physical strength that can instantly inflate or deflate us.

A test: We establish a subject's base strength. Then we ask the subject to think of a negative event in their life and test again. Their strength noticeably decreases. When asking the subject to think of a positive event, they retest considerably stronger. Are you aware of your own strength shifts during different moods and states of mind?

Past events are not just benign reveries located in our head, like old files in a dusty cabinet. Whether positive or negative, all thought patterns influence our Biofield. When positive, the Biofield yields strength and health advantages. When negative, it depletes us. This is clear, empirical evidence in support of the power of positive thinking. Think positive, become stronger—instantly. A consistently applied positive attitude builds a stronger person. Alladin and his magic lamp tell a story about the capacity of the human entity to exceed its limitations when one's thoughts, desires, and intentions are pure and strongly focused.

27* Depending upon the circumstances, your mind, physical body or Energy Body can dominate your actions.

I was teaching a private session one evening to an intermediate student named Len who was working on the Neihanchi kata. At one point Len became flustered when he accidentally reversed a movement sequence. He cursed aloud at his mistake. On a light-hearted whim, I quipped, "That's right Len, tell your body who's boss." Shortly after, Len nearly tripped while making a lateral cross over step. To which I stated, "That's right Body, don't let Lenny boss you!" The situation was quite amusing as his visibly rising frustration released a lot of pent-up Ki, making Len even more agitated and his performance riddled with mistakes. It was a perfect example of a mind, body and spirit at odds, all vying for control.

Sometimes the physical body overrides the mind. Suppose you don't want to break away from an event on the TV but you have a strong desire to pee. You will only be able to suppress the sensation for so long before your body overrides your desire to sit still by making you antsy with a burning feeling in your bladder.

I find it most interesting when such overrides occur as a result of acting from an inauthentic base. An inauthentic person is some-one who acts or behaves based on false information and beliefs. Such a state reveals an ignorance about, or insensitivity to, one's true needs, and the rightful means to acquire them. Inauthenticity binds one to a perpetual state of unease and discord by inviting unnecessary conflict.

The best examples of dominating forces are those rare events of superhuman feats of strength performed under extreme stress. My interpretation is that the Energy Body overrides all prior phys-ical limitations imposed by the ego with an abundant release of Ki into the system to lift the car off the child or sustain otherwise fatal wounds or horrific conditions, and live.

By contrast, I've witnessed well-trained minds override oth-erwise instinctively fixed energy patterns. The right kind of train-ing, for example, can recalibrate one's hair trigger for violence. It takes time, but some angry individuals with touchy emotions have learned to override their amygdala hijack and avoid descending into the *Red Zone*, my term for that primitive, animalistic impulse-driven state of 'seeing red' that cannot find any other alternative beyond the utter annihilation of their opponent.

From a practical standpoint, and with proper training, you can bring these three dimensions of self into accord allowing you to strike harder and faster, uproot stances, and overpower locks placed upon you in a manner previously unable to accomplish. Many unwanted behaviors or circumstances can be changed when you rid yourself of habitual, negative or chaotic patterns of self.

28* Your Energy Body always seeks to maintain internal homeostasis consistent with your state of consciousness.

Understanding the relationship of Ki manipulation to homeostasis and your Bandwidth of Being will enable greater control over your Biofield.

The term *homeostasis* refers to the body's tendency to maintain relative stability between all its interdependent parts, particularly in regard to your physiology. Your body constantly monitors itself to function within a self-prescribed comfort range; not too hot/not too cold, not too hungry/not too sated, not too much potassium/not too much sodium, not too acidic/not too alkaline, not too agitated/not too sedated, not too active/not too sedentary, not too insecure/not overly secure, etc. Meridian channels regulate Ki by a continuous mind/brain/body matrix of hormonal, neural, circulatory, enzymatic controls, each cross-checking one another.

Our involuntary mind is located in the brain's limbic or Reptilian system. This system regulates Ki flow without our knowledge. But like breathing, mental control can be either unconscious or conscious. Maybe it's doing a good job regulating your body unconsciously. Then again, maybe not. In five decades of teaching, I've met some very smart people, yet all but a rare few of them were aware of any heightened control over their body outside of its biomechanics until they were introduced to Kiko. It was as if they discovered a secret circuit board of the self. Kiko challenged their current paradigm by giving them a corrective lens to witness their unrealized potential. The external side of training is half the story—a cup without contents. The contents of the cup, subtle energy, is the missing other half of the equation. This is what authentic martial arts is all about.

Biological systems evolve by degrees. To adapt to higher level functioning, our systems and structures must acquire and install upgraded, more optimal self-regulatory mechanisms. The transition from old to new however, comes with a period of vulnerability. Like the snake shedding its skin, we are most susceptible to attack or upset during these changeovers.

Homeostasis places a firm boundary around our life possibilities, beliefs and actions. This balancing act runs across the entire gamut of our being from regulating our emotional states, musculoskeletal actions, neurochemical processes, right down to the subatomic level where molecular bonds are created or broken as our physiology necessitates. Most of this regulation occurs involuntarily, below consciousness. These controls kick in automatically and instinctively. But based upon one's level of individual awareness, we can also exert significant control over this process.

We each have our own frequency, our own vibe, our own privately regulated inner thermostats with different settings, different formulas, for maintaining our individual baselines. Some of us tend more toward order and health, while others in the extreme, dwell in chaos and friction. When you are clear about what actions produce what results, you get to choose your life's arc. When you change your diet, your living space, your work, your workout routine, your thought patterns, you tinker with your bandwidth. Simply put, healthy practices upgrade us. Unhealthy ones degrade us.

It is a challenge to change your frequency. Most people don't initiate deep lasting change. This is why people vacillate, sometimes moving forward, sometimes moving backward, but mostly remaining the same. This seesaw movement creates the illusion of growth or advance. People's personalities and behaviors change little over time. Martial art training parallels this reality. No one becomes an instantaneous fight expert. To develop expert skills, you have to break pre-martial art patterns and replace them with new habits and practices. You have to alter the factors that define you as non-skilled or less skilled. It takes real effort to push through the resistances that bind you to your past way of being.

If faced with a physical threat you might choose to run or fight, to kick versus punch, to dive for the legs, or throw a chair.

All these multi-layered interior functions taken as a whole, whether regulated involuntarily or voluntarily, define one's *band-width of being*. This bandwidth is the energetic expression of all our habitual patterns, all our self-regulating cycles, that keep us vibrating within a specific frequency range. Although this bandwidth is not rigidly fixed, internal and external forces confine us to general parameters to maintain our ways. In a collective sense, this bandwidth also generates a specific consciousness whose primary goal is to reinforce its reality. Another way to say this is that our bandwidth of being produces a consciousness that projects a reality that reinforces itself.

How does our bandwidth of being manifest on a day-to-day level? Most of us have habitual thought patterns, specific sleep, eating, rest and activity cycles. We dress in a particular fashion; prefer a certain style, certain colors, even certain clothing pressures. If you were to step back from your daily actions and look at your behavior in terms of patterns and cycles, you might be surprised to see that you vacillate within a fairly well-defined parameter. Stepping outside of it can feel unfamiliar, perhaps, even uncomfortable. People do not like too much change on a core level because a certain threshold of change alters one's self-identity. When people are not sure who they are, they can easily fall back to familiar ways to reinstate their identity and feeling of security.

What does all of this have to do with the martial arts and the manipulation of Ki? Your bandwidth of being with all its self-regulations, continually presets your Ki field to behave within a prescribed spectrum. And nothing will alter this flow until significant change is imposed upon it.

Kiko offers a broader selection of choices by widening our awareness to include the Energy Body. Kiko training immediately challenged the status of my current way of being and seeing. As I gained more control over the influences of my inner life, I discovered a new field of previously concealed potential.

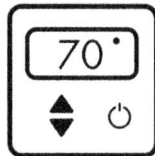

Our body functions similar to a home thermostat. Say you set your thermostat for 70 degrees in the daytime, 60 at night. No matter what the outside temperature, your furnace will do everything it can to maintain the interior climate you set. Our physiology modulates our frequency. Our frequency in turn modulates our physiology. Each keeps a check on the other. Much of this process is pre-coded in our DNA. Your entire metabolic system sloshes back and forth until it gets everything just so. Just as it takes time for your furnace to respond to a cold snap, it takes time for your body to warm up, cool down, excite or calm, shift from feeling to thinking, from offense to defense. Neither your house furnace nor the living furnace, your body, can adjust on a dime. It takes time to shift resources to meet and match all your internal and external demands.

How did this regulatory system get established? How much flexibility does our system have for change?

Traditional martial training, specifically the Asian Dō-based arts, were designed to change one's Bandwidth of Being. A change in frequency, is a change in the Ki flow in your body. Your presets get rewired, paving the way for new patterns, new cycles of behavior. In regard to Ki manipulation, the critical change is making oneself more sensitive to, more conscious of your actual, not imagined, Biofield currents.

When I say traditional martial arts, I need to qualify this statement. In modern Western culture, the average person is being disenfranchised from his and her true legacy powers. As I have previously established, the lower dantien is being cut off from the upper dantien by a protracted, perhaps, self-inflicted campaign aimed at shifting the psycho-physical center of the human being into the upper dantien (the head). The Dō arts, whose traditions contain transformative practices like kata, provide both an anchoring counterweight and a pathway to maintain or restore the true power center of the body.

Traditional martial arts, not the current MMA, not progressive stream-lined, stripped down systems like Krav Maga, or the sport-emphasized variants like Tae Kwon Do or Kick boxing, offer an antidote, a counter weight, to the divides currently shifting our reliance away from the heart and gut to the head. The profiteers of the world want our insights offsite, under their control. They want our total reliance on their bankable outside resources.

Kata is one of the three pillars of traditional training that will firmly anchor the mind to the body, allowing insights to flow freely between them.

Fixed habits do not change when subjected to random, minor, or occasional influences. Old patterns change only when intersected by new patterns whose charge is equal to or superior in intensity, effort, and time spent in the current ways. And these changes must be practiced consistently and consciously until the old patterns are overridden, or should I say overwritten?

We hear stories of people who suffer acute traumas going through life-altering changes. The intense charge of a trauma is often significant enough to displace the weaker charge of prior behaviors. This strong charge can happen suddenly, or gradually with consistent effort.

The monastic masters recognized that in order to upgrade your Energy field (my term, not theirs) there needed to be consistent repetition of highly integrated movement/energy patterns until the influences of the old field were replaced. These integrated patterns encompassed four dimensions; physical practices (kata), nutritional dietary changes, repatterning thoughts (meditation), and re-assemblage of the surrounding environment to make room for sacred space (dojo).

Traditional *Repatterning*

Once the Dōka has committed to his or her path by acknowledging the desire to upgrade, it's time to expend the effort to make lasting and fundamental changes to their Bandwidth of Being. Traditional Dō arts lay out four engagements to bring this change about:

1. A change in surroundings. In traditional schools this process starts by donning new garb and entering the dojo (Way Place): When you don the monk's robes (gi) the old you is symbolically left at the dojo entrance. The dojo is the *tabula rasa*, the clean slate, an open space to new possibilities.

2. Ritual: Proper ritual opens a portal to the unconscious allowing access to the spiritual/quantum world. Ritual takes the student out of their ordinary secular realm into the liminal. Ritual invokes the sacred or divine nature of life. When your ego yields its attachment to the mundane world to embrace the unseen world of higher vibrations, you have entered sacred space. The goal of ritual is to make known that which cannot be known through the rational mind. We don't want just a random change of patterns. We want to upgrade both our beliefs and behaviors and make sure they take root.

Most rituals are designed to conjure, manifest, or enable one's entry into sacred space. Bowing casts off the shackles of inattentiveness to the spiritual fields. It is humbling to discover that there is more than what is immediately known or perceived. A beginning and ending class ritual creates boundaries not commonly acknowledged in Western culture, like bowing, facing north to initiate kata or facing east in yoga. Rituals create a psychic partition separating the sacred from the everyday to reveal new perspectives. Thereafter, the mundane can be reinvited back into a richer fabric of reality. Initially, the mundane drops to the background and the sacred takes the foreground. At the very least, students are asked, by way of ritual, to reassemble themselves for a psycho/physio-spiritual adventure.

Where military ritual reinforces the power of control and dominance, spiritual ritual awakens one's highest nature to the power of compassionate cooperation.

3. Physical practice: The practice of highly integrated movement patterns is designed to restructure you right down to the subatomic level. Kata fulfills this function with its integrative kinetic repatterning. Kata practice becomes a frequency resonator, a kinesthetic tuning fork, for harmonizing oneself.

4. Meditation: Inward directed, contemplative practices will restore your psychological grounding and improve your interoception to reveal and quell the enemy within and to realign discordant thought flows. As selected physical practices ground the body, meditation grounds the mind. Meditation is a unifying activity aligning all aspects of the self into a functionally cohesive unit.

You get out of an activity what you put into it. Achieving amazing breakthroughs with part time effort is for the rare few. The mainstream media's mantra, 'You can do it all,' is a false path.

The Three Second Strength Wave: Homeostasis and Ki flow

A critical point about homeostasis is that the average person's Energy system cannot instantly restore that which it expends. The Biofield system moves in pulses, waves.

The researcher, Margaret Moga, cited earlier, has been developing scientific measures of 'energy healing' and other bioenergetic phenomena. In Moga's study of the neuroanatomy of circadian rhythms and the central autonomic nervous system she has observed, working with exceptional healers, a unique magnetic field waveform associated, with the 'charge-discharge' characteristics of Reich's *orgone*.

Wilhelm Reich (1897-1957) was a medical doctor and psychoanalyst who believed that traumatic experiences blocked the natural flow of a primordial life force which led to physical and mental disease. In 1939 Reich claimed that he had discovered a massless, omnipresent substance, a biological or cosmic energy more closely associated with living energy than with inert matter. He called it "orgone energy". Could we say that Reich's orgone was his attempt to define Ki?

My anecdotal observations theorize that our Energy system overshoots and undershoots until settling within preset parameters. If changes in your bandwidth alters your fundamental Ki flow then the Kiko student must become sensitive to these shifts and learn to adjust appropriately. Beyond any unknown circumstances, the charging and discharging of Energy takes place on one of three levels:

Level 1

In our testing, when the average or untrained person discharged Ki, the strength surge took place within a three second window, after which the person experienced a drop in muscular charge of about 10-30% for the next three second cycle. This was followed by an undershoot/overshoot, recharge/refill cycle in sine wave fashion until the Ki system settled, usually in under thirty seconds. (note: the return to equilibrium varies amongst individuals for a variety of factors).

Level 2

Consciously generated strength gains derived from Hard or Soft Gating in initial training stages also lasted approximately three seconds. This was followed by a drop in strength commensurate to the charge gathered. This could be anywhere from a 30-100% drop in strength. This means the amount gained from Gating for three seconds was lost for three seconds, restored for three seconds, and so on in this alternating scale until settling at the subject's normal homeostatic range in roughly under thirty seconds.

Level 3

At advanced stages of training, subjects showed strength gain was simultaneously replenished after discharge. There was little spilling back and forth within the system because the adepts had rewired their Biofield to continuously balance and refresh the charge/discharge cycle.

29* Ki is regulated through voluntary and involuntary processes.

Years ago, I came across the work of Dr. Harold Painter, a long-term internal practitioner. Painter concluded from his lengthy experience that Ki was mostly the result of self-suggestion, a form of self-hypnosis. That is, if you believe strongly enough in a certain event occurring, you can bring that phenomenon about through the strength of your conviction. I'd like to unpack this idea a bit further.

Suppose Ki flow is entirely a matter of self-suggestion, a form of self-hypnosis. You simply say to yourself, "I will be stronger," and voila, you are stronger. This theory does not explain why every single person I tested with no prior knowledge of Kiko failed to increase their strength using this method, until they were shown how to manipulate their Ki. Often subjects were not told anything about the effects of their physical posturing on bodily strength, nor were they told the objective behind the experiments. I would just ask subjects to assume various postures and then conduct an assortment of strength tests.

This harkens to the story of Christopher Columbus who bested all challengers to balance an egg on end. Columbus cracked the egg's base, then stood it upright. None of his competitors had thought to do that. It's easy once you're shown how to do what otherwise appears an impossible task.

How does the mind convert a thought or belief into physical reality? How does a suggestion travel through our body to make us physically stronger? Do we assume thought alone is what makes a muscle stronger or are there other processes at work?

I can stand all day in front of my computer and suggest that it turn itself on. But it will not start until I press the power button. My computer does not function solely as a result of my suggestion to switch it on. I must physically press the power button to trigger a series of internal events built into the computer. My intent to compute opened one gate, leading to my finger pressing the power button (the second gate) that activated a process sending juice to the computer with its own internal gating mechanisms. I believe the Mind and Ki work similarly.

If the mind, exclusively via self-suggestion, is capable of bringing all that we desire, everyone on the planet would be healthy, wealthy and wise simply by desiring such. Look around. This is far from the case. People are sicker than ever. The U.S. for example, spends more on healthcare than Japan, Germany, France, China, U.K., Italy, Canada, Brazil, Spain and Australia combined. The average person cannot, by sheer will alone, increase their physical strength merely through suggestion. Not one person in all my years of research tested stronger when asked to 'suggest themselves stronger', compared to the strength they acquired doing additional, simple, but specific, physical motions to free up and direct their Ki. Only then did they trigger the appropriate internal mechanisms to direct their Biofield/Ki.

Our desire to fulfill a goal is only as effective as our ability to clear the internal communication channels letting that desire flow on a strong Ki current.

The Power of Mind

The mind often dominates our body through self-suggestion. Consider the flowing outcomes during a series of Kiko tests I conducted with Tian Zhua, a man with forty years of martial experience and high skills in Kiko. You should quickly see the complexity of mind and body influences in this exchange.

Test 1: We both assume a neutral state of mind. I ask Tian Zhua to push me out of my fighting stance. He cannot easily uproot me. My body feels heavy to him.

Test 2: I ask him to either Hard or Soft Gate. I am easily uprooted.

Test 3: I ask him to say aloud, "I cannot push Hayashi out of his stance." Suddenly, he cannot push me, even though he knows he can do it from the prior test.

Test 4: I ask him to either Hard or Soft Gate and push while I say to myself, 'Tian Zhua cannot push me from my stance.' Even though he was successful the first time via Gating, he can no longer push me easily.

Test 5: We both say to ourselves that we will be successful in the test, Tian Zhua pushing and I resisting his push. The outcome is similar to the first test. We have neutralized one another, although on a higher plane.

When given a direct suggestion, our unconscious will summon that current through our body. Our pushing tests above became a cat and mouse game of competing energy dominance. How efficient is your circuit board?

Playing or Fighting in Key/Ki

A novice musician hears a distinct melody in her mind but is unable to play it because she lacks finger dexterity, strength, control and familiarity with her instrument. Liken Mind as player and Body as instrument. Assuming that the mind (instrument) is not broken, or out of key, which speaks to the root problem, minds and bodies functioning sub-optimally become poor mechanisms to carry any intention (music) to its desired outcome. Western society is grossly out of key. Even worse, some people stew in frustration when their desires do not bear fruit. Many of them may lack the understanding that a mind can be at cross purposes with itself, producing a canceling cross-current.

"If one does not understand the nature of mental processes they will remain in a perpetual state of suffering and restlessness filled with conflict."

Krishnamurti

Self-suggestion functions well when your desires supersede or transcend the regulatory nature of your ego to filter inner events. I call this level of self-suggestion, a *Pure Mind* intention. As long as your ego filters your thoughts, it will redirect necessary energy away from fulfilling your desires. It takes energy to filter thoughts when your Energy Body could be fully directed instead toward accomplishing your goals.

When a self-suggestion comes from the Pure Mind, a mind devoid of counter thinking, your actions will lead to an unimpeded Ki flow and a successful manifestation. Consider this when executing martial technique. You can desire your techniques to be powerful, even suggest they be so, but any counter thought or counter purpose will undermine the outcome. Such thoughts could be as subtle as the need for your fellow students to validate your worth, wishful thinking, or ungrounded wishes or expectations that do not match the reality of your current skills.

30* The Chinese internal energy model recognizes three primary power centers.

Centuries ago, the Chinese adopted a three-tiered energy model for their internal practices. Their model differs from the Hindu Chakric model, which denotes seven to nine primary Energy centers. The Chinese sought an ideal flow among what are called the three dantiens (Jap. *Tanden*): the Lower, Middle, and Upper elixir fields. When fully functioning, these three dantiens support one another, charging and discharging Ki as each center needs. Our lower abdomen is considered our root dantien, our physical center of gravity. It holds the greatest charge. Like the roots of a tree, the lower dantien provides the power for the trunk (heart) and canopy (head) centers above. The lower dantien powers our physical nature and acts as our taproot to the organic world.

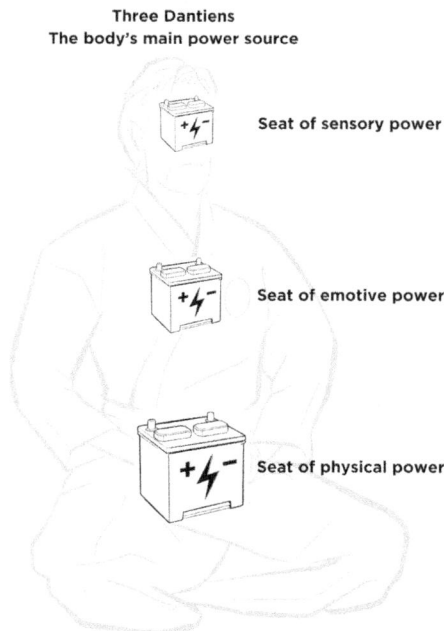

Three Dantiens
The body's main power source

Seat of sensory power

Seat of emotive power

Seat of physical power

The Metaphysics of Ground Grappling—Or Grappling with One's Grounding

In light of the revolutionary changes witnessed in the world today, it was not surprising to me to see the current cultural shift away from traditional standing systems to ground fighting systems. As society propels itself further into the head, an unconscious, counter-balancing response has been to get us lower to the ground. The trending of Earthing practices, Yoga and ground-grappling popularity could be viewed as one antidote to the excess of modern headiness.

Even within traditional martial arts, I've seen a major shift from purely ballistic technique to more close-quarter, grappling routines. This has led to a revival of Asian Push Hands practices in some dojos. These are subtle, instinctive attempts to get closer to one another as social controls push us further apart.

In the past, the feedback loop between the body and the mind provided vital information for how to proceed with any physical action. Healthy proprioception and muscle memory reinforced confidence to go full throttle in physical activities. I contend this feedback loop was stronger generations ago. For example, when the body says, 'It's okay to jump', we leapt with confidence because we had jumped successfully before. However, with the new center forming in the head, I see increasing evidence of diminished body communication leading to erroneous decisions. A perfect example of this upside-down system can be seen in our attitude toward mathematics. Years ago, I remember reading that the U.S. ranked in the 25th percentile in math, but number 1 in confidence in math abilities. I got the picture of an upside-down snowman. As our heads draw in ever more energy, our base battery in the lower torso draws less charge. Society is becoming energetically top heavy, over-heady.

Now, when the mind asks if the body should jump, scant body wisdom returns to the head. We haven't jumped enough in real life to get strong feedback of our success. This may contribute to the tremendous increase in anxiety amongst today's youth who must rely on their heads to decide how to act because their actual physical confidence is lacking. Perhaps, a head-centric person recalls a video game involving jumping. Or they see a movie star jump off a cliff and survive. Based on what I call *virtual* facts, the head-centric individual might falsely conclude, "Okay, I'll jump." This illusion of a mind guessing it's okay to jump can have disastrous physical consequences.

31* The body's three power centers distribute their charge as the need arises.

The mind prepares. The body executes.
The emotions add E-motive charge.

The three dantiens route our Ki among mental processes, emotional release and expression, and physical action in order to maintain our regularity of being. One theory I've been investigating is the possibility that our legs act as the primary fuel or conduit for the lower dantien, arms for the middle dantien, and our five base senses for the upper dantien.

When attempting to solve a mathematical problem you aren't particularly engaging your emotional system. And hopefully, no one is doing mathematical equations during sex. The more head-centric the action, the more passive the body. The more active the body, the quieter the mind. No action is completely exclusive of the other center's involvement. You can observe the shifting energy using this simple, three-tiered template. Know the proper purpose, function and relevance of each center in your training.

32* Society is reorienting the upper dantien to be the dominant energy center.

The human center is shifting

Two social currents are reshaping the course of martial arts today. The younger generation is losing their basic connectivity to their bodies. Their primal instincts are not activating because modern kids rarely get to be primal. The second, whether inadvertent or intentional, technology is culling centered and confident physicality out of the human herd, save for the elite, professional athletes. The American middle class is not the only shrinking strata of society. The middle grade athlete is diminishing. A gap is widening between physical and mental athleticism. The digital world is breeding a once highly prized physical coordination trait out of us. Driverless cars are a good example of the trend in bodily pacification. You need only be a passenger, from the concept of 'passive'. You don't have to do anything. You won't have to pay attention to the road, move the steering wheel, coordinate your feet and eyes to the brake, etc. The digital world beckons the mind, not the body. Consider the World Economic Forum's hope that the metaverse someday will find your digital avatar more important than your physical body. You won't have to move your body at all to be happy. Long term pacification will entrance the body, addicting one to further physical passivity which will destabilize the normal functioning Energy Body. The current extent of our non-physical activities is causing profound shifts of energy away from the lower to the upper dantien.

Fueling or Fooling Ourselves?

In the past, when one spoke of a centered person, it was understood such an individual exhibited a balanced mind and body. We are rapidly retreating from this once vaunted and admired ideal. Trending societal habits are abdicating lower dantien influence to the upper dantien. Just as we are witnessing the American middle class disappearing due to a shrinking and shifting economy, I see parallel divides occurring between elite and mainstream martial athletes, and between our own minds and bodies.

Upward Melting Snowman

Imagine a snowman with its three customary snowballs of varying sizes. The largest ball forms the base. The middle forms the chest. The smallest forms the head. This triangulated structure creates a physically stable pyramid. The wider the base, the more topple proof the structure. Our energy concentrates in the three dantiens like this snowman. The strongest concentration of Ki is found in the lower dantien. This arrangement is also the best topple proof Biofield structure because the lower dantien fuels the upper two centers. The mind does not fuel itself. The mind can only fool itself into thinking all the excitement it creates is energizing, when in fact, it is expending energy. By analogy, the government (head) doesn't gather energy. It spends it, while the people (body) must divert resources necessary for maintaining its own vitality upward to the ever-expanding, ever-spending ruling faction. Everything is interconnected.

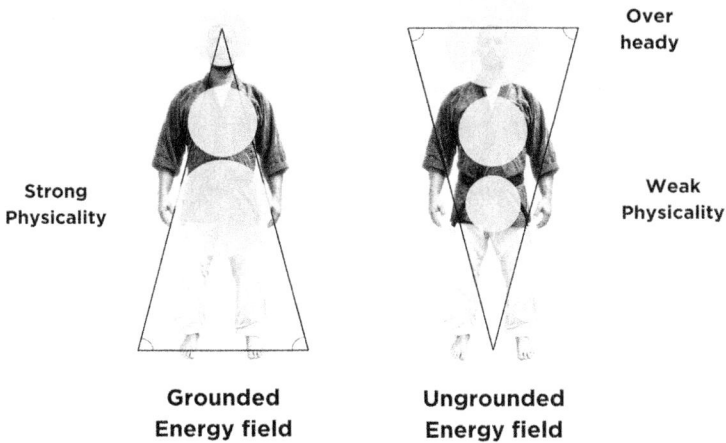

Strong Physicality	Over heady
Grounded Energy field	Weak Physicality
	Ungrounded Energy field

As modern culture moves further from physical life, the Biofield will shift a greater charge and value into the head/mind. This will come at the cost of a reduced charge to the body. As the digital world diminishes our need and desire for physical activity by re-shaping our priorities and interests from physical to mental ones, this will decrease our body connectivity and the energy-storing capacity of the lower dantien. This shift may come with critical, perhaps even dire, consequences. Notice the current parallel push away from earth-based fuels (lower dantien) to wind solar and electrical-based energy sources (upper dantien)

One practical indication of this shift is a disconcerting rise in sport injuries. As of this writing, the CDC estimates we will have up to two million high school athletic injuries per year, accounting for the second leading cause of emergency room visits for children and adolescents, and the second leading cause of overall school injuries. It was estimated that eight million youth were seen in hospital emergency rooms and by medical professional for injuries and sports-related harm. And these numbers don't account for injuries not seen by physicians.

University coaches have lamented to me that incoming, fresh-man athletes are arriving with more injuries and less attentiveness to proper training protocols, even though the coaching practices and protective equipment is at an all-time high for safety. The lack of physicality is rendering simple, sport-like activities ever more dangerous.

I've taught thousands of children since 1970. Today's youths, in general, are noticeably less agile, less graceful, less fit and more prone to injury and illness. Their lack of physical activity renders them less coordinated overall. They may be mentally agile, but they lack emotional and physically maturity. A 2022 research study from the University of Georgia found that 75% of U.S. teens aren't getting enough exercise. The statistics point to a less body-based, body-centered generation. Another study concludes that one third of American youth are obese. There are geneticists raising concerns that we appear to be irreversibly devolving as a civilization. Some psychologists believe we are not maturing our youth until age thirty. This is a far cry from our great grandfather's time when little men and women were formed by age twelve. I'm not making a judgement so much as noting a seismic cultural shift.

I believe the effects of our fast-growing technologies on the development of the body are making young students head rich but body poor. And this shift is impacting martial training. Young students have already begun to mistake cognitive knowledge for realization. How many sensei have found themselves in an uphill battle with ever-younger students who, after doing a few reps of a technique lament, "I know it!"

Should the head become the dominant energy center it will cut people from their intuition, their unconscious, and the wisdom of the spiritual/quantum world. As one commentator observed, 'Your new power source will be derived from a cell tower!' Is this why we are seeing an exponential rise in cell towers?

Will such a gross transformation occur? Will future martial artists be a mix of enhanced brain, decreased brawn, and embedded technology? In just over a quarter of a century, we have become tightly strapped to and unduly dependent upon our electronic devices. What value will the lower dantien have in a metaverse where you will be able to work, shop, create, play, and train martially, in a virtual world? Our physical nature is literally being chipped away.

On the flip side, there is a growing counter trend seeking to enhance physical connectivity. There are martial teachers interested in teaching meaningful integration of the mind and body, who know how to cultivate this habit to help others awaken to its value. While plenty of body-robbing currents are de-evolving us by diminishing and degrading our physical assets, this counter movement is pushing back with paths to evolve them. Until someone comes up with an acceptable replacement for my body, I will continue to promote more bodily awareness and activity. Kiko presents a sensible study to fuse Mind, Body and Biofield. Which direction are you headed?

DIRECTIONALITY

33* Physical strength is influenced by the direction one faces.

There is an old Okinawan Fighting Form called Chinto. One interpretation of its kanji is, *Fighting to the East*. This translation was my initial impetus to ask if the direction we face when performing a kata had any impact on strength performance. I was in for a surprise. Directionality plays a major role in martial performance. As my research dug deeper, it became evident from our testing that the Earth's geomagnetic field exerted an influence on Ki flow as the body rotated through 45-degree arcs starting from any cardinal direction. We knew the meridians influenced muscle contractability but we were surprised to find the direction our bodies faced also caused noticeable peaks and troughs in muscular strength. Most of us are not conscious of the geomagnetic stimuli we encounter every day. Yet, many migrating and homing creatures are sensitive to the Earth's magnetic field. To see if there was any science in support of my theory, I came across the work of Joe Kirkshivink at Caltech who has been testing humans for years to see if they have, what he calls, a subconscious sixth sense.

Mounting evidence for magnetoreception has largely been behavioral, based on movement patterns or tests showing that changing magnetic fields can alter animals' habits. We know animals can sense magnetic fields, but not how these fields function at the cellular and neural level. There is no obvious sense organ to dissect the magnetic fields that constantly sweep through us.

Kirschvink proposes that miniature compass-like needles sit within our receptor cells, either near the trigeminal nerve behind animals' noses or in their inner ear. The question of our magneto-sensitivity remains open ended. Kirschvink thinks we retain a vestige of it. Michael Winklhofer, a biophysicist at the University of Oldenburg in Germany feels civilization may have lost this sensitivity.

If we possess magnetoreceptors as a primal sensory mechanism, and if we discover these receptors signal our muscles, this offers a plausible explanation why a kata's directionality of moving in precise compass directions, usually 45 or 90-degree arcs, factors into kata performance. Perhaps, this is one reason why, during fight competitions, one competitor suddenly feels the impulse to attack or retreat. The latter may not always be determined solely by spotting a physical opening, but by sensing an energetic opening or weakness, felt as either a dip in the opponent's Biofield and/or a surge in one's own. From the Kiko standpoint, the best time to attack is when the other's Ki field recedes or shifts to one's advantage. An opponent's Ki field is generally the weakest at the end of their exhale.

To prove that Ki fluctuations resulted from the directions we faced, I set up a series of strength tests using the four cardinal directions and recorded strength shifts too important to disregard. For example, the majority of subjects north-facing (at least, in the northern hemisphere) tested noticeably stronger resisting a slow wrist takedown or being uprooted from a strong stance than facing south.

An excellent analogy offered by one of my senior yudansha explains how we might be affected by the Earth's geomagnetic fields. Imagine you are submerged in a river up to your neck, and told to perform a kata. Going directly against or with the current would require very different muscular actions, as would performing in various other directions. Now, instead of a water current imagine a similar, if not highly nuanced affect from surrounding electro-magnetic field currents. We are fairly certain, after decades of testing, this will prove to be the case.

Synchronicity: When Luck Strikes Wisdom

Over the years, individuals would ask me how I figured all of this out. They had never entertained the idea of Kiko principles and thus found it rather incredulous that I had managed to lay down so many pertinent inroads. I have already explained in detail my first encounter with the strange phenomenon of the effortless wrist release. The directionality breakthrough had to do, in part, with the coincidence of where and how I teach. In my private studio, my *kamiza* just happens to face near compass North. By sheer happenchance, most of my testing was essentially done with students north-facing. If this factor had not been so consistent, I might never have noticed directionality as a variable in the Kiko equation. I recall a training moment with Stone where I realized if my studio had a different layout, we might not have discovered Kiko at all, or arrived at the same conclusions.

I have consistently observed that Ki naturally rises and falls in a sine wave fashion, like ocean waves or tides. Our testing reveals that every 45-degree change a person faces alters the Ki flow by charging muscles groups unique to the direction chosen and the manner in which it was arrived at. That is, if you stood facing west, you could turn left or right to arrive north. Rotating the body clockwise versus counter-clockwise leads to different strength outcomes. Were the originators of some fighting arts aware of the effects of compass directionality on their Energy Body? Do our bodies act as capacitors?

A **capacitor** is a device that stores electrical energy in an electric field. The internalist who speaks of packing Ki is likely referring to our ability to store an electro-magnetic charge.

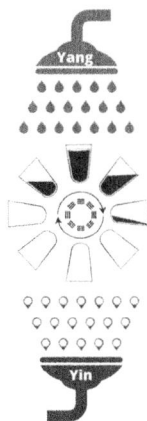

Imagine an upright glass of water placed under a shower head. The glass naturally fills. Consider this filling a Yin state. If the glass were to rotate clockwise, and we paused every 45-degrees to inspect its contents, we would see the water spilling out on the right side. At 90-degrees most of the water will have run out. At 180 degrees, the glass, now upside down, has no chance of water getting in. Consider the emptying glass a Yang state. As the glass rotates to 271-degrees, it starts to take in water again. We must not ascribe no value to the empty glass until it catches water again. Value is determined by the state of the glass at each 45-degree arc along the circle. This parallels the Bagua's trigrams (A diagram consisting of broken and unbroken lines). Each Trigram is unique in purpose by virtue of its positioning on the circle. The Bagua could be understood as a graphic commentary about the nature of Ki in different *guas* (locations).

Rather than holding water, imagine our glass holds two kinds of charge. A Yang charge (emptying) and a Yin charge (filling or potentially receiving). With the exception of the glass at zero and ninety degrees, we have Yang and Yin actions happening simultaneously, with one or the other dominating. I believe this action illustrates what is happening to our Energy Body when we physically rotate 360-degrees. Geomagnetic field signals are likely being picked up by our Biofield which redistributes charge/Ki to the muscles. Ki is discharged through muscular contraction and metabolic activity. Even though the glass is empty at 90 thru 270-degrees, the state of the glass content has radically altered. One state has released water while the other is about to receive water. The earth's magnetic poles function in similar fashion. One pole exerts while the other receives the exertion. The exertive pole is Yang. The receptive pole is Yin. Yin leads. Yang chases. Emptying leads the filling. Filling chases the emptying.

34* The role of directionality in modulating physical strength may have influenced the composition of key kata so its performers moved along the strongest Ki pathways.

In the KATA section of this book, I detail a movement set from Okinawa's Seisan kata to explain why certain directions may have been selected for the performer. It is not coincidental that many kata patterns have practitioners move in 45/90degree arcs. We have witnessed that Energy polarity shifts with every 45-degree arc of the torso and limbs. Every bodily configuration falling within the correct directional parameters represents a formula to charge a technique.

Early in my training, I often wondered why kata turned in such precise directions. The best rationale came years later when a noted U.S. expert claimed that kata's turns were not indicating the direction of a new attack, as I had originally been taught, but were taking an opponent in front of us and maneuvering him or her to the finishing angle. This was a fair and accurate revelation. But I would amend his statement. We turn on such angles because the kata's indicated direction falls in alignment with both the Earth's geomagnetic field flow and our Biofield's receptivity to this influence. Kiko supports kata bunkai. I do not know how many world-wide practitioners of ancient fighting forms considered directionality a key to understanding their bunkai but I can present compelling evidence why the direction you start a kata, and/or execute specific technique, is critical for understanding any essential fighting Form.

Combatants cannot always control the directions they face. But they can develop the sensitivity to gain internal advantages in regard to these directions. Kiko teaches us how to configure the body to avail ourselves of these directional influences. The best fighters move by feel, by a visceral directive. What do you think this feel is based upon?

Wansu kata's two throws

For the longest time I had trouble figuring out what T. Shimabuku had in mind as a bunkai for a sequence where he repeats what looks like two crescent steps in Seisan dachi followed by two vertical fist strikes, with the latter strike in each set directed across the body. There is no apparent blocking action. One day I realized these two sets were likely demonstrating the energetic difference when doing a leg takedown on the right versus left side of an opponent. To trip an adversary by stepping behind their right lead leg, one should turn left 90% to maximize the tactic. To trip the adversary going behind their left lead leg, one must push near backward to utilize Kiko correctly. Reversing these actions becomes much harder to succeed.

Kata's change in direction

Changes in kata direction often indicate a polarity shift, meaning that energy flips from Yin to Yang or Yang to Yin. You are not just engaging a new opponent or taking an opponent to an off-angle to break their structure, but learning how to control their Biofield when the polarity reverses. (Observation 40)

Seiuchin kata's split into a Y

In Okinawa's Seiuchin kata, there is a section where one turns right 45-degrees and executes several moves, then turns left 90-degrees and repeats the set again. These angle changes represent polarity shifts in Biofield functioning. Things are not what they seem with essential kata. Hidden lessons found in Biofield functioning explain these precise angles.

Directionality and Ki flow is a meaty subject. For the purpose of illustrating the importance and power behind an internal move, when I write about the Seisan dachi Crescent step I will be referring solely to north-facing movement. I will reinforce this technicality throughout the book. Facing other directions creates a different set of variables. This is likely one of the main reasons martial artists get baffled about Ki's existence. They may try a simple strength test and fail for lack of grasping all the variables at play.

SIDEDNESS

35* The lack of understanding how sidedness influences martial technique has led to widespread misassumptions, distortions and improper use of common martial technique.

This may be the most controversial statement in this book; Any martial system that executes its basic techniques or sequences of techniques equally on both sides of the body, or repeats identical sequences in two different directions, whether moving forward or backward, as in mirror images, is likely violating Kiko principles. From the perspective of advanced martial arts, mirror image actions are mediocre exhibitions. A simple example could be the use of the palm strike. Some schools hold the fingers straight, others insist on bending the fingers at the middle knuckle. There is a significant enough difference between these methods that they need to be better explored.

36* Your Biofield functions differently on the left and right sides of your body.

Most people have a dominant limb, a more coordinated arm or leg. Maybe your right arm feels stronger, denser, fuller, more organized, more present to you. This is why we hear some teachers insisting their students do mirror kata exercises to even out any imbalance. Logically, this makes sense. But from the Ki standpoint, the right and left sides are not equal, not in the way generally believed. The sidedness I am referring to is a bioenergetic sidedness, not whether you are conventionally right or left-handed. Bioenergetic sidedness refers to how Ki flows through the limbs and which direction and intensity it flows at any given moment.

We all possess bilateral Strength Channels (meridians) ascending and descending through the limbs and around the torso, but the amount of charge or volume carried through or to the limbs differs significantly.

I had assumed, given the nature of our limb/meridian connection that Ki flowed equally on our two halves. My premise turned out false. For I consistently observed that Ki flowed variably on the right and left sides. This discovery led to the observation of Energy Body sidedness. Fighting forms demonstrating mirror movement sets were not just implying that one be able to execute identical bunkai on right and left sides, but showing that mirror-sided performance needed to account for and adjust to this critical interior difference. This sidedness nuance is entirely absent in modern martial curriculums. From school to school across the U.S. I have witnessed mirrored martial sets performed identically. This confirms to me that most mainstream martial practices, from a deeper technical perspective, are done in a subpar manner.

Consider a North-facing body. The left side of the body is Yin. Yin channels on the inside of the left leg and the outside of the left arm carry a stronger Ki charge than the Yang channels on that side. The right side, Yang, exhibits the opposite characteristic—Energy (Ki) out, or discharge. This is likely how our Biofield regulates our overall energy needs. The Energy tide comes in and the Energy tide goes out, with few exceptions. Even observing how you prefer to stand next to certain people reveals your Energy preference in that moment. Someone walking alongside you on your right side will more likely pick up a Ki charge from you. Conversely, someone walking on your left side will more often give you a charge. This affect is not absolute, but it suggests an underlying order or pattern to Ki functioning influencing our choice of body posturing.

Think of the meridian system as a network of pipes. The diameter of the pipes, and the volume of Ki flowing through the pipes, varies from person to person, moment to moment. Similar to the way a blood vessel can change its diameter via vasoconstriction, our bioenergetic conduits appear to share a similar flexibility. The diameters of these pipelines can be altered by physical and/or mental means.

I arrived at the sidedness conclusion after evaluating the effectiveness of various kata sets from both a tactical and energetic framework. If I didn't know why a kata sequence stepped with a left versus a right foot forward, how was I going to figure out Ki flow in a complicated series of steps, breathing patterns, and limb postures? I decided to dig into a single action; a left foot forward step into the Seisan dachi.

The Seisan dachi is unique to Okinawan karate. It is taught as a half-circle stepping pattern called a Crescent or C-step. I began with several questions; Does stepping naturally with the right or left foot lead to an equal strength outcome? If not, what is the reason for the difference? What is the proper way to Crescent step? Finally, does using this stance yield a consistent result throughout a kata?

Given the shortest distance between two points is a straight line, a half-circle step is an inefficient way to move forward. If the masters took this truism into consideration, they must have had a sound reason for arcing their step.

In our Seisan kata we move the left foot forward on a left diagonal line from a natural stance to a shoulder width, one-foot length position ahead of the other foot. My first test was to see if taking a normal, linear, casual walking step with my left and right foot yielded equal strength results. To find the answer, I needed subjects to test my hypothesis. I recruited volunteers to assume a resistant posture. I would push them several times to establish their baseline resistance. Then I would take a normal step forward, first with my left leg, and test my strength, then with my right, test again, and note the results. Stepping with my left, I gained marginal strength, perhaps a 10-20% increase. Stepping with my right foot and pushing, I generally lost the equivalent strength. I repeated the test again with a Crescent step. Half-circle stepping with my left foot ramped up my pushing strength to well over 50%. A Crescent step with my right foot weakened me by the same degree.

The strength difference I gained between a normal, forward walking step and the Crescent step was roughly a three-time increase. Doing the same comparison on the other foot, I lost about three times as much strength crescent stepping with my right foot versus a straightforward step. I wondered what other factors might add to my strength increase.

After testing many subjects, it was clear that stepping with the left foot offered a superior strength gain. This was not about one's dominant limb. I tested many right and left-handers with the same results. This outcome provided a vital clue why a fighting form might initiate with a left foot. The next question was to determine the optimal way to Crescent step. Of all the actions I explored, Crescent stepping proved the best method and strongest affirmation for footwork in general.

The only possible explanation for this dramatic strength increase was that Ki or Biofield charge flowed differently on the left and right side of the body. Furthermore, if the meridians are the same in every person, these tests implied that in a resting state, Ki does not flow through the right and left legs equally.

This conclusion was explosive in its implications. I had never previously heard or read about this sidedness trait in martial technique. I concluded that Energy must be flowing up the inside of the left leg in greater volume (or charge) than up the inside of the right leg. Conversely, Ki must then be flowing down the outside of the right leg in greater volume or with greater charge than down the outside of the left leg. This could explain why certain kata moves initiate with a right or left limb. I could already see in this discovery a means of testing the efficacy of any martial art technique.

I eventually created a Kiko template to test the combative sequences from any system. I described the fluctuating Ki flow as either dilating or constricting the Strength Channels using Hard Gates initially, and later, testing with Soft Gates. (Observation 16).

I consulted an acupuncture chart and noticed coincidentally, that each leg has three Yin channels rising up the inside of the legs and three Yang channels descending along the outside of the leg. Without complicating Kiko functions, a Crescent step appears to utilize four separate muscular actions to move the leg through a full arc; the leg must lift slightly upward to reduce friction with the ground. The leg moves forward. The leg moves outward on the last half of the arc, and the foot itself can move in a small arc. This last action is seldom seen today. This partial foot rotation only becomes evident when the rear leg is slightly turned out before stepping forward. I postulated that all three strength channels were being activated with a Crescent step thus accounting for the increase in strength and the reason this action was included in kata. I still hold to this theory. After much experimentation, I narrowed the step down to its most optimal arc.

The awareness of energy sidedness completely changed my thinking about the technical terrain of the fighting arts. I am speaking broadly, not just about a single class of technique, style or system. If sidedness was showing a major difference in physical power between right and left limb actions, it is likely that the basic techniques of soundly constructed martial systems were to be performed differently left and right, rather than the current, one-size-fits-all mentality.

A left or right limb technique, regardless of system, carries a different energy value depending on the direction the torso faces and where the stepping foot lands relative to the opponent's stance. I have contained my observations in this discussion only to north-facing practice. Although each of us has bilateral channels flowing up and down our limbs, evidenced in any acupuncture chart, I have observed a consistently remarkable anomaly from decades of testing. The average person facing north, conducts more energy up the inside of their left leg then down the outside of that leg (at least in the Northern hemisphere). Conversely, the right leg conveys more energy down the outside of it then drawn up the inside of it. The arms function slightly different, but adhere to the same principle. The average person conducts more energy up the outside of their left arm and down the inside of their right arm. Conversely, the right arm conducts more energy down the inside of that arm than down the inside of the left arm.

This observation strikes at the heart of the confusion amongst martial artists how to best perform basic techniques. Energy sidedness suggests that the majority of the world's mainstream practitioners are not extracting the most power from their techniques if they adhere to doing both sides identically or when facing opposite compass directions.

I realized that I would be confronting a wave of resistance and surely, criticism, if I made this information public to the mainstream martial community. Yet, proof from hundreds of hours of testing shouted this fact. My research suggests that the world's instructors are doing their stances, blocks and strikes sub-optimally. Even if you observe someone performing a kata with these nuances intact, unless you were aware of their purpose, you would likely either overlook them or chalk them up to individual quirks, for you would have no idea why they were done in this manner. I believe this wisdom makes Okinawan karate-dō Kiko a unique contribution to the world of martial Qigong.

Energy-sidedness is one of the lost subtleties of martial kata and probably most other fighting arts. The father of modern karate, Gichin Funakoshi, stated that karate was too complicated for the average Japanese so he modified the Forms to make them broadly accessible. In so doing, I am pretty certain the issue of sidedness was abandoned or lost, if Funakoshi himself even knew this about his own art. I don't mean any disrespect to his enormous contribution to the spread of the arts throughout the world, but the current evidence stands. There is no question in my mind that commercialization has diluted many martial systems.

Mediocrity Reigns

Decades ago, I took a serious turn toward developing my writing career after I was told I ought to write children's books and find a collaborative illustrator. Through my extensive student network, I came across the accomplished children's book artist, Larry Ross, who shared a profound observation; "Mediocrity sells." In his opinion, the vast majority of children's books were written by C-grade writers, read by C-grade readers. I have since found his statement a truism within the martial arts. Few dojos are run by the likes of a Kano, Funakoshi, Uyeshiba, or a Gracie.

My research discoveries are for those who want to better understand their martial arts for their own personal growth and empowerment. I invite those who would like to learn more about the internal aspect of their arts to join our search and advance this dialog. I am however, fully content to just work with my own devoted core student body.

Using the insight of the Kiko principles behind a single step, my attention turned toward strikes, blocks and locks. The sidedness principle pervaded every movement, every technique, every fighting set or sequence. Sidedness shed a clarifying light on why our fundamental fighting forms were constructed with such detail.

I have proven that strikes performed with slight nuances from one side to the other leads to a substantial rise in power. Blocks became a particular fascination with me. Traditional blocks can be divided in Yin or Yang parries, each paired with a specific breathing pattern. Just as I had witnessed how stances, properly adopted, charged one for pushing, uprooting, pulling or pressing, the same holds true for parries. Blocking in a Cat stance (*Neko dachi*) causes a major energy draw, weakening a partner even with the lightest of contact, but usually only when stepping backward while inhaling. Its forward counterpart turned out to be the T-stance (*Shiko dachi*). Previously, gross stance distinctions, like wider, narrower, or lower, gave way to more precise postural definitions maximizing the stance's energetic value for better leverage with locks and more penetrating striking power. Everywhere I peered through the Kiko lens I found more answers, more potential. I have never experienced a scarcity of insights to this day.

If you are a *kyudansha*, below black belt grade, or hold an equivalent rank in a non-belt system, little technical ambiguity may have come your way. But when you have been in the arts over a decade you will surely come across fighting styles doing basic moves differently. This should make any intelligent person wonder if one way is better or equal. Kiko dispelled some of the confusion for how a technique ought to be performed, for we now had a means to put our technique into proper context.

Take a high block, for example. Some schools execute a high block rotating their arm outward so the ulna bone (pinky side) makes first contact. Other schools rotate the forearm so that the flat back of the arm makes first contact. Another school exposes the ulna, but additionally cocks the wrist toward the pinky side. From the Kiko perspective, all three methods work best if the block with the left arm is performed differently from the block with the right. Mainstream systems however, have standardized their blocking techniques, choosing methods easier to teach, easier to execute. However, this leads to suboptimal execution.

I had a conversation years ago with a high-dan, four-decade, East Coast, career Shitoryu sensei. I wanted to know if he had discovered such nuances in his Forms. The fellow stated he didn't want to look any deeper and wasn't going to change. End of conversation. He was not the only expert who assumed this attitude. It was as if these professionals held their hands over their ears, which I found odd.

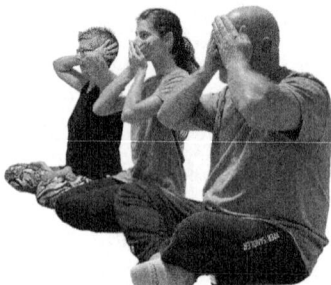

Does the natural curiosity that draws us into our arts wither with age? This has certainly not been my case. I have only become more curious. After I had established the sidedness formula, it was time to take a deep dive into Kata.

37* Physical movements on the left side of the body generally initiate an 'energy-in' action while movements on the right side generally initiate an 'energy-out' action depending upon the direction faced.

Maybe we have limb dominance all wrong.
Maybe it's right side for putting out Ki,
and left side for drawing Ki inward.

If we liken our physical form to a body of water with inlets and outlets representing Ki flow, then whenever you inhale and exhale, a large wave of Ki enters your left limbs, passes over the torso and out your right limbs.

Unlocking Ki's complex functioning has been hampered by its overly broad definitions. When Ki is understood as the underlying energy for every bodily function, it is easy to get lost in a maze of endless possibilities making it hard to tie Ki down to any one effect. On the other hand, if Ki is understood as an energy functioning on different levels of being, then we must separate out, and define each dimension.

Imagine the difficulty of assembling the puzzle of a Biofield in constant flux. It's no surprise people get exasperated with Ki's elusive nature and decry in frustration, there is no such thing as Ki. Kiko presents us with a streaming, four-dimensional puzzle. Nothing is fixed. Everything is moving as a result of endless forces tugging at us. My mission was to define the primary behavior of these forces.

Several advanced students suggested I nail down the most essential Biofield behaviors the majority of our test subjects could duplicate with the highest degree of success.

Don't take it personally, but everything is personal!
Tian Zhua

The longer I taught, the more I realized I was giving mini privates with each and every student in my group classes. Everyone was hearing something slightly different, and not always the message I was trying to convey. No matter how direct a demonstration or explanation of a technique or concept, it will only be received at the level of awareness of the listener/observer. I know this, because I would ask members of the class to explain back to me what I had demonstrated. Every teacher's hurdle is conveying information accurately.

All Choked Up

I was teaching a front choke escape one evening to an adult, coed class of mixed skills. I impressed upon the students the need to do the release exactly as shown. I demonstrated the technique slowly, multiple times. Shortly thereafter I noticed that about a third of the class had not listened, or misinterpreted what I had shown. So, I demonstrated again. Remarkably, there were still a few holdouts who did not, or could not, follow my directions.

I told the group that to escape this choke effortlessly, the proper details must be adhered to. To prove my point, I had the class do the escape with their partner with a slight change from the correct way. I let them decide between the two methods.

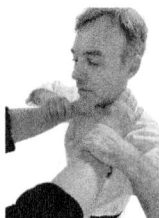

METHOD 1: Grip by enclosing your fingers around the wrists as shown, inhale and pull.

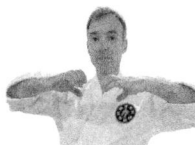

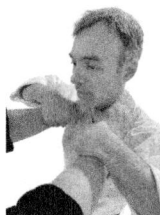

METHOD 2: Grip by placing all your fingers atop the wrists, inhale and pull.

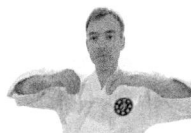

Imagine someone clasps your throat with both hands to choke and their arms fairly extended. In the first method of escape (the incorrect one) students placed their fingers in a circle around the choker's wrists and attempted to slowly pull their hands apart horizontally.

In the second method of escape (the correct one) the students placed their fingers, including their thumb, over the top of the choker's wrists and again attempted to pull the hands apart using the same lateral action.

Students were surprised at the results. Although the two methods appear nearly identical, the incorrect grip made it extremely difficult for them to escape the choke. The correct method made the technique feel unrealistically easy.

I did not wish to explain the Kiko rationale that night for I had a number of lower belts who needed to focus their attention on less subtle training dimensions. So, I asked everyone to just stick with the physical details.

After class, an intermediate student named Andre, approached me asking why this escape had worked so well. I knew if I answered his question, it would induce a slew of follow up questions. Kiko is a deep, involved subject. 'For a later time," I told him.

Unbeknownst to me, Andre asked my fourth dan, senior assistant, to explain. The value of loyalty had the assistant ask Andre if I had okayed a discussion on Kiko. Frustrated, Andre turned to yet another teaching assistant and asked him to explain the rationale. Not getting anywhere, he provokingly announced that if no one gave him the answer he would find it on Google. The senior assistant, overhearing his challenge, was prepared to bet Andre $200 that he would not get to the bottom of the mystery, but he bit his tongue.

Some people have the notion that if information exists, it is theirs for the plucking at their whim. And further, that Google is a kind of Akashic library containing every known worldly fact.

I do not purposefully withhold knowledge from students. I have learned that information meted out at a realistic pace most often yields the greatest benefit. Analogize the situation to a college freshman wanting to skip directly to fourth year, senior studies. Unless this student is a genius, skipping three educational levels will likely be detrimental to his education. There is a time and place for certain knowledge to be imparted and assimilated. Base first. Walls second. Ceiling last. Our entire Western educational complex is built upon this premise.

Andre's quest died down that week. Zoom ahead one year. During a private lesson, Andre confessed that he had gone to another dojo where he offered to pay the instructor "the price of one private session," if the sensei could answer why the choke release demonstrated had worked so well. Coincidentally, Andre visited a dojo run by a former student of mine whom I knew did not know the answer.

Miles to Go!

In similar fashion, a man named Miles would occasionally drop in to observe my classes. As a younger man, Miles had been a noted tournament competitor in Tae Kwon Do. One day I showed Miles the Kiko choke escape to whet his appetite for future training. Naturally, he asked why it worked so well. "I can't tell you," I teased him. Miles knew several seasoned teachers and told me he would ask them.

The first teacher he queried immediately wanted to fight me. Respectfully, Miles withheld my address. The second teacher bluntly answered, "Pressure points," to which I asked, "Which ones?" The teacher hadn't a clue. "It isn't pressure points," I told Miles. Miles then said he knew of a highly regarded older master. If anyone had the answer, he surely would.

Months later, Miles dropped by the dojo again. He had indeed spoken to the old master about the choke escape. "What did this master say?" I asked. "He hadn't a clue," Miles answered. That was a man I could respect. No ego, no pretense, just straightforward honesty.

When it comes to Ki work, personalization is a necessity. The more advanced the student, the more tailored the teaching must become. A one size lesson does not fit all. For each student is like a constantly shifting Rubik's Cube. Teacher and student must form a symbiotic relationship as they try to match all the colorful technical variables for optimal understanding and performance.

KATA

38* Soft Gate principles and techniques were not included in Western Hard style martial curriculums.

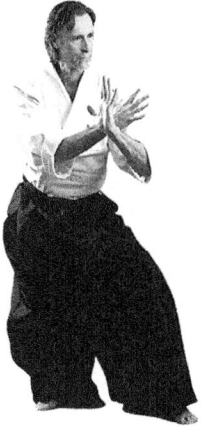

I suspect a rare few, first-generation, Hard-style, Western teachers received detailed instruction in the use of Soft Gate Energy principles in their arts. The subject still remains relatively closed to Western ears. Even many Soft stylists are unaware of the intricate workings of their own disciplines due to a long held Asian tradition of doing without questioning.

The effortless wrist escape I experienced with Frogman had raised a big question about how much our martial ancestors knew about Ki and how to employ it. If so, I felt the evidence should be found in their kata. But this question presented a major hurdle. If I didn't know a kata's intended bunkai, how could I possibly determine if Ki was involved in its creation? I would have to work backward and attempt to determine kata's function and efficacy by a careful analysis of its Form, then test my hypothesis.

I first had to understand what role if any, Ki played in individual martial movements. For example, is a simple block/punch action a Ki-filled action, a ki-less action, or a hybrid? Does everyone's Ki move in the same manner when they block/punch? If so, what determines an internal technique from an external one? If not, what is the difference? Can we look at someone perform a kata and determine if they are moving Ki correctly?

I would build my hypothesis one move at a time, then reconstruct the entire movement sequence to see if any effortless power formula emerged from this testing, all the while not knowing if this was at all intended by the kata founders.

One thing we professionals understand about our kata is when we change the emphasis of a move or movement sequence, we change its potential bunkai. This is one reason why katas vary from system to system, even within single fighting arts. Different perceptions lead to different conclusions. I don't believe there should be one bunkai (application) for any particular kata sequence. But I am convinced, no matter what bunkai you settle upon, it must be in accordance with two principal systems to express authentic power—correct biomechanics and correct bioenergetics.

I never had to look beyond the opening moves of Okinawa's Seisan kata to conclude the Asian masters were aware of Ki's importance in the construction of their Forms. All essential kata, in my opinion, share a common element:

> On the most fundamental energetic level, kata done
> correctly builds up tremendous muscular charge.

My research revealed that proper kata sequences charge and discharge Ki in continuous energy-in/energy-out cycles. I am not talking about repeatedly cocking an arm or leg back to strike. There is another action happening beneath the obvious. As Ki is expelled in a punch, it is redrawn back into the body by means of a precise, Hard Gating formula. Cases where a performer stops or slows down in a kata sequence, for example, are often done to draw in further energy or to allow Ki to backwash to the appropriate musculature.

This rise and fall Ki cycle opened up a new level of kata bunkai, many times matching the external action. Of course, I have already pointed out that the majority of Western students either did not get the correct internal sequence, misinterpreted how a set was to be done, or altered the sequence to fit their own physical needs or comprehension. (This later phenomenon has occurred with far more frequency than is commonly recognized, admitted to, or discussed). In the everyday world, mediocrity fights against mediocrity, believing this to be the highwater mark of skill. Kiko far exceeds this standard of technique.

When you perform a kata that has been passed incorrectly, or interpreted incorrectly, along with a teacher's added eccentricities, you have the recipe for subpar, distorted application, even if the application trumps your opponent. So, let's start with a simple line of reasoning about Ki's relationship to any martial art.

Why Move Martially?
If you do not move effectively, you will likely experience pain

and loss, failure or death. We move to avoid pain and injury and to enhance pleasure or victory. The movement away from one is the movement toward the other. It's a rare individual who doesn't feel any pain getting struck or cranked. In an interview, decades ago, with the man who introduced Kung fu into Manhattan, Grandmaster Wai Hong stated, 'When you damage another's structure, it doesn't matter if they feel pain or not. They will be incapacitated.'

What's The *Best* Way?

Martial arts were built around three foundational questions; How do we do it? Why this way? And, What if? All technical and tactical issues will fall within this line of inquiry. We can start with the influences of the immediate external environment. Is there a wall at your back? Are you standing on icy ground? Are you on an incline? Your internal environment will also affect your decisions. What if you are wheel chair bound, blind, one-armed, in a cast, ill, nine years old, a senior citizen, an overly fearful/anxious, paranoid, hyper-excitable or distracted person? You are going to respond differently under all these conditions. The Fighting Arts were never construed to be a one size fits all preparatory intervention. Kata addresses all the probable existing variables. The ancient masters took careful inventory of their possibilities and potentials and tailored them to their strengths.

Why Move One Way Over Another?

Biomechanically correct movements will make you stronger. Bioenergetic alignment will make you stronger yet.

Meaning

Meaning is the personal value we attach to our experiences. Our teachers share their meanings to guide our experiences, but ultimately, we must live the martial experience to fully grasp its meaning for ourselves. There is a great variety of purpose in what different people strive for in their martial arts. The sheer volume of world martial styles and systems, guesstimated at over 6,000, suggests this alone. This isn't a new problem. It was much the same in Asia a hundred years ago.

Some MMA fighters consider traditional Form practice less meaningful because it lacks the test of real combat. Conversely, some traditional Form practitioners find the MMA fight indulgence overly focused on fighting. To each his own. What's important is that you find meaning in your endeavors and allow others to find it in theirs. Meaning is not an inert value. Meaning expands as you mature, shrinks as you immature, and is influenced by the culture you live in. The philosopher Ian Hacking points out that there is a circular relationship that exists between our bodily processes and our sociocultural meanings. Body interacts with cultural meaning systems, which create behavioral patterns, which create body experiences and so on, round and round. And do not assume because you are aging you are maturing. The world is populated with many adult babies. Look at the unsportsmanlike behavior of Conor McGregor in 2018, a world class MMA fighter. He descended into a childlike, abusive tantrum when he did not get his way. His was a disgraceful display of good sportsmanship. What actions nourish you? What actions make your life relevant and full? What is it about your art that nourishes you?

When it comes to understanding a martial art, its kata, and bunkai (applied value), we have a mostly top-down hierarchy of perception and attitudes. The sensei's attitude is passed to the student like hand me down clothes. It shapes the student's mindset with a specific focus of attention. A sensei's rules are either in or out of sync with the students, other schools, other styles. Martial arts are ripe with turf wars. Walk into any dojo and mention that you checked out the instructor down the road. You'll often get an earful.

There is an enormous diversity of opinions about the meaning of many aspects of martial technique and methods of training, even within the same systems. Some proponents of these differences can get downright testy, professing theirs to be the ultimate way. Go on the Internet and read the comments from any martial Youtube demonstration. You will usually find someone denigrating the performance and/or the performer no matter how superb their display. It's unavoidable. But it should not be your concern. Everyone is entitled to their opinion. Don't waste your energy worrying about what someone else is doing if you know what you are doing?

Your treasure lies at the end of your own shovel.

Meaning is tied to logic and intuition. Thoughts spring from your ego. Some believe intuition emerges 'before ego'. Meaning forms your beliefs expressed as feelings and actions. You feel good when you are getting something out of your training. You feel less good when you are training improperly.

A radical shift in martial perspective occurred when the monastics of Asia intermingled their practical study with their spiritual pursuits. Knowledge of underlying energy currents were woven into their external training patterns. For the majority, the Kiko arts were so subtle they only reached highly intuitive and sensitive disciples.

When I use the word '*Energy*,' I don't mean energetic, in the sense you had a good night's sleep and feel rested and awake with abundant pep. I mean that you possess an immaterial nature that can be controlled to enhance your physical strength beyond basic body mechanics. In this context, Energy is synonymous with Ki.

People generally do not think of their lives in terms of patterns but rather as a series of individual patchwork actions; wake, clothe, wash, drink coffee, go to work, text your friends, etc. Kata prods you to think in patterns. This is what makes kata important. Instead of looking at your responses to the world as an endless string of random events; I punch, I kick. I eat. I work. I scratch my head. I play. It asks you to look at the pattern of your eating, working, training, head-scratching and playing. Looking at your life patterns compared to thinking in terms of single events reveals fixations and habituations exposing imbalances and disorganizations that can be more readily addressed.

Let's Get Practical

When I introduce new shodans to internal practices most of them are clueless about what Kiko study entails. A few expect a quasi-mystical teaching, cryptic koans or perhaps, a display of wizardly power. On the other hand, there are those who prefer their art remain one-dimensional, not too complicated. They might quip, "Just teach me how to fight! I don't want that *kata* stuff."

Most everyone is surprised when the information presented turns out to be straightforward, not hard to understand at all, though it requires effort to learn. What baffles most of my clients, and they are a very smart group, is how they didn't see the subject coming. Even after years of training, few had anticipated their art's internal venue.

Why Kata?

Do not look for one rationale in any kata. The better katas present multi-agenda, multi-level lessons. Look instead for progressive lessons and compounding rationales as your awareness expands. Essential kata are rarely ever black or white. On the high-end, things are not what they appear.

> Without **tools** the **tactics** are limbless
> Without tactics the **strategy** is hollow
> Without strategy the **state of mind** is aimless
> Without a clear mind the **energy flow** of the body
> remains unbalanced.
>
> Five layers of kata study

Kata's presentation in the United States has been all over the chart. Instruction ranges from, 'you can't change a single move,' to 'edit where necessary,' to 'no bunkai provided,' to 'figure-it-out-for-yourself', to systems with well thought out, multi-tiered applications. Failure to gain a consistent foothold in kata's full import is a part of its mess.

As kata is integral to the martial puzzle, a fighting art is integral to one's life puzzle. To fully grasp kata, you must interface it with a partner to unlock its true value. If you retreat to the mountains and practice nothing but kata, you will not return an accomplished fighter. You may achieve other significant goals, but fighting efficiency will not be one of them. Partnered bunkai is the glue that reinforces kata's solo practice as a combative discipline. Enlisting a willing partner to realistically role play your opposer allows you to engage in a critical energy and information transfer. This is the essence of the concept of *kumite*, literally, an exchange of hands, broadly implying an even exchange with others.

Solo kata reinforces bunkai by working on your own kinetic orientation. All this must become ingrained through consistent and focused repetition. Similarly, to truly understand life, you must live it fully and fearlessly engaged.

Mainstream American kata schools have been handicapped by a lack of knowledge about their kata's inner structure. This value was seldom conveyed and rarely articulated in any meaningful entirety. You can only take away from the fighting arts what you can make sense of. In the West, we left out everything we could not see of these arts. Some believe the art's internal face was purposefully omitted by Asian masters who decided to keep this information for their own selective community. This has contributed to modern practices becoming one dimensional, all about the fight, the kill. Such mentality develops technique without spiritual or compassionate grounding and leads to an exhibition lacking a balance of peace, wisdom, and inner serenity.

Think Big/Dive Deep

Take the common lay description for a martial art; the Art of Self-Defense. Martial curriculums obviously possess physical techniques of defense and offense. Where is that same clarity regarding the mechanics of the self? My early concept of 'self' felt flimsy, ambiguous, amorphous. I get the world isn't just filled with good guys, rainbows and lollipops. Where I got tripped up was attempting to answer 'who am I?' or "what makes me a self?" If I could answer either of these questions, I might know more precisely how to better defend this 'self.'

In Buddhism we have an understanding that the self is an aggregate of constantly shifting attributes. The idea of nothing being permanent, everything in flux, made my search more elusive. For how do you define something that isn't fixed, whose 'true form is no form' as the Buddha's Heart Sutra suggests? I felt like I was trying to catch a river with a fishing net. Maybe the Taoists have it right. Chill!

The martial arts provide us with three pillars of study to answer these questions and to literally re-shape our Form:

1. **Solo practice**: The integration of kata's biomechanical proficiencies with our own kinetic pattern.
2. **Cooperative partnered, hands-on bunkai:** the refinement and grounding of kata's combative lessons into a practical reality. Partnered kata is the only practice that allows one to test a fighting form's bioeneregic efficiency through trial-and-error rehearsal.
3. **Free style kumite:** testing kata's application efficacy with a partner who agrees to act as opponent using full force attack speed with clearly defined parameters of engagement.

A fourth level could be added with the *caveat*, you might get hurt—an actual fight, sanctioned or otherwise.

Solo Versus Partnered Kata: Exercise Vs. Exploration

Several interlocking characteristics define the current trends in the traditional fighting arts which could benefit from better articulation; the value of complexity vs. efficiency (how much detail is enough?), the value of kata vs. kumite (what's the best fit?) and the value of exercise vs. exploration. Going into the intricate details of a technique versus just pumping it out, performing a solo kata versus engaging in partnered applications, or exercising versus exploring movement, may initially seem like night and day practices with different aims but they all share the same end goal—effectiveness.

Katas are preset sequences of movement, breath and concentration. Some kata were developed from the earlier Indian *Nata*. *Nata* is an ancient Indian Buddhist term describing the earliest form of an art of ritual movement practiced for spiritual cultivation. The Nata was used by *Vajramukti* practitioners in India. Vajramukti was an Indian movement meditation, healing, and martial art based upon static and dynamic principles perfected by the Ksatriya warrior caste of ancient India. Practitioners of early esoteric *Chuan Fa* (Jap. *Kempo*) were called *Vajranata*.

Whether you practice kata alone or apply its techniques in a partnered exchange, rote rehearse techniques on a gross or fine level of detail, or explore dimensions of your rehearsal, each method develops a particular type of insight. In Japanese, types of insight are termed *Ken*. Kata develops *jiken*, insight into your own being. Solo training turns the eye inward to your own intrinsic energy currents and coordination. Kumite develops *taken*; insight into another's being. Partnered practice, inclusive of bunkai, and its free form expression in kumite, turns the eye outward to the exchange of energy with another to attune you to your partner's Energy field. Each has its own special provenance, particularities, and relevance that works in different ways to pierce fictions of your ego, induce inner harmony and develop confidence born of real self-understanding. Both are as indispensable as your right and left hands, and are the best forms of confidence worth attaining. Achieving a high degree of *jiken* and *taken* results in a state termed *naiken*. Before either of these two insights can be developed, or the practices to do so are seriously engaged, it is necessary to begin from a state of physical and mental health. Exploration leads to the understanding of what comprises proper practice. Exercise is the repetition of these practices for their benefits.

Martial bunkai is as varied as you are creative, as relevant and grounded as you are realistic, and as connected to the fight as you accurately perceive the nature of a fight. There is no right or wrong interpretation, no ultimate single way to do a kata that trumps all others. No arbiter will call out your ideas unless you are contested in the martial arena or on the street. You will only be as inspired as the information matches your goals, and as insightful as your consciousness is clear, expansive, and flexible.

A student's understanding of kata rarely goes beyond the sensei's (or you are not long for the dojo). If a martial organization were like a room, your sensei would represent its ceiling of information. Students form the floor. The teachings make up its walls. This is how the house of martial learning is constructed. Look around. There are lots of housing projects out there; tiny homes, substandard rentals, multi-million-dollar mansions, dilapidated wrecks.

Don't get upset about differences in your version of a Fighting Form from another school's quirks of performance. Your study is not a competition between methods. It's an inquiry into the nature of movement, focusing on the essence of conflict and how deep the Asian perspective, relevancy, and meaning went into their research to penetrate this subject. It only matters that you choose a starting point and move from there. Each kata offers a special lens to peer through. I put one genomic strand of kata under the microscope of inquiry to discover that each strand contains the essence of all bodily movement.

Some katas were imbued with a therapeutic value along with their practical aims. Others were crafted to cultivate one's Ki. As one Zen monk stated: 'The whole moon and the entire sky are reflected in a single dew drop on a blade of grass'. I could add, in a single kata or single action of the body.

Our body can be used as a mobile laboratory to exhume wisdom through calculated experience. When the body is trained, cleansed, purified, awakened, opened, we can peer with greater clarity into our inner world and see it as a perfect reflection of our outer world. For everything going on inside us has a corollary to what is taking place outside of us. If you want a clue to how well your life is going, look at how in sync your inner and outer worlds are. That will fix your position on the Joy scale. Why a Joy scale? Joy is the feeling that you are exactly where you should be at any given moment.

Use your emotional grid to get to the heart of yourself.

39* Solo kata performance may require a slightly altered movement pattern than its application against a partner.

Should a solo kata performance identically match its bunkai? If not, why not? Evidence from my research supports the idea these two modes of expression may need to be different at times. The reason lies in the fact that when doing solo kata you are dealing solely with your own Biofield energies. When performing with or against a partner, you are engaged with another's energy field altering your flow and thus may require adjustment. This question should be placed on the debate floor to help professionals get a better understanding of the nature and purpose of their own kata. Let's look at various ways kata and its bunkai are currently understood:

1. Kata is a performance-centric conditioning act with little to no concrete bunkai. It is merely a facilitator of solo skill and character development, which can be liberally or loosely applied to an opponent.
2. Kata is a starting point of possible engagement scenarios. Like a dictionary, the performer selects and arranges the most meaningful sentences/ideas. Thus, kata becomes a general blueprint of reaction/response combinations.
3. Kata is a precise, methodical, and meticulous record of cause-and-effect outcomes that requires little to no modification in either its solo or partnered expression.

Solo kata performance maintains a separate identity from partnered bunkai even though their mutual aim is to advance combative skills. Think of these two activities like a bridge being built simultaneously from opposite shores toward connection. One end of the bridge builds and strengthens internal insights and talents. The other reinforces external insights and talents. An example from the Wansu kata below illustrates the kata/bunkai dilemma:

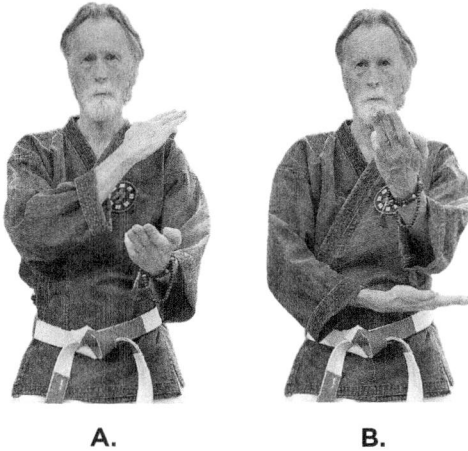

A.   **B.**

Wansu kata:

There is a sequence in the Wansu kata of isshinryu where a performer crescent steps forward with a right foot, executes a right open hand mid-block, followed by a simultaneous cross hand action and a palm's up spear hand. (image A.) There are many applications for this action. Taken entirely at its solo value, regardless of its bunkai, if the move is executed in image A, the performer should test stronger than other modifications. However, if we take a simple bunkai of deflecting, grabbing, and circling the attacker's limb to control their elbow, we would need the spear to pass *above* the crossing arm (image B), not below it as expressed in the solo version. You might suggest the kata then be done in the latter fashion. By pairing the solo version to the bunkai you solve the problem. However, when we tested subjects with these adjusted arm motions in their solo performance, it reduced overall body strength. Logic suggests we reverse our thinking and spear *below* the crossing arm in the bunkai. Unfortunately, this action against an actual partner weakens the application. The lesson seems to be that solo kata may have been designed to emphasize a practitioner's internal controls while the bunkai was designed to emphasize external controls, thus the reason for the minor alteration in solo versus applied technique.

The above example is not an absolute. There are cases where a solo kata set fits partnered bunkai to a tee. I suggest some divergence however, may have been necessary to preserve the continuity of Ki flow.

239

Understanding kata's biomechanical (external) principles is not enough to properly engineer improvisational bunkai. If you engage in bunkai without activating bioenergetic principles there is a likelihood, in the face of a powerful and willful opponent, your bunkai might fail. There is also the possibility that you may have completely misperceived the nature of the technique entirely. An example below illustrates.

Oops!

In master Shimabuku's video capture of his Wansu kata there is a sequence where he demonstrates a 90 degree turn followed by what looks like a mid-body shuto/knee strike/punch. This set is repeated in the opposite direction. Critics have decried Shimabuku's video performance as 'old man' kata. Perhaps, they cite that he doesn't lift his knee full height in the above-mentioned sequence. But I believe these knee lifts are not strikes. The emphasis is on the opposite action, placing the leg back on the ground. A lower lifting knee causes a backwash of Ki to precisely charge the lower torso to magnify the torsion necessary to complete a powerful takedown over the back leg.

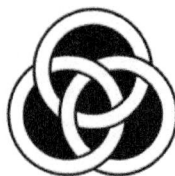

Sando: The Three Ways of Kata Practice

In our monastic training we consider three ways to perform any fight sequence. They are called the *Hayaku, Kime* and *Shinkokyu* methods. These three practices constitute the main foundation of monastic Form training.

Hayaku Kata

This method stresses quick movement combinations or sets. A set is to be understood as the initiation and resolution of an attack. Its purpose is to achieve unity and smoothness of action along with heightened body control and balance. Practice in this method can lead to *Bushin*, or *Warrior Mind*, typified by a feeling of confidence in your abilities.

Kime Kata

The Kime (power/focus/decisiveness) method of kata stresses slow, restrained and calculated tensions against your own body. This is the original dynamic tension principle taught by Bohidharma at the Shaolin. Sanchin is an excellent example of this type of practice. Kime kata leads to *Fudoshin*. The character *shin*, can mean heart, mind, spirit, vitality, or inner strength. It carries the connotations of imperturbability, unshakable calmness, and courage without recklessness. We can interpret Fudoshin to mean *'immovable heart'*. Only this method can lead to an intuitive certainty about your life and actions, and a belief and solidarity in your way of thought.

Shinkokyu Kata

Shinkokyu (mind/breath/step) practice is the method of deep breathing in kata, a principle greatly ignored today. Practice is done in a relaxed, soft manner. Concentration is placed solely on the flow and depth of the breath. In this form of practice, the breath leads the movement. This method leads to *Mushin, empty-mind*, a complete non-awareness of thought and the realization of the oneness of being.

In addition to the above methods, physical movements may be performed along a straight, circular, or curving path.

Straight moves are initially the quickest. Most striking arts use linear actions. Practicing straight moves alone however, does not fully utilize the body's muscles.

Circular moves form the basis of many Indian and Chinese martial arts. They are initially slower, using much bigger movements. Because larger and far more muscles are used, these actions are stronger. Practicing circular blocks builds up *chikara* (power).

Curved moves are intermediary actions falling between the straight and circular methods. Their principles apply equally to the circular and straight extremes. The master uses curves as a natural result of infusing power into straight moves and to activate Ki currents. More simply put, technique is considered:

Straight for Speed *(Choku)*
Circular for Strength (*Mawashi*)
Curved for Coordination *(Kake)*

Everything done on the physical plane will also have its mental correlates:

Strength *(Sen No Sen)*, the mental fortitude to defend and strike back

Alertness *(Sen)*, the ability to anticipate the battle

Initiative *(Go No Sen)*, the ability to defend and strike simultaneously

Many precious refinements in Asian kata were lost in translation as they moved across time, cultures, and generations, from the country of their origin to cultures with different social interests, values, needs and strength preferences. Not only were martial systems poorly interpreted by early Westerner adoptees, their Kata, like any other commodity or service, fell prey to commercialization. This resulted in many kata becoming overly standardized, weighed down by dogmatic views, or wrapped in extraneous mysticism, marketing hype over functionality.

A common characteristic found in many kata are movement sets repeated two or three times. As previously discussed, many 'repeats' were never meant to be identical. For example, in Kiko training, a left mid-body block is repeated with an important nuance from a right mid-body block. Few students are trained to move at this finer level of skill or perception. No one is likely to even spot or consider the difference in their arms block-ability because they wouldn't know what they were looking at. At best, they might view it as a fluke—until you test its efficacy.

40* As evident in their postural arrangements, all essential Kata store a record of Hard Gate, Energy Body principles.

A Biofield Resource in The I Form, Seisan and Neihanchi katas

I did not invent martial kata. I entered its arena like the many generations of disciples before me and dutifully rehearsed its patterns for five and a half decades. Each year I persisted raised more questions about kata's structural arrangement and integrity. I now believe, no matter the Form or its originating culture, all fighting forms possess a Kiko subflooring.

Young martial artists today are unaware how little Western cultures were initially exposed to Asian kata interpretation. Nor is there a universal agreement how a particular Form should be approached or explored. Some students, given only their form's exoskeleton, are left to figure out its applicable value. Others are provided with exacting formulas with zero wiggle room. Few U.S. schools in the 60's practiced move-by-move kata bunkai. If they did, their bunkai was often presented in a simplified parry/punch format. It was rare for inner details to make their way into the applications. Katas were regularly drilled with the attention on their surface detail.

First and second-generation sensei naturally taught the way they had been taught. Few were encouraged to look beyond their teacher's pointed finger. It never dawned upon me for an instant whether my fighting forms had been passed along properly. There was no way as a novice or intermediate student I could have made such a determination. I took it on blind faith they had. Asian kata, plain and simple, were foreign, unfamiliar practices to Westerners.

How many move-specific athletic disciplines consisting of a string of twenty to forty moves does the average Western boy or girl learn during their entire school life? Outside of dance, gymnastics and skating routines, where one can learn choreographed sequences easily exceeding the average number of kata movements, there are few Western sports requiring the learning of so many precise techniques in a row.

Obviously, fighting forms have fighting applications that require a handle on the basic skills; speed, control, endurance, flexibility, balance, timing etc., to match a real time exchange. Below, I will lay the groundwork for some not so obvious aspects of martial Formwork.

'I Form' As Eye Opener

Around 1970, under W.S. Russell's instruction, I was introduced to a series of four I or H patterned exercises blandly called, *I Forms*. There are many martial systems that utilize a basic I or H-shaped floor *embusen* (lines of movement). The most familiar and perhaps, the most practiced of these patterns are the *Taikyokus* (First Cause) found in the Japanese arts.

In the early 1970's there was no Internet, no mobile phones, no DVD/CDs and few books published on the martial arts. One relied on their sensei as the main source for any and all substantive information. I mistakenly thought Sensei Russell had made up these I Form drills as preparatory routines for the more formal kata to follow. Years later, I found out that Tatsuo Shimabuku, Isshinryu's founder, taught a basic I or H pattern as part of his training curriculum, which Russell must have adopted. Shimabuku's I Form was most likely a modification of the Taikyoku from his early Shorinryu training days.

Russell's presented these I Forms as a basic training. The first pattern combined the Seisan dachi with stepping, blocking and punching techniques. Breathing was completely ignored. His stated purpose was to teach us how to manage simple fight controls through the Form's eight sets of block/strike actions. The exercise appears straightforward. You walk all sides of a serified 'I' floor design. You begin with low blocks, middle blocks moving up the centerline, high blocks at the top, then finish the pattern retracing your moves in the opposite direction, finishing with low blocks back where you started.

The I Form

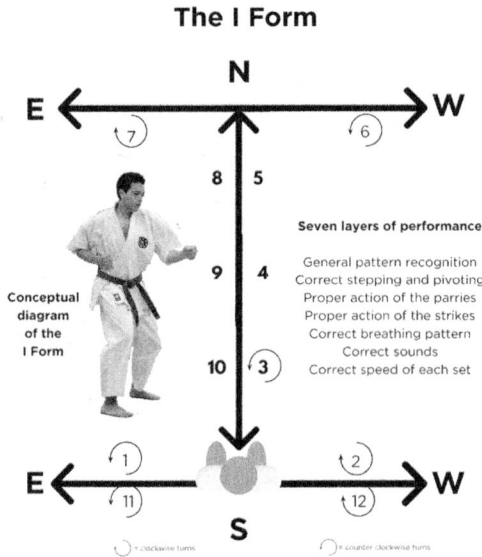

Seven layers of performance

General pattern recognition
Correct stepping and pivoting
Proper action of the parries
Proper action of the strikes
Correct breathing pattern
Correct sounds
Correct speed of each set

Conceptual diagram of the I Form

Bow

Turn left 90 degrees/low block, punch
Turn right 180 degrees, low block, punch
Turn left 90 degrees, middle block, punch, step punch, step punch
Turn left 270 degrees, high block, punch
Turn right 180, high block punch
Turn left 90, middle block, punch, step punch, step punch
Turn left 270, Low block, punch
Turn right 180, Low block, punch

I admit, I find reading technical breakdowns bland. But bear with me. You should find the outcome illuminating. For three decades I never questioned Russell's rationale. Then one day, the sequence piqued my curiosity. In almost every I or H Form, the opening moves begin by turning 90 degrees to the left. Given that the creator(s) had a 360 degree freedom to move, I wondered what rationale validated their initial left turn. I could not find anyone to explain this clearly. Three other oddities in the Form jumped out. There were four low-blocking actions, two left-handed middle blocks, and an awkward 270 degree turn followed by a high block. The pattern wasn't as balanced as it appeared.

Months of deductive reasoning led to two astonishing revelations. This drill was far more than a 'basic' pre-kata drill. Gichin Funakoshi himself commented that the Taikyoku's were patterns which advanced students would return to over and again. I began to see his reasoning.

Revelation #1

A novice in a ballistic art will initially learn their martial alphabet of basic strikes and parries from stationary postures. The next logical progression is to put these building blocks into simple, moving step/block/punch sequences. Think of it like the elementary words and sentences constructed in a grammar school manual; See Jane block. See Jane punch. See Jane block and punch.

I was no longer satisfied with the See Jane block/punch explanation. My investigation led to an unexpected conclusion; the first two movement sets were wrong! From a combative perspective, I was convinced the opening 90-degree turns were incorrect. I could not say who erred; my teacher, Russell; Isshinryu's founder, Shimabuku; or the supposed creator of the Taikyokus, Ankoh Itosu, Funakoshi's teacher. The initial two turns should be performed at 45-degree angles, tracing the shape of an arrowhead on the ground. I realized my assessment was going against the grain of historically sound, hundred-year-old, martial art systems that incorporated these patterns. I imagined how that would go over in the professional martial art community when I made my allegation public? Lead balloon came to mind.

Then something extraordinary occurred. Call it a serendipity. A student had gifted me the book, *Shotokan Secrets* by Bruce Clayton (Black Belt, 2004). I was floored when I read that Funakoshi had changed Ankoh Itosu's (Funakoshi's teacher) original moves of the Taikyoku to 90-degree angles. In Clayton's words they were originally in the shape of "arrowheads". My 45-degree angle theory was correct! I was so excited reading Clayton's confirmation of my theory I eagerly called the author to see if he had more information on the subject. You may ask, what's the big deal about the angle of the turns in this basic form? Precise angles in form work are fundamental for understanding personal combat and Ki flow. For me this was a clear example of a brilliant simplicity built into this Form.

Revelation #2: Tactical Lessons

Once I adjusted the angles, the I Form revealed one of the strongest arguments for why kata was crafted by the masters. In just the first three sets, this rudimentary pattern, with its modified angle change, suddenly made sense as a virtuoso lesson in **tactics**:

Set 1: Step out on a 45-degree angle with your left foot, cross block, punch. Return to center

Set 2: Step out on a 45-degree angle with your right foot, cross block punch. Return to center

Set 3: Step forward with your left foot, middle block, punch, step punch, step punch.

(Traditional styles with similar I or H patterns will often take a full step forward after turning. The Isshinryu is a modified variant of those patterns where only one step is taken).

I assume those premodern fight masters understood that any assault would likely consist of random technique. That is, most defenders will not know what an assailant will do until he does it. Although an assailant could do anything, we experts understand it is highly probable they will do some expected things.

In a random attack, what is the likelihood an assailant will kick versus punch as their initial move? The answer—punch. The average person is not an experienced or confident kicker.

What is the likelihood they will punch or initiate with a right hand versus a left hand? The answer—right hand. 70-90% of the world's population is right hand dominant. The remaining 10-30 % is either left-handed or ambidextrous.

What is the likelihood this right-hand punch will be aimed at your torso or face? The answer—very likely that it will be aimed at your torso or face. The torso is the largest body target, easiest to hit.

What is the likelihood they will step forward with a right or left foot when throwing their right punch? The answer—right foot. Striking off the back foot is often a trained response.

So far, we have deduced in a random assault there is a strong likelihood you will be initially attacked by a right punch, push, or grab, thrown off the lead right foot at your face or torso.

What is the best defense against such an attack? Run? Stand your ground? Duck? Charge forward? Dodge left, dodge right, dodge left forward diagonal, right forward diagonal, left rear diagonal, right rear diagonal, dive for their legs? Stand still? The lay public would be guessing. To gain the best tactical advantage, the traditional martial answer is to move the left foot forward diagonally. The reason: Most people are right-handed, which goes for the defender as well. In the martial arts, the left arm is used primarily for defense, the right for offense. The left hand is sacrificed to create an opening for a strong right hand counter strike. Additionally, when you throw a strike with your right hand it's up to 30% more powerful if launched off the rear leg while generating forward momentum. Also, by positioning yourself on your attacker's right side, he or she is in the worst position to continue to effectively attack with any limb. And it gets better.

The Internal masters must have been aware that a forward arcing left foot motion drew the greatest amount of charge into them and away from their opponent. The left leg action becomes like an energy vampire 'if' one steps to the outside of the other's lead right foot while inhaling. This action literally sucks the Ki streaming down the outside of the opponent's leg.

If I just lost you at the vampiric, ki-sucking step, or you think you're clever and have trapped me by telling me the opening move is a low block/punch and I already established the punch will probably go to my torso or face. How is a low block going to stop a high strike?

A traditional low block is prepped by drawing it across the chest, prior to its downward sweep. This preliminary drawing across action is the actual block, which makes it a middle-blocking action, concluding in a downward strike, not a downward block.

What about a face-high punch? Unless you are fighting a giant, your opponent's strike will likely rise up toward your face. A middle-blocking action will deflect it as it rises.

I believe the creators of this pattern didn't think of their three-step routine exclusively in terms of individual technique but more broadly in terms of its tactics. If this I Form had been created foremost as a tactical resource then its initial three turns could be broken down into a hierarchy of three primary maneuvers in order of importance:

Tactic 1: Go Left

In every circumstance where you are physically assaulted, your primary tactic is to advance on a left forward outside diagonal, 45-degrees to your opponent, regardless if the assailant attempts to kick, grab or strike with either their right or left limbs or both simultaneously. This opening set covers all these eventualities. Students were to drill this first tactic until it could be executed without thought. This tactic will give anyone an instant advantage and reduce potential injury to you.

Tactic 2: Go Right

Failing to step to the left diagonal, the next preferred tactic is to step to the opposite side of the opponent, 45-degrees to your right diagonal.

Tactic 3: Go Straight

Only if you are unable to go left or right you are to go straight ahead using a neutralizing tactic. This move, in my opinion, is one of the best neutralizing sequences in the martial arts. Those that understand it place themselves at a great self-protective advantage.

It is possible the 90-degree turns in this basic routine were designed as a teaching aid to remember primary versus secondary tactics? 1. Left. 2. Right. 3. Straight ahead.

This routine, with its simple hierarchy of tactics, is not just a See Jane block/punch routine, but a life-saving, See Jane kick Jack's predatorial butt and live to tell her friends.

It is a given amongst fight professionals that the fewer decisions you have to make under duress, and the fewer techniques you know, the easier it is to learn and apply them. You do not want you to be burdened having to calculate that an opponent throwing a right hand is remedied by your left block, but if they throw a left hand you have to use your right block, and so on. This thinking over complicates. It's unlikely your mind will be clear enough under the stress of a serious assault to remember such detail. You must focus instead on time-tested tactics. Use the left middle block regardless of what is thrown at you and cut to the left on a forward diagonal. Failing this tactic, go to the opposite side of the opponent. If unable to cut left or right, go straight ahead. All the world's militaries embrace the fundamental strategy of a few good techniques done well.

Then why not have one simple, universal kata? Why not just do this three-set drill—one and done? You could. But the martial arts open up the inquiry to all the other what ifs an assailant or competitor can hurl at you; What if the fight continues? What if you're grabbed from behind? What if he shoots for your legs? What about that badass energy sucking move? The possibilities are endless.

Revelation #3

Though my initial 45-degree angle deduction was correct from a combative, tactical perspective, it turned out that the former 90-degree turn, and subsequently, all the turns in the form, concealed Kiko principles. I don't think we will ever know if the I Form pattern I had been taught had been stripped of this prized quality when it arrived on Western shores, but the I/H embusen appears to be the template of a quintessential Kiko pattern whose roots may extend 11,000 years into the past to the *Star Walkers*.

Recognizing that bountiful crops appeared during certain celestial arrangements, some ancient star gazers recreated the celestial star patterns on the ground then walked their diagrams in the hopes of conjuring that same bounty. These Star Walkers offer us a possible link to the earliest development of kata. Star Walking is still practiced today in specific Taoist alchemist lineages. Either way, I made it my personal mission to restore or insert the Kiko principles we discovered into the I Form pattern I had been taught. This has resulted in a sophisticated, seven-layered, Ki-cultivating practice.

Fighting Out of Narrow Contexts

Within the structure of the fighting forms I examined, I found, with some tweaking, uncanny power formulas that could not possibly be coincidental. Whether past masters consciously, instinctively, or intuitively understood correct Ki flow, I have concluded the reason they meticulously preserved and passed their kata on to successive generations was not just to save their kata's obvious biomechanical lessons, but to convey their bioenergetic, Ki-based wisdom. For this reason, Kiko must be considered a vital component in all essential Fighting Forms of Asia. Kiko's multiple formula platform is the reason the better systems possess kata with its nuance intact. Why does one system block with the flat side of the forearm while another uses the bone edge? Why does Shotokan prefer punching with a near fully extended downward fist, while Isshinryu keeps the palm sideways and the arm ¾ extended? Why does Wing Chun strike with the bottom two knuckles while traditional karate systems focus on the top two? Kiko fills in the picture beyond the conclusion of different tactics. Correct Energy flow must align to match the technical focus.

Each classic or traditional stance moves Ki in sync with its intended configuration and application. When a Neko dachi (Cat stance) is called for in a kata, replacing it with a different stance will alter the Ki flow required to effortlessly apply the move. But, here's a problem, except for the top tier masters, mediocracy rules. If mediocrity gets the job done, why look further?

Ask a master, 'What if I change my stance?' The knowledgeable ones will reply, 'You change the outcome'. This is why martial Forms are taught with such exactness. The originators strove for maximum results.

When the noted, Okinawan Shorinryu master, Shoshin Nagamine exclaimed, 'If you are not doing Kata, you are not doing karate,' he was likely referring to the Kiko principles embedded in karate's essential Forms, though he never outright names them. Of course, India and China have also given us tremendous fighting knowledge in their respective arts but again, we see little explanation of their internal mysteries. Was it many tight lips or an intuitive-based Kiko that explains its lack of articulation?

The problem Western cultures faced opening the Asian warrior's technical gift box was the absence of a cipher or Ki-code to interpret these arts to their full depth. Were Asian fighting forms to be taken at face value or were there layers of technique within technique? How much latitude should or could one take in interpreting a Form without losing its intended value? Once the West got its hands on these exotic combat choreographies, it proceeded to under-interpret them. We reduced their techniques to simplistic blocks, kicks, and punches; topical remedies oblivious to any additional wisdom contained within them.

We may never know why certain fighting forms were created in the exact sequences presented but we can glean many answers from investigating these sets under the Kiko lens by reverse engineering them for an accurate sense of their bunkai.

Seisan Kata: A Tale of Two Sets

While analyzing the opening sequence of Isshinryu's Seisan kata, as I explained in the Sidedness section, I realized there were too many external actions going on to determine what influenced what. We have a left foot moving forward with a simultaneous right hand, reinforcing parry moving across the chest, followed by a left middle block, concluding with a rising, right vertical fist strike with a slight pop upward at the end.

For the majority, these moves boil down to a bread and butter, block/strike counter. At my stage of training, this surface level bunkai felt off the mark. I did not believe that a hundred years of martial knowledge encoded in the likes of Seisan kata had culminated with the masters wanting us to block and punch.

To discover if and how Kiko worked in this Form, I narrowed my inquiry to Seisan's opening step before tackling strings of moves. I would isolate the Ki effects of individual Hard Gates in single limb actions to see how each functioned.

This process proved highly productive. It yielded far deeper tactics beyond its commonly taught interpretations. Proper stepping and breathing boosted both blocking and striking. I noted further that the left forward step was only powerful if it ended up on the outside of an opponent's lead right foot. Seisan's opening step was not just closing distance, ending up chest-to chest with an adversary. The maneuver was avoiding an unwanted body collision while setting up a shoulder lock by maneuvering to the opponent's right side. This observation opened a critical new front for understanding kata bunkai. Energy Body transactions between adversaries offer a rare set of crucial controls. Cutting to the left forward diagonal changed the kata's defensive tactic from block/punch, to a block/grab shoulder lock submission. It didn't matter if the opponent attacked with a right, left or both hands. This action was worthy as a master Form, and a powerful testament to the dynamism of our Fighting Forms. I believe all the essential kata of Asia possess this underlying Kiko functionality.

To reiterate, when it comes to the distribution of Ki to the musculature, we have two systems in play; The Hard Gating system only requires the correct physical action or bodily arrangement. You don't need to know anything about Ki, Energy Body, or Biofield. You just keep your body relaxed, your mind rooted in your body and focused on the task at hand. The Soft Gating system, by contrast, requires conscious volition aided by your attention on the correct Ki flow for the chosen outcome. These two systems, when applied individually, are really a matter of emphasis. Ultimately, we want both systems in accord.

Break Down

I am going to break down the Kiko principles in the opening two movement sets from the Isshinryu/Isshin kempo Seisan kata to show you how Kiko underlies a well-constructed internal Form. If you are a kata devotee these principles should appear in your own techniques and Forms. You can skip the detailed description below if you are unfamiliar with Seisan kata and pick up the overview several paragraphs later.

In my book, *Internal Karate: Mind Matters and Seven Gates of Power*, I point out seven distinct stratifications of martial technique, regardless of style. Ask the professional what is behind their basic punch and you will get a more detailed response than any novice could provide. Superficial knowledge, like rolling the fingers into a fist and propelling your arm forward is the obvious strata. When you dig into the earth however, you don't just find dirt. Less obvious layers and substances exist. Additional rationales will emerge if you keep asking, "Why?" like an inquisitive child never satisfied with the answer. The first six steps of Seisan kata reveal fascinating lessons in Ki manipulation.

Seisan kata is one of the most widely practiced fighting forms on Okinawa. It is used in multiple karate systems. Its many variations alone would perplex even advanced level students. For you would soon discover that you can't get three people on the mat to perform the kata identically, no less break it down the same. The better Seisans adhere to Kiko principles. The lesser ones do not. Because there are different purposes, understandings, and martial formulas for success, it is only natural we find variants in the world's fighting forms. Barring the anatomical nuances of students, it matters less if someone else's style does their kata with a different move or emphasis, but rather your teacher's objective in transmitting the Form to you. If you train in a technically sound school, this fact should not concern you. A deep dive into these distinctions is best saved for post-shodan study or a minimum five to ten years of experience.

The Technical Skinny on Seisan

SET 1

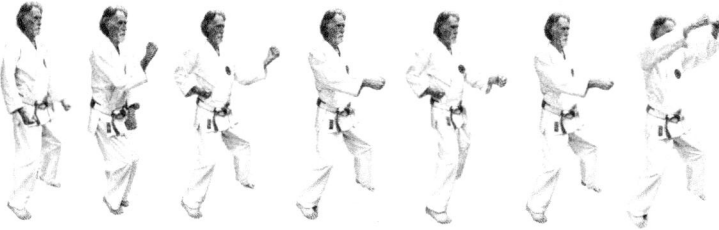

Assume the *Yoi* (Ready position) by sliding your right foot to the right. directly under the shoulders ending with the feet parallel. Because Ki flows naturally from left to right, this opening action draws Ki into the torso to be used by the limbs.

Next, arc your left foot forward and execute a left, reinforced forearm middle block followed by a right vertical punch. Step again and do a left vertical punch. Step for a final, third time, and do a right vertical punch. Slip step forward and execute a double hand rising high block. Twist to the left 180 degrees, moving thru a Reverse Cat into a right leg back, Seisan dachi. Cross your two open hands at the wrists in front of your chest, left in front of the right. Swing the arms downwards to the sides with simultaneous knifehand chops (shutos).

SET 2

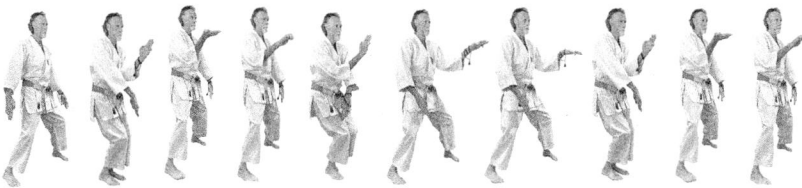

Now facing the opposite direction, crescent step with your right foot and execute a reinforced mid-body, open hand, palms up, hook block. Flip the hand over, bend the middle knuckles and slowly pull your hand back toward you, exhaling. Pull the arm back to where the elbow rests a fist width between your elbow and waist. Crescent step forward and do a similar, but not exact sequence with your left hand. This time extend your deflecting left arm away from you, straight-wristed and open-handed as you exhale. Then flip your hand over and quickly retract it on an in-breath while bending your wrist outward toward the pinky side (crane or snake hand). Conclude by repeating the identical sequence as your initial right foot step.

If the above description has some Isshinryu folks yelling, "Hold on!" This is because mainstream Isshinryu executes all three sets the same.

I interpret Set 1 as having no punches, even though most karateka would swear the action consist of three, mid-body straight punches. They certainly look like vertical strikes. And they could be interpreted as such to keep things tidy, but this isn't the complete story. From the Kiko standpoint, it is technically incorrect to perform the set identically. Seisan's bunkai reveals why.

Kata is a record of what worked on the killing field, and later, within the monastic circles, what worked on life's broader battle-fields. The monastics concurred that living in a world of whirling matter, it is impossible to avoid threatening collisions from time to time. Conflict and its resultant suffering therefore, is simply the natural consequence of being part of this universal flux. The word, conflict here is not meant to have a negative connotation, but rather, implies its Latin origin as a 'coming together.'

The five pillars of traditional Okinawan martial arts; *kihon, kata, kumite* (inclusive of bunkai), *kokyu* (breathing patterns), and *kime* (focusing on Ki direction) present us with an intriguing puzzle. How do we seamlessly weave these five aspects together in a practical and effective manner? Each pillar gives clues to the other's value. But if you don't know what the finished product looks like, it will be nearly impossible to solve this puzzle. Let's take a closer look at the puzzle pieces and peel the veneer off these two kata sequences:

In **Set 1** we have three Crescent steps forward; left, right, left, coupled with three closed hand punches. In **Set 2,** moving in the opposite direction, we have three Crescent steps forward again, only now it is right, left, right, coupled with three open hand moves.

Do you think it coincidental that the hands are closed into fists in one direction and open in the opposite direction? What rationale might exist for structuring the sequences in this manner?

To learn to fight properly, you want the most tried and tested patterns with their explanations up front so you can practice correctly from the get go. Most Westerners did not find such explanation included in their kata box.

The easiest interpretation for the first sequence would be to simply block, then punch, punch, punch your adversary. Do you think the best answer the world's fighting masters had to offer us was to block, punch, punch, punch? How often have you seen anyone execute three punches with two Crescent steps in any competition or street fight? It's not a realistic recourse.

In my book, *The Soul Polishers Apprentice*, I wrote a chapter entitled '*What Quadrant Are You In?*' It is a fictitious story of a novice who meets a series of progressively more talented fight masters each insisting they understand the essence of kata. Each expert gives convincing, logical reasons why the sequence is done in such and such a manner. Each succeeding master trumps the former revealing deeper insights.

As your awareness of kata broadens, your actions will follow suit. Your kata performance and bunkai should evolve with more meaningful, more realistic applications and tactics. In Kiko-emphasized kata, every physical and mental action is dissected to its quintessential Ki flow to optimize its power.

Assertion 1

As discussed earlier, my research uncovered compass directionality as a major factor in kata work. Therefore, we begin Seisan kata facing compass north to attune meridian channels to the Earth's geomagnetic fields. Facing north, in this kata variant, requires we step forward with a left foot into a Seisan dachi. Only the north or west-facing, left foot forward Crescent step enhances the body's capacity to draw the maximum charge. Stepping with a right in this direction will cause a discharge of Ki.

Energy fields in the immediate training environment, coupled with the earth's geomagnetic field influence will cause a kata to morph or reshape itself to adapt to shifts in the Biofield. This is why you will always see variations of the same Forms throughout the world. Kata changes are not just due to anatomical quirks or personal preferences. Kata should morph to accommodate the influence of surrounding Energy fields.

Stepping with the left crescent opens the Yin meridians on the inside of the leg, causing an electro-chemical charge along a precise neuro-muscular pathway. To accentuate this charge, you must inhale into the lower abdomen when stepping and blocking.

Next, the parrying action of the mid-body block must draw the opponent's arm toward you as you contact it. This is referred to as a drawing block, meaning in our case, absorbing Ki, not just the obvious visual retraction of the arm. When done correctly, the opponent should experience an overall drop in physical strength. This decrease in strength will simultaneously add more damaging force to your strikes and locks.

Seisan kata teaches how to engage in a covert, electro-magnetic duel with an opponent's Energy Body in advance of the limbs making contact, or at the instant of contact. Kiko teaches you how to subvert energy by drawing a charge off the adversary while simultaneously charging yourself.

This initial, north-facing, three step sequence offers a solution for dealing with a right, left, or double-handed upper body attack.

The second sequence, moving compass south, presents the energy formula for dealing with a right, left, or double-hand attack when engaging with a right foot forward and parrying to the outside of the attacking arm.

Stances not only establish physical equilibrium and tactical positioning for strikes, blocks, locks, supportive moves or set ups, but function as Energy depleting, charging and grounding maneuvers.

There is nothing random about Seisan's opening tactic. If you had a simple method to neutralize just these three primary limb attacks; right hand, left hand, both hands, when being struck or grabbed, you will have considerably narrowed the attacking field, because the majority of strike threats often pass through a narrow target area from the brow to the groin as indicated below. Seisan kata's first two fight sequences address this concern head on.

Strike Zone

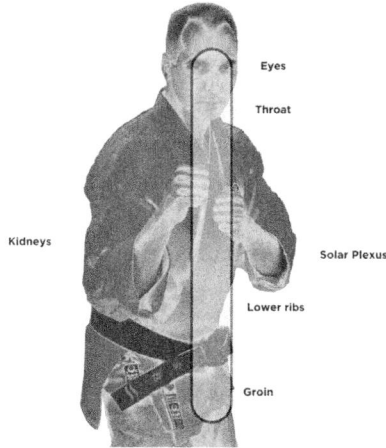

The I Form's three-step sequence and the Japanese Taikyokus may have been considered so significant to some of kata's founding fathers that this pattern was either appropriated from their Taikyokus/*Pinans* (also *Ping Ans*) and added to Seisan Kata or appropriated from Seisan kata and added to the Taikyokus/Pinans. In either case, the three step forward motion is a signature trait in many traditional Forms. It should be noted that in Asia the number three and its multiples are considered auspicious numbers, while in the West 'two' completes a binary or balanced set.

In our system, all of Seisan's punch-like motions are set ups for standing locks. I am not advising against strikes in this kata's bunkai. I am suggesting the opponent, at this level of control, is judiciously subdued when appropriate to do so, in alignment with the Buddhist precept to avoid taking a life.

For those who study Okinawan Isshinryu, every opening sequence of every Isshinryu kata is designed to instantly deprive the opponent of any electro-magnetic advantage. I do not believe this function was unconsciously included in the creation of these kata. How many other fighting forms were crafted with this in-built refinement?

No matter what kata you practice, you still need basic skills in speed, timing, endurance, coordination and strength. You still need to be vigilant. You still need the necessary biomechanical control and conditioning. Kiko adds an additional technical tier; a sophisticated, electro-magnetic counter-action to compliment the proper biomechanics.

Crescent stepping with the left leg (a stance and direction-specific statement) increases body charge. Crescent stepping with the right leg discharges or decreases muscle charge.

The Crescent step was placed into Seisan kata as the best means of optimizing your strength. The arcing of the foot activates all three leg meridians simultaneously giving your technique maximum charge. Stepping straight, minus the arc, only sends the charge up one meridian, generating roughly one third of your potential strength. Mainstream teaching has been lax in defining and expressing the ideal Crescent step in systems favoring this dachi.

Ki channels open and close, or metaphorically, dilate and constrict, with every physical motion. Just as your circulatory system pumps blood, and your limbic system shunts lymphatic fluid by means of physical motion, your limb actions generate electromagnetic and/or photonic currents. Your body does this to maintain your system's Biofield balance. These two sequences demonstrate how this charge/discharge system functions. Lessons are learned primarily by doing, by feel, and complimented by a sensei's verbal explanation of the correct rationale. Kata is first and foremost a kinesthetic experience.

Therapeutic Posturing

If we had the instrumentation to evaluate a person exclusively by means of their physical actions and correlated these actions to various illnesses, I believe we would see a relationship of types of illnesses to physical movement patterns. This is why yogic and martial disciplines will often have a positive therapeutic effect upon a practitioner's health. Anyone properly performing martial arts or yoga may see a reduction of some health concerns and certainly an increase in strength.

Pumping Ki

The first three-step set in Seisan kata activates an energy on, off, on, Yang expression. The second, south-facing three step pattern, beginning with a right foot forward, reverses the effect to an off, on, off, Yin expression. A different muscle chain is activated. Here, the hands must be open and soft (relaxed) to optimize Ki flow. Directional changes in kata were indicators of a polarity change, or a reversed Biofield current.

North-Facing Energy Draw
using an inside block

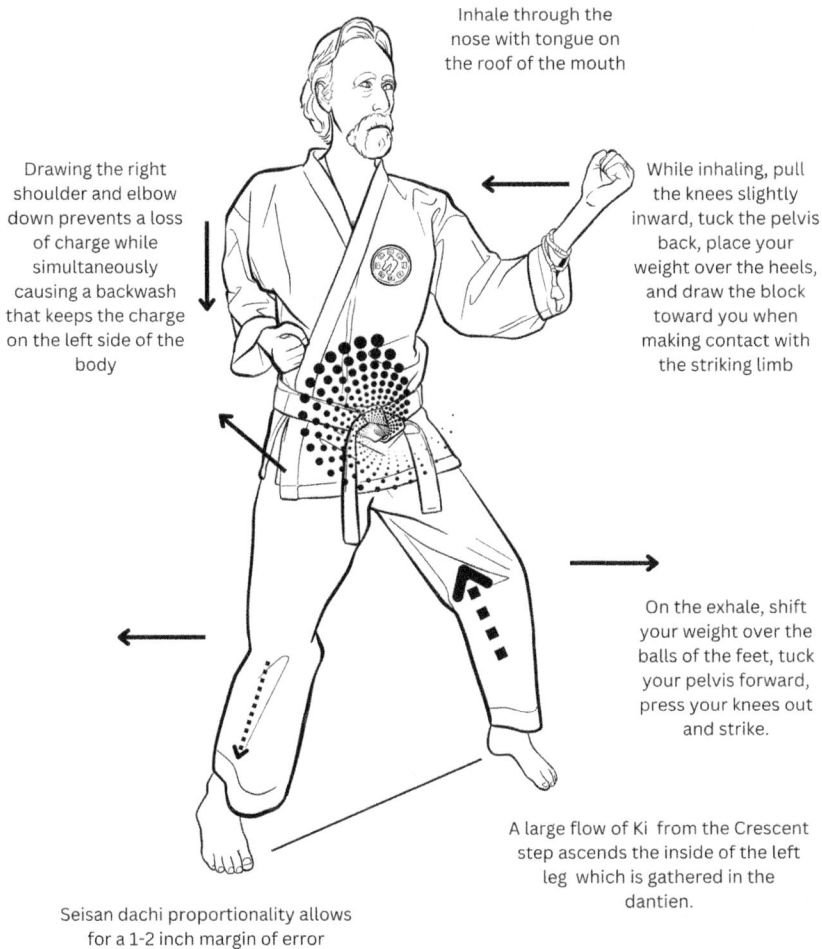

Inhale through the nose with tongue on the roof of the mouth

Drawing the right shoulder and elbow down prevents a loss of charge while simultaneously causing a backwash that keeps the charge on the left side of the body

While inhaling, pull the knees slightly inward, tuck the pelvis back, place your weight over the heels, and draw the block toward you when making contact with the striking limb

On the exhale, shift your weight over the balls of the feet, tuck your pelvis forward, press your knees out and strike.

A large flow of Ki from the Crescent step ascends the inside of the left leg which is gathered in the dantien.

Seisan dachi proportionality allows for a 1-2 inch margin of error

Ki flows up the inside of the left leg with greater charge then up the inside of the right leg optimizing the left side as a more suitable energy inlet. This is one reason many kata begin stepping with the left foot, or turning to the left, which yields a similar effect.

South-Facing Energy Draw
using an outside block

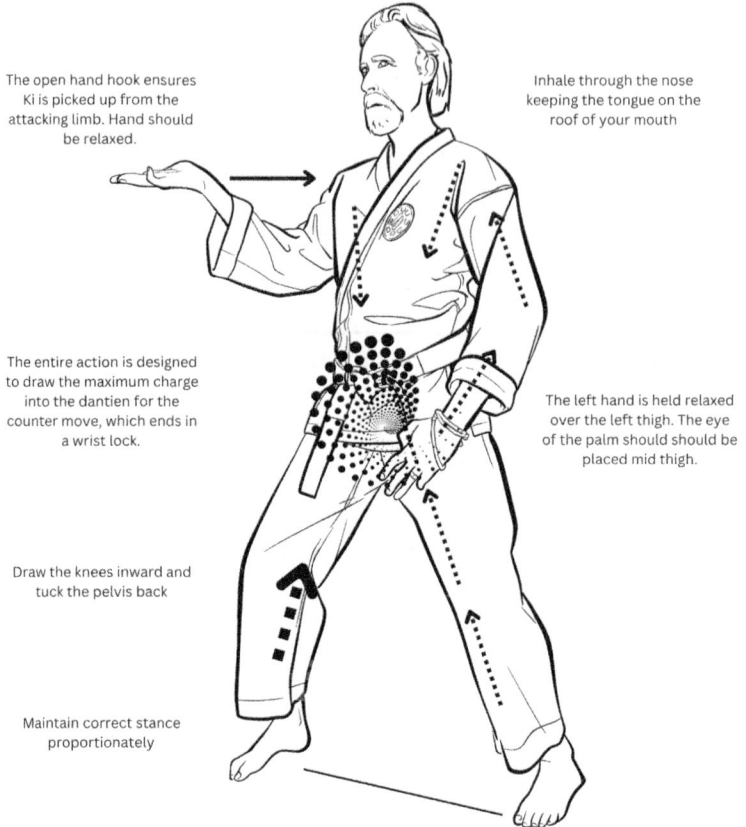

The open hand hook ensures
Ki is picked up from the
attacking limb. Hand should
be relaxed.

Inhale through the nose
keeping the tongue on the
roof of your mouth

The entire action is designed
to draw the maximum charge
into the dantien for the
counter move, which ends in
a wrist lock.

The left hand is held relaxed
over the left thigh. The eye
of the palm should should be
placed mid thigh.

Draw the knees inward and
tuck the pelvis back

Maintain correct stance
proportionately

Ki flows down the outside of the right leg with greater charge
then down the outside of the left leg. The right leg is more suitable as an energy outlet. This also holds true in normal, everyday
activity. These actions can be altered or reversed.

Energy rising up the inside of the legs will gather charge in the
lower dantien, assuming two conditions are met; the abdomen is
relaxed and the attention is held at the base of it. The strongest
charge amasses in the densest part of the torso, the center of
physical gravity. However, it's not enough to just gather this fire
in your belly. The charge must be directed into the limbs. You can
mentally lead Ki to the appropriate muscles using visualization
(Soft Gate) or pump Ki solely by limb actions complimented with

the correct breathing method. You can switch methods or combine them. But any conflict between these systems will lead to a degree of self-canceling.

If you were to perform Set 1 with open hands and Set 2 with closed hands, you will have created an unwanted discharge of Ki in your system, weakening your technique. This explains why the hands must be closed in Set 1 and open in Set 2.

These subtle energy effects on strength are only obvious when correctly tested with engaged subjects. External, well-conditioned technique can get the job done. Kiko's value is that it excels against significantly stronger opponents. The mainstream martial community does not incorporate Kiko refinements because they do not see any limitations with their Hard style applications that cannot be remedied with more conditioning. Kiko masters might say that's all well and good, but there is another level to technique that can magnify the outcome—*instantly*.

What happens to your Ki once it's drawn into the dantien with closed versus open hands?

When the left foot steps forward, energy rises into the dantien where it is plugged at the left wrist due to the sealing of Ki from the closed fist. Ki does not flow through contracted muscle tissue. The fist stems the Ki from leaving the torso. If, instead, you hold your left hand open and soft (absent of tension), the energy rising up the left leg is expelled as an energy wave out the left arm. On the right side, the opposite event occurs. When you step forward with the right foot, energy is sent down or discharged from the torso through the right leg into the ground like a lightning bolt absorbed by the earth. If your right hand were closed, no energy will be drawn into the right arm to replenish the lost charge through the leg. But if you hold a soft, open right hand, you will draw energy from the other's right arm into the torso and down the right leg. When the channel(s) from right hand to right leg remains open, a continuous recharging occurs.

Set 2 shows how this charging/discharging cycle is used with open hands in a reversed polarity.

The tactical lessons of many fighting forms are multi-tiered. Students begin with basic fight controls then progress to more advanced manipulations. Set 1 teaches you how to organize Ki using an inside mid-block. Your left arm contacts the opponent's right punch on the inside of their attacking arm. Set 2 teaches you how to organize your Ki to deal with a parry to the *outside* of their arm, that is, your right arm blocks to the outside of the opponent's right arm— because the polarity has changed.

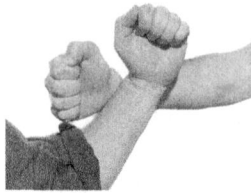

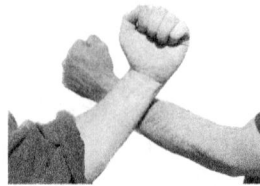

Inside block   **Outside block**

Essential Kata always offer dual-level lessons. The obvious, overt application might be a block/hit, or block/lock. Kiko reveals the covert application to be used against the entangled Biofields. This lesson involves managing the electro-chemical charge/discharge transfer that your adversary is likely unaware of. It is the main reason for the many variations in the wrist and finger formations of traditional blocks. Keep in mind, when facing North: the left side receives. The right side, sends.

The Hook Block
Let's look at the hooking hand action in Set 2. In the section on blocks, I explained why a hooking block is chosen. Let me go into more detail.

Application of the first step sequence in Set 2
I refer to this bunkai as the hook/block/pull sequence. As a right punch comes toward you, weave your right foot toward the opponent's right side (the weave slips the strike) and block to the outside by hooking your right hand over the striking arm or wrist. Next, turn your hand palm's down, grab their arm and yank. This action initially raised several questions; Why hook with palms up then flip the hand over? Why not just have the hand already turned palms down to grab? Secondly, what happens after the pull? A pull does little to neutralize an opponent. What if he's a heavy dude?

I do not believe hooking someone's arm to pull them concludes this movement set (a common application). You hook with palms up to draw a charge off the inside portion of the attacker's arm. It is reasonable and probable to assume that a striker will punch with a fist held somewhere from vertical to palms down. Regardless, draw your hooked hand toward you to siphon Ki. Once you've gripped the opponent's arm, apply a wrist lock using the arm actions of the second step.

This opposite side action will differ because Ki does not flow equally on the two sides of the body.

In many traditional kata it is not unusual to find overlapping bunkai sets. In our case, step 1 and 2 resolve one attack. Step 2 and 3 resolve the same attack against the opposite arm.

Ki Flow in The Arms

Every aggressive right arm motion toward you is likely preceded by a strong Ki flow extending past the aggressor's arm. A weaker charge flows down the left arm, which runs a stronger current in the opposite direction, that is, toward the shoulder. This is crucial information. When you engage someone's left arm you must overwhelm their system by sending a fast charge up that arm. By contrast, you underwhelm a right arm attack by drawing the charge off them. This is why Kiko blocks are done as draws against right arm attacks and sends against left arm attacks.

In the second set of the second sequence, you shoot out your left blocking arm with a straight wrist, palm's up, to deflect the left strike by sliding up and along their arm while exhaling, then turn your palm downward, tilting the wrist toward the pinky side draw the arm back while inhaling. Both of these actions are done quickly.

Set One: North Facing

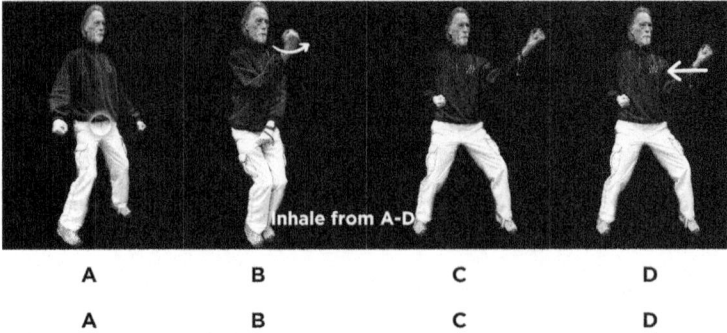

Inhale from A-D

| A | B | C | D |

| A | B | C | D |

Set Two, Sequence One: South Facing

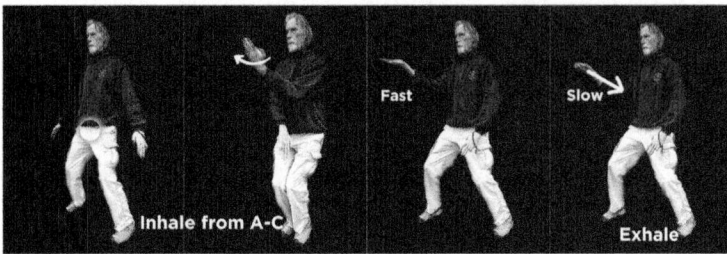

Fast Slow

Inhale from A-C

Exhale

Set Two, Sequence Two: South Facing

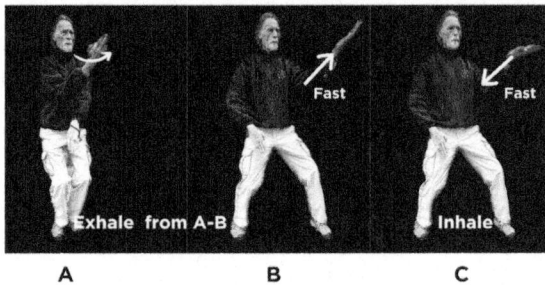

Fast Fast

Exhale from A-B Inhale

| A | B | C |

Seisan kata Step 1 shows the correct pattern to maximize a Ki draw and Step 2, a Ki send, assuming the proper breath is coupled with each action.

In my early research, we paired forward thrusting motions with exhales. Breathing out felt intuitively correct when extending a limb outward. When retracting a limb, we inhaled. Seisan kata upgraded my thinking. This Form was demonstrating how to withdraw a hand while still sending Ki. It is possible to take in another's Ki when breathing out and to send Ki when breathing in.

Advanced Forms rarely, if ever, teach one to just block and move on. We don't want an opponent to remain a threat. All decent kata bunkai should terminate an attack.

To resolve the first right hand attack in Set 2, we deflect and hook over the striking arm to draw the charge. We continue to draw the charge as we flip the palm down and grab the opponent's wrist. This is followed by a second step. Using our free hand, we reach under their right arm and draw it toward us by slicing with the cutting edge of the radial bone across their triceps. This action displaces their triceps and shuts off Ki flow for resisting a bend to their arm. Once their arm bends, we apply a wrist lock.

Deflect   Hook   Push/Pull   Lock

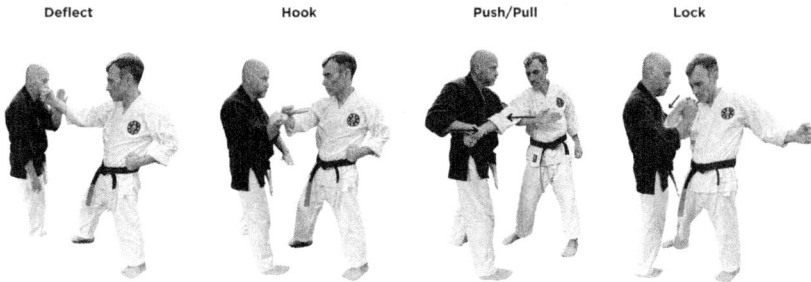

In the second overlapping sequence of this Set, we defend to the outside against a left punch by sending a fast charge up their left arm even while grabbing their wrist. We also finish with a wristlock. However, the sidedness equation compels us to reach over the top of their bicep with our free arm and cut across it with the edge of the ulna (pinky side) bone, and finish with a Figure Four wrist lock. Drawing or sending of Ki is done by the correct limb and breath action.

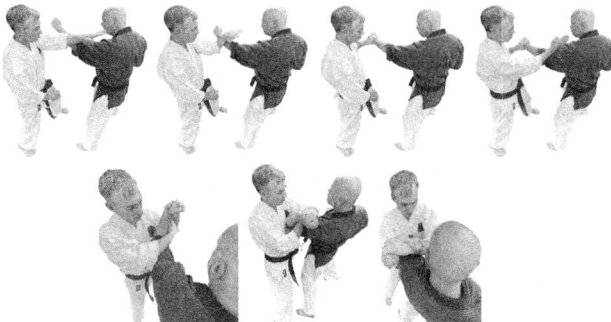

If you were to reach over where you should reach under, or reach under where you should reach over, the opponent's arm strength jumps dramatically, assuming you didn't surprise or overwhelm your adversary with superior gross strength.

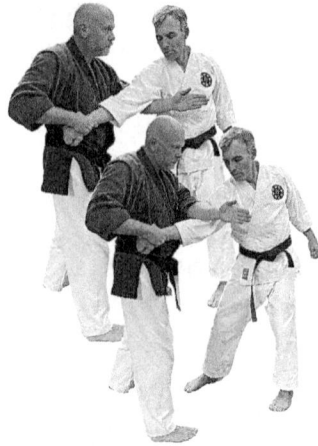

A test: One subject grabbed another's right wrist with their right hand as illustrated. They were asked to compare two methods of applying a wrist lock. They reached under their partner's arm with their left, then drew it toward themselves as if drawing a violin bow, and attempted to fold their arm. This was followed by reaching over the top with their left arm bending their opponent's arm. Many found the latter action much harder.

ナイハンチ

NAI-NEI-NO-HAN-FUAN-FAN-CHI-CHIN

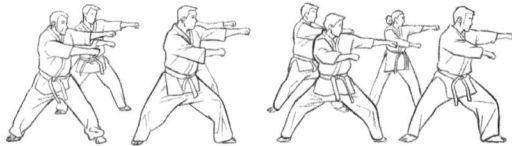

INNER-INSIDE-INTERNAL-WITHIN-ARCH-BEND-CURVE-COMPLEXITY-CONFLICT-BATTLE-SET-PERFORMANCE

Neihanchi Kata's Combat/Ki Relationship

While writing this section, I happened to be reading a book by a Western academic skilled in Okinawan karate. The author convincingly asserted that the Japanese altered Okinawa's early karate forms. In doing so, they rendered the kata less lethal and exposed practitioners to certain vulnerabilities in a live combat situation. The author substantiated his position with commentary from noted Okinawan masters and drew examples from movement physics to prove his point. In every regard, at this author's level of understanding, which was clearly elevated, he is right. My observations of Neihanchi however, diverge greatly. I work within an entirely different system of the Form's expression and purpose.

I'd like to use the synchronicity of this author's example of what he calls *dentou* (genuine) Okinawan karate and the Japanese modifications to Neihanchi kata to present another viewpoint. I agree the author is spot on in noting the Okinawan sequence is combat-centric while the Japanese variation is not only focused on character development but primarily ballistic-centric. At first glance, the latter appears a dilution of combat value when contrasted to its Okinawan predecessor. But we must dive deep to catch the full import of either variation.

Neihanchi kata typically begins with a short, lateral cross step (one foot crosses tightly over the other) into either a:

Neihanchi stance, Okinawan version as illustrated in the stance section. My Neihanchi stance aligns with the narrower Okinawan variant.

Kiba dachi (traditional Horse stance)

Tekki (Iron Horse stance), Japanese version.

I frame out my divergent thinking with several questions; What is the compelling reason for anyone to practice Neihanchi kata? Is there an essential lesson conveyed through all its variants? If we were to ask these two questions in most Western schools, the majority of its sensei will be hamstrung for a clear answer. I would also like to challenge the notion of absoluteness when using any Western scientific metric (movement physics, or biomechanics) to evaluate the structure of any Asian Fighting Form. A story seems appropriate:

Years ago, I was introduced to an accomplished Tae Kwon do and ninjitsu adept named Jonathan. Jonathan, then in his forties, was fit, confident, intelligent and articulate. By happenchance, he was the friend of a visiting guest of mine, the head of the Wu Hsin Tao, North America, Arakawa Mitsugi, a highly skilled, Japanese-trained, Aikibudo master. The three of us began a lively discussion. At one point, Jonathan asked if he could demonstrate a technique on me from the SPEAR method of martial training. SPEAR is an acronym for Spontaneous Protection Enabling Accelerated Response. This evidence-based, scientifically proven method uses reflexive action in threatening situations as a basis for defense. Its founder, Tony Blauer, developed the system in Canada during the 1980s.

Jonathan asked me to extend my right arm, palm's up, hand fisted, and try to prevent him from bending my arm. I obliged. I was unable to hold my arm straight against the force of his bend. He explained, that with my hand balled into a fist I would unable to stop the bend. But, if I opened my hand, it should be impossible for him to bend my arm. He was right. I resisted with little effort. I asked to try the test again with my hand in a fist. This time, I moved Ki into my triceps, a simple Soft Gate technique. No matter how hard Jonathan tried, he could not bend my arm. Baffled, he asked how this was possible.

Jonathan's evidence-based SPEAR method worked. However, this is not the only means available, nor is the current method applying movement physics. I have read books expounding various scientific principles lying behind martial postures replete with elaborate diagrams indicating vectors, levers and fulcrums highlighting the absolute science behind a posture needing to be just so. But body physics offers an absolute only within the parameters of that system. While such measurements can accurately determine joint stress and optimal positioning to avoid such pressure, a martial art, any art, cannot be solely contained within this scientific framework. This would remove the possibility of other dimensions of expression extant beyond mathematical or scientific certainties. It would kill the spirit of every martial Dō. I have witnessed Kiko trump movement physics or perfect biomechanics numerous times. The biomechanical principles get turned completely upside down, implying that there is a superior subsystem at work contrary to the Western 'absolutes.' Kiko reveals a *meta*-physic in the invisible clash of Biofields. Kiko does not exist outside science. It exists outside the current scientific framework being applied to our techniques. I'm happy to guide any reader through simple tests to prove my point.

In my examination of Fighting Forms, and in the light of this concealed subsystem, I feel it necessary to make some general observations:

1. Never assume any kata has been transmitted perfectly from its original state.
2. Consider that some degree of kata nuance has been lost, forgotten, willfully or innocently omitted (possibly to be reintroduced when one is at a higher skill level). That is, assume the manual (oral, visual or written) explaining kata's every dimension in detail has been, at least, partially excluded.
3. Kata with short, tight, linear and/or circular movements can

generally be considered either a grappling/gripping/lock-ing-centric or an Internal Form.

4. Kata with elongated limb movements and thrusting strikes, coupled with wide, deep stances, are generally considered ballistic-centric.

5. Kata done slowly and/or rhythmically is assumed to be an Energy cultivating, meditative Form.

6. Kata done at a single, fast-paced speed can be assumed to be an External, or Hard form.

Analysis of Neihanchi Opening Sequence.

You do not need to know the Neihanchi kata to appreciate the following breakdown. The kata has no turns. Movement is solely side to side, which led to the erroneous interpretation [my take] that its bunkai was selected for when your back is up against a wall. Neihanchi is performed in two mirrored sets. Kiko's sidedness principle dictates these sets not be identical. I should point out that Tatsuo Shimabuku's Isshinryu Neihanchi is the only Okinawan variant that initiates stepping to the left instead of the right.

In my early years, I was given a ballistic interpretation for Nei-hanchi's bunkai (striking, with or without takedowns). I do not believe this represents the essence of the Form. I contend that Nei-hanchi kata is a sophisticated *Push Hands* Form, in alignment with the British author, Nathan Johnson's, research but with a different interpretation. I believe Neihanchi is teaching a vital weave among three combat fundamentals; striking, grappling, and Internal (Ki) work, the latter function being my emphasis, not Johnson's.

What technical benefit is offered by assuming a Neihanchi stance, or by stepping across the supporting leg in the opening sequence? For me, the answer lay far east of closing distance, pro-tecting the knee joints, or widening the zone of defense. (See the diagram below).

I do not believe Neihanchi's bunkai is responding to any attack 90 degrees to one's right or left side, which you move toward to close distance. It is precarious to cross step in the midst of a strong attack mounted against you. Advancing toward an attack only accelerates its force, making it more lethal. I find this interpre-tation tactically questionable.

There's only one primary target for an attacker at right an-gles to you—your head. You could just as easily wait for the strike, then parry, lock or counter-strike. Why put yourself in a vulnerable state? Unless of course, the kata is suggesting the attack is coming from elsewhere, or perhaps, not ballistic at all. Let's also look at the curious idea of the initial palm's up, or sideways parry, to meet the attacking arm which we saw in Set 2 of the Seisan kata. One would need to understand the Biofield effect of a palms up, hand posture. Also, why would anyone choose to over-torque, that is, rotate the torso to an extreme 90 degree side angle? This flies in the face of essential kata logic of efficient, lethal and *natural* responses.

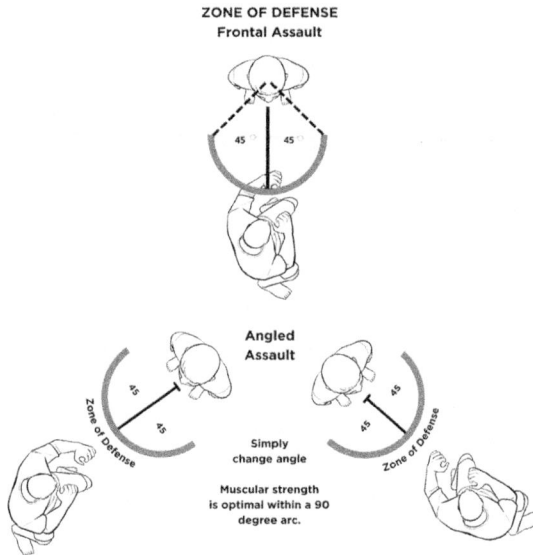

ZONE OF DEFENSE
Frontal Assault

Angled
Assault

Simply
change angle

Muscular strength
is optimal within a 90
degree arc.

Zone of Defense

One's zone of defense in a Neihanchi stance can easily cover a natural, 90-degree arc split into two 45-degree angles from the centerline of your body. Any action requiring you to extend beyond this zone calls for adjusting your stance to shift the zone. In this manner you never compromise the optimal muscular output or positioning of your arms, spine and knees.

Purpose of the Neihanchi Stance:
The mainstream understanding of the toed-in, Okinawan Neihanchi stance is that turning the feet inward increases the range of body rotation left to right, while reducing undue torque against the knee joints. More importantly the Neihanchi stance distributes substantial strength into the rising motion of the arms and lateral movement of the torso. What kind of threat would require such actions?

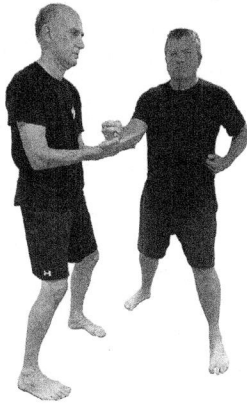

A test: We had subject A stand sideways on the right side of Subject B in a natural stance, feet forward, with their right arm extended in a loose fist as illustrated above. Subject A placed their palms under subject B's arm and slowly lifted as B resisted. The test was repeated with subject B's feet turned outward, 45-degrees, then inward 45-degrees into a Neihanchi dachi. Subject A's lift-ability increased noticeably when rotating his heels outward.

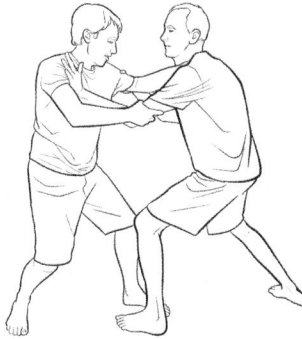

Neihanchi's Push Hands Foundation

The world's fighting arts grew out of two learning environments; close-quarter grappling inquiry and mid-to-long-range ballistic inquiry. We can define a martial artist as any student actively investigating how to deal with violent or competitive physical conflicts. Grappling versus striking actions have often been misconstrued as mutually exclusive fighting systems in the Western martial mindset. You clearly see this bifurcation between Western wrestling and boxing where the other style's techniques are forbidden in the sport's arena. We must credit the rise of the

MMA for re-merging these systems closer to the more realistic fight scenario of *vale tudo*—anything goes. The majority of karate systems, introduced into the U.S. in the early 60's, were primarily presented as striking arts.

Push Hands (Ch. *Tuishou*) emerged out of grappling and centering inquires. Push Hands is to standing grappling what rolling is to ground fighting. In Push Hands you start close quarter with a partner and slowly begin to unravel the intricacies of weight, balance, strength, posture, deflections, grips, locks, escapes, timing, coordination, breathing, Ki flow, etc. as you slow tussle.

We can see then that martial art fighting skills developed along two main ideological branches; those that used partnered push hands to develop the contact reflexes, and those that strictly adhered to ballistic, kick/punch style motions, which primarily developed the visual reflexes. The latter defines mostly modern and western style martial arts. 'Push Hands' refers to methods of physical engagement by means of 'crossing arms' or maintaining contact, also referred to as the exchange of 'hands', that is, limbs/ bodies in continuous contact with one another. This type of exercise builds an intuitive contact sensitivity, and generally progresses from complimentary (working with your partner) to oppositional skill sets (working against your partner). Push Hands works on the theory that 'contact reflexes' offer faster reactions than the 'visual reflexes' needed in most ballistic-style training.

The art of Push Hands also possesses the combined elements of play and fight. Play fighting is what children do. Competitive matches are what young men do. Killing is what warriors do. In modern warrior education, we can't go around killing our partners to see if our techniques work, so we must work within the confines of the play/fight arena. Sometimes the emphasis leans more to the fight side, sometimes to the play side. Out of this investigatory, live-action role play/fight state emerges certain universal truths about valid techniques and their underlying principles. From my perspective, Okinawa's Neihanchi kata is a Push Hands Form, for it bears a close relationship to a Push Hands interpretation from start to finish. Japanese modifications to the Form have elongated the techniques of the Okinawan version to make it more amenable as a mid-to-long-range striking art. This postulate is supported by the author Bruce Clayton in his excellent work *Shotokan Secrets* (Black Belt Communications, 2004). Clayton contends that the Shuri Castle's unarmed defensive strategy, maintained by

Okinawan's political elite, stressed long range, one-strike-kill, or knock to the ground techniques. According to Clayton, this was the best tactic for the Castle's open-floored blueprint, and the fact that its protectors had been dispossessed of weapons.

One critical factor missing today in the Japanese and Okinawan versions is a discussion of Neihanchi's internal fundamentals. Even the distinguished master, Choki Motobu, noted for his command of the Neihanchi kata, in his 1932 seminal work, *My Art and Skill Of Karate*, makes no mention of any internal fundamentals. Yet, I believe these fundamentals provide the most convincing rationale for why this kata's moves are arranged so precisely.

I don't suffer the illusion that I am offering readers the absolute interpretation of Neihanchi bunkai. I am an unabashed outlier. There is a great deal of diversity in the bunkai of this kata from many fine experts who all see something different in the Form and make compelling cases with decisive applications. I toss my bunkai hat into this ring to present a refreshing new perspective.

Like most professionals, I've sought to understand the how's and why of my Fighting Forms. Let me share and perhaps, clear up what I perceive are some misunderstandings and misassumptions in regard to the Neihanchi stance.

We all want to know why past masters chose a particular stance over other postures, which should bring us to our own experiential confirmations or validations of a stance or footwork. First, there is what we are trying to do with the stance and second, how we are trying to do it. We have multiple historical, sometimes conflicting, perspectives that, at the very least, give us a springboard for our own trials.

There are a number of hurdles to leap looking at the past use of the Neihanchi stance(s), as they vary amongst styles. To illustrate one of these obstacles, I again reference the 2020 translation of Choki Motobu's, *My Art and Skill of Karate*. Anyone who translates the work of a highly skilled expert, who is not at that same level of skill or indoctrinated in the 'house' language of that art's community will often experience 'the curse of a lack of insider knowledge,' or what is referred to by certain researchers of Asian works as 'Twilight' language. I could analogize this situation to a Cartesian scientist translating the high-end work of a quantum physicist.

My expertise lies in the internal structure of a martial art. Neihanchi stance is the externalization of a principle regarding Ki manipulation for specific strength increases relative to the kata's bunkai. This principle can be expressed through multiple formulas, which is one reason we have variations of this stance. Some Neihanchi katas do not adhere to any bioenergetic formulas. Their success relies entirely on gross, external strength to successfully execute its bunkai.

When you assume any martial posture, there is an immediate shift in the body's electro-magnetic field. This field, existing as positive and negative currents, will distribute a charge to specific muscles for a specific task. Foot positioning is part of this distribution system. All footwork follows an internal proportionality formula. Neihanchi stance, begins with its narrowest posture assumed from a Musubu dachi or v'd feet on a 90-degree angle, accompanied by moving the heels outward until the toes point inward no more than 45-degrees. Beyond 45-degrees results in a polarity shift, leading to a weakness in application. Done correctly, this posture will distribute a strong current in support of either/or both arm(s) rising upward and rotation of the torso. The debate I see some engaged in, trying to determine if the Kiba dachi or narrower Neihanchi variants are the correct postures, is moot, if you do not understand how the body's Biofield is affected by the footwork. Without a Ki decoder, it will remain a guess for many. This is not the language of the old-world masters. This is an emerging new language to describe, on the quantum level, what is going on beneath the surface technique.

Regarding Motobu's bowed legs and their possible influence on the kata, this might be of interest; I have bowed legs. While pursuing body work with a Structural Integrationist (formally called Rolfing) we discussed my "cowboy" legs. The therapist was convinced my structure was the result of years of karate stance work, particularly the Seisan dachi, which is best applied by pushing the knees outward when striking. I found his observation peculiar, for I have many three-decade plus senior students who do not have bowed legs. The bow does make certain stances easier for me, but this does not infer my technique is superior as a result, nor have I found that certain physical anomalies definitively negate other's abilities. The body's electrical system appears quite adaptable. A physical anomaly may direct that person's internal energy by an alternate route, allowing them to be just as potent.

I have been investigating martial postures and their energetic polarities for three decades. My observation is that Neihanchi stance is a principle which can be expressed in, at least, three manners; the narrow posture I have described above, a less wide Kiba dachi, which I call Funakoshi's Tekki or Iron Horse posture (also Motobu's)—as long as one puts pressure on the balls of the feet pulling inward [my emphasis]. (The feet themselves do not move. They remain parallel), or a full Kiba dachi, as long as one puts pressure on the heels of the feet pressing outward. Between the widest Neihanchi formula and the narrowest, different applications may be implied. The narrower stance suggests a grappling exchange, the wider stance, a ballistic response. All the above is easily testable, if you know what you are testing for. The outcomes of these positions are task specific and will result in dramatic strength increases.

In regards to translations of meaning, Motobu states he disagreed with Itosu's tightening the soles of his feet, for he could easily push someone over doing so, may have been the wrong test altogether. We don't know if the translator captured Itosu's house language as to the precise nature of this tension or if Motobu over-generalized his observation. Tensing one's soles is a subjective statement. Exactly how did Itosu tense his feet? And what was the sequencing of this tension, which would make a difference? Did the tension begin focused on the inside, outside, balls, heels, etc? Isshinryu's Shimabuku, for example, outlined a specific tension sequence for performing Sanchin kata, indicating one could cause problems, probably meaning weaknesses, when done out of sequence.

We don't know if Itosu's kata and bunkai was exactly Motobu's, because moves preceding any foot tension will affect the strength in the upper limbs. We also do not know if there was some level of bias or competition between the two men that might mislead our comprehension of their kata performance.

It would be too lengthy to break all this down here, so I will conclude that Kata's internal technique is a mostly lost art which I would like to see restored and reinfused back into traditional Forms with more accurate explication.

The toed-in Okinawan Neihanchi stance triggers increased upward strength against any downward pressure on your arms, along with rotational strength in the torso. What might such a pressure be? Perhaps, an arm or pair of strong arms pressing down on the defender, trying to tie him up, common in a fight. We want torque-ability in the waist to rotate and/or to deflect those strong arms or reverse the tactic on the opponent.

Neihanchi kata can be broadly viewed as an investigatory practice between two parties in a martial give and take hoping to gain more knowledge and skill about personal combat. When practiced solo and properly, Neihanchi will trigger unseen Biofield events affecting muscular output. When practicing with a partner, Push Hands Neihanchi will acquaint the players with three common fight controls, which follow the well-heeled Okinawan maxim; *strike to seize control, seize control to strike*. Control is seized using an overhand grip. This Neihanchi bunkai leaves the opponent with only a few untrained reactions; pull straight back, thrust their arm forward, raise or lower their arm to break the grip. The idea is not to force your opponent into any of these positions but rather to follow their natural reactions when gripped. Neihanchi presents the means to essentially place the opponent metaphorically up against a wall by anticipating their reactions, thus systematically narrowing their responses.

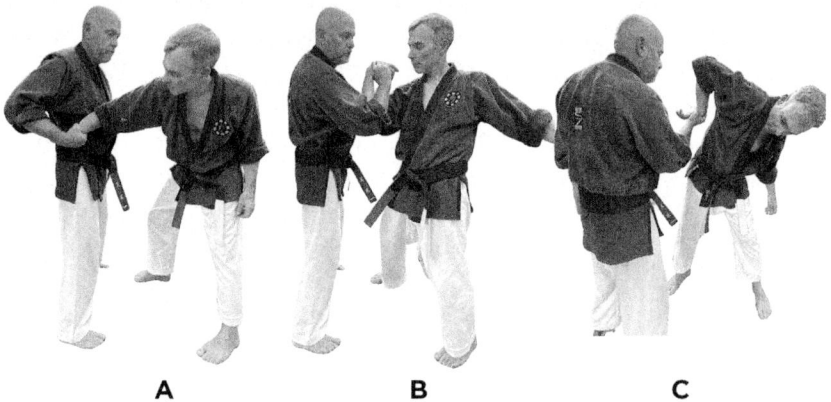

A   B   C

A. Catching and holding an opponent's arm at the chamber using an overhand grip.
B. Controlling the opponent's wrist when their arm retracts backward and upward.
C. Controlling the opponent's wrist when their arm retracts backward and downward.

Neihanchi Bunkai

1. The bow, salutational hand position and opening footwork, where one moves from a Musubu dachi into Neihanchi dachi, charges the upper body with Ki. The central purpose of the bow is a 'return to center,' the gathering of Ki through physical and mental composure.
2. An opponent compromises both your arms.
3. You step left on a slight forward diagonal to gain control of his left arm as illustrated (A right step is used in other variants).
4. You execute a palm's upward, hook-hand parry.

Let's look at the initial left hand hooking motion. Ask the average person to grab your arm and they will clutch your wrist one hundred percent of the time by reaching out with their palm down. I've never observed any untrained person turn their palm upward first then flip their hand over to grab. You saw this action in Seisan kata. As I explained, the palm up, hooking hand, when laid across the outside of an incoming strike will immediately draw a charge from the attacker, weakening his arm while instantly strengthening the defender, provided one breathes in when hooking and keeps their hooking hand relaxed. Relaxing the hand allows for unobstructed Biofield flow.

If you are gripped, and wish to activate Kiko to break the grip, you can imagine (Soft Gate) your gripped left wrist rotating counter-clockwise before you cross step. This visualized rotation will enhance your arm's energy draw. The crossover step will biomechanically throw the opponent's arm and torso off center to compromise his grip strength. Second, it causes his left (weaker) arm to reverse its polarity to send rather than receive energy on the left side of his body. Remember, in the Isshinryu variant, Neihanchi kata opens to the left. We hook with a left arm stopping at a forty-five-degree angle, (not a 90 degree angle) with the hand held roughly shoulder height. There are two reasons for this precise positioning. We want to rotate the opponent's arm pinky side or ulnar bone facing upward to shut off his Ki, weaken his grip, and expose the underbelly of his arm for gripping.

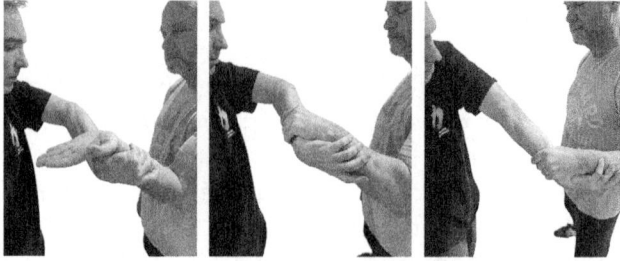

If you grip as indicated below in the first image, the opponent remains lethal, strong, and can strike with his free arm. If you grip as illustrated in the second image and pull the arm to your chamber, the opponent will find it impossible to strike with his free arm, not to mention that you also control his legs. Pulling downward will prevent a kick from the gripped side. Drawing their arm toward you will negate a kick from their opposite leg.

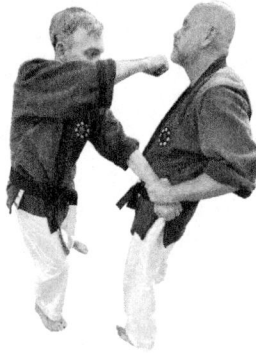

Failure to rotate properly allows the opponent to remain a threat.

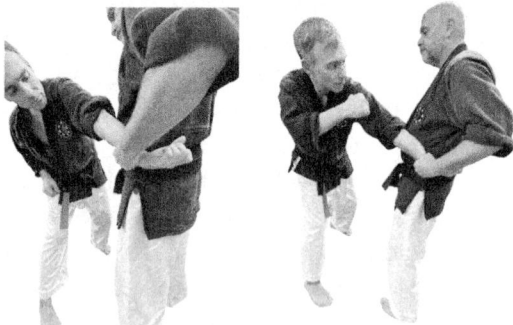

Proper position. The opponent's shoulder is restricted
from any severe strike

I have proven this effect hundreds of times with many sub-jects. And this is just the beginning of the Energy 'dialog' between the players in an internally-focused, Neihanchi Push Hands. The entire kata, from my vantage, begins as an investigation of what to do when your arm(s) are compromised and later expands into striking. Neihanchi opens with both your hands gripped and con-cludes with a dual wrist and shoulder lock. This drama is played out on both sides of the body, in near mirror image.

The second half of the Form starts with the same compromised hands. Because the defender's Ki flows differently on the two sides of the body, the action varies to take advantage of this fact. The goal of Neihanchi is to teach a student that the moment you are cross-gripped, you can immediately deflate the other's Biof-ield as you flow through one of the three controls outlined earlier. This is a far more potent and practical lesson about Neihanchi's value then memorizing a random string of eccentric bunkai, for as soon as one or both of your arms are grabbed you will succinctly know what to do. When your technique transcends into principle, your body will move fluidly in the moment. By contrast, if you have learned that technique A must match attack B, and something goes wrong, it is unlikely you will be able to transit fast enough with a matched defense without years of training. You cannot suc-cessfully fight by numbers. Our Neihanchi bunkai differs from the well-researched and published work of Nathan Johnson. We use a simpler, more natural response to the dual hand grip.

As a sidenote, one grappler told me these moves cannot be realistically pulled off. I told him a solid blow to one's face will of-ten do the trick. He agreed. Let's put these moves in proper con-text. If you're going into a cage match with a professional fighter, you're going to need far more skills. From a civilian self-defense standpoint, however, these techniques offer an excellent starting point to understand how joints move and how an opponent can be physically manipulated.

41* Each and every kata is a five-in-one form

The Five Element Theory & Kata

I gained a major Kiko insight sparked by a critique from a first-generation British Kempo teacher. Sometime in 2000, I crossed paths with the author, Nagaboshi Tomio (Terrance Dukes) in his hefty tome, *The Bodhisattva Warrior*. This book, not for the faint hearted, is considered the Bible of the British Mushindo Kempo organization. Nagaboshi carried a vital seed of monastic martial art training into England during the early 1970's. As I was pinning down kata's internal principles, I was also dialoging frequently with Nagaboshi's future successor, Arakawa Mitsugi, who passed along a comment from Nagaboshi that when I understood Sanchin's five-in-one nature, things would fall into place. His cryptic message whet my curiosity to search in earnest for this dividualized kata trait. The implication being that there isn't just one way to perform the kata but five different methods, best viewed in the light of the Chinese Five Element Theory. As I had done previously with the I Form, I applied deductive logic to figure out what Nagaboshi might have been referring to.

I asked myself if there were any manner or method of performing a kata that readily lent itself to a logical, interconnected, five-in-one overlay. My focus was to apply this formula to Okinawa's premiere Form—*Sanchin*. I set out with three critical questions; What might be five different ways to perform Sanchin kata? How might the Five Elements be matched to each of these methods? What would be the purpose of doing the Kata in this fashion?

With some prior and fortuitous internal discoveries pointing me in the general direction, I eventually arrived at a satisfactory answer. Although, it took years of foundational work to build a framework of perception keen enough to allow me to see the internal mechanics underlying Nagaboshi's suggested hypothesis. I will walk you through my reasoning process.

First, I felt two criteria had to be met. Simply choosing random variables for performing a kata only makes sense in a narrow context that perhaps there are only five irreducible methods for performing any kata. I did not believe this to be the case. The five-in-one theory had to be logical and the Elements had to be interconnected in a meaningful way during either a solo or partnered performance. I sensed the former was the case. I also surmised that the Kata's outer form would have to remain intact, that is, the visible structure of the kata would have to be done exactly the same way (or with relatively subtle variation), otherwise I'd be doing five different kata, not a five-in-one kata. Readers interested in this topic should investigate the evolution of the Chinese Five Element Theory or Five Element Phases, and how this theory came to pervade the country's philosophical, martial, and medical thinking.

I selected seven functional characteristics sought in any kata performance to see if any fit a five-sided definition. I list them randomly as;

1. Speed
2. Distance, proximity
3. Directionality
4. Form – the outer structure of a kata.
5. Breath: the respiratory action during a kata.
6. Mental orientation: i.e., where your mental focus and concentration is placed.
7. Energetic orientation: The internal Form or what your Ki is doing.
8. Offensive or defensive modality; techniques, strategies and/or tactics

Speed

The **speed modality** did not fit the five-in-one theory box. Its boundaries have essentially only two primary variables—fast or slow. In between speeds would be arbitrary, too subjective to make sense of significant value if, for example, we were to list 3/4 speed versus 5/8's speed. At best we could add mid-speed. There is a value to changing speeds within a kata, but I did not see the relevancy of five speeds.

Distance/Proximity

The **Distance/Proximity** modality also did not fit smoothly into the five–in-one Theory. Proximity, like speed, have only two highly subjective endpoints—near or far. At best I could accept mid-distance similar to the speed modality. I did not see the relevancy of five proximities for performing kata. I was already anchored to the idea that the physical movements of the kata likely remained unchanged, that the five-in-one distinction must be embedded in a relatively fixed outer structure.

Directionality

Directionality in kata bunkai carries some significance. Outside the relevance of standing in front, to the left, to the right, behind, above or below an opponent, these distinctions carry little weight in a solo kata performance because there is no concrete variable around which we can orient to five directions, save direction itself, given that we could begin at any point around a 360 degree circle. Such a broad choice of angles led me to believe that the five-in-one theory held little relevance in directionality. Besides, the short variant of Sanchin kata is performed in one direction—straight ahead.

External Form

The **Form modality** clearly did not fit the five-in-one theory. If I had to change the physical structure of a kata for each performance it would no longer be the same kata. If mid-blocks were to become high blocks, right turns to become left turns, narrow stances to widen, or single arm motions to become double arm motions, I would be creating altogether different forms with completely different combat dynamics.

Bunkai

The **functional/applied dimension** of Form initially offered the best fit of the five-in-one theory. This variable was my first, solid, enthusiastic stab at understanding the theory. Five-in-one might represent five different types of attacks or defenses; blunt trauma, nerve strikes, cavity strikes, torquing or grappling actions, and Ki strikes. If this were the case, then the value of the five elements would enter by way of the type of strike or lock for each movement sequence. But this thinking quickly turned problematic. No single kata move or sequence 'always' lends itself to being applied five different ways. The perspective had merit from a combative value if you are investigating a broad range of potential fight controls, but it too fell into my category of too subjective to smoothly fit the theory. I discounted the offensive/defensive application modality as relevant.

Breathing

The **breathing modality** did not fit the five-in-one theory without forcing it to work. We have *in* and *out* breaths done at various intensities and holding breaths at various time intervals, but selective breathing patterns do not all support the mechanical expression of the kata's technique. Without changing the external pattern, I could be imposing energy-weakening strategies on the musculoskeletal system, for example, by reversing the breathing in a simple strike. Breathing in while punching outward is generally counter-productive. I saw no benefit for implicating the Five Element system solely within the respiratory sphere.

Mental Focus

Only one performance mode met my criteria of being logical, interconnected and would not alter the kata's outer form. This was a focus on manipulating the Biofield, the body's Ki system.

I could clearly see why a normal person might be baffled with this modality. They would either be looking at an acupuncture chart wondering how a conceptual, five-in-one, framework fit a kata performance, or be trying to come up with a match for five different energy states for performing any kata. I liken this to a cook reading a chemistry chart of Elements wondering how to bake a pie.

Energy Orientation

My foundation in Kiko had given me firm grounding in practical martial applications. I understood different meridians were equated with various elements. But this fact offered little guidance in performing a Fire Element kata. It did beg me to think about the different elemental meridian pathways while going through the Form. But I wasn't sure if the five-in-one theory implied I was to think of the specific organ equated with the Element, as each element is also associated with a bodily organ or part. For example, I could do a Sanchin kata thinking of my heart, a Fire Element organ, or intend on my kidney; a Water Element organ. This might explain the therapeutic side of kata, but I felt I might be better served to pair my heart intent with physical movements and postures that supported heart meridian flow, rather than the prescribed kata moves. As Nagaboshi's successor, Shifu Mitsugi, would say, "You are in the right church, but wrong pew."

By happenchance, a crucial informational interface loomed over the ensuing months. During our normal Hard and Soft Gate practices I had observed some testing inconsistencies and anomalies. Tian Zhua, a senior-most karateka, was not getting the same results as the rest of us, until I questioned the postural anomaly of his neck. His neck craned forward noticeably more so than the rest of us. I wondered if this postural trait affected his Ki flow. Oddly, when I asked him to retract his neck, his Hard Gating results fell more in line with the group responses. This led to my theory that personality may be the result of our human shape/structure and that this shape/structure was probably built from an energetic root. This observation led to an *Ah! Ha!* moment resolving the five-in-one kata puzzle. We all possess not only a psychological

persona or identity, but a structural personality, and most importantly, an *energetic personality*. Each of us possesses a primary
Biofield persona or Ki flow pattern drawn from the Five Element
womb. This is similar to Western astrology's understanding that
each of us is born under a specific astrological sign within a scale
of twelve possible signs each with a dominant characteristic given
our birth date.

The Five Element Theory had been staring me in the face
all along. I sat in front of the acupuncture chart in my studio and
contemplated the idea if you were born in a particular year, in a
particular season, you adopted an inherent Elemental energy orientation. These 'orientations' are best understood doing basic Ki
work to fully grasp their distinctions.

Why should this intrinsic, five-in-one, energy orientation matter to martial artists? If you know your opponent has a Fire Energy
persona, the Five Element Cycle of Destruction reveals how to
destroy his Ki flow on a fundamental level and quash his physical
attack with a Water element counter. I am not referring to a physical action representing a Fire technique, but an underlying orientation that can be activated in any selected physical technique.

The five-in-one kata principle explains how to move your Ki in
one of five prime directions. Used in conjunction with any technique drawn from the Cycle of Destruction, the correct elemental
activation has the potential to cut effortlessly through an opponent. In summary, we perform kata in five different energetic ways
to acquaint ourselves with both our own and/or our opponent's
elemental energy persona. This rationale is logical and interconnected. I have since tested it thousands of times successfully. The
five-in-one theory is a means of training our Biofield (Ki) by taking
it through a range of five different orientations to sensitize ourselves how each orientation feels, and then to select and direct
one of the five Ki frequencies to destroy or repel any attempted
hostility.

Here is a simple breakdown of the Energy Body's five internal movements, which I call the *Five Orientations* or *Five Attitudes*:

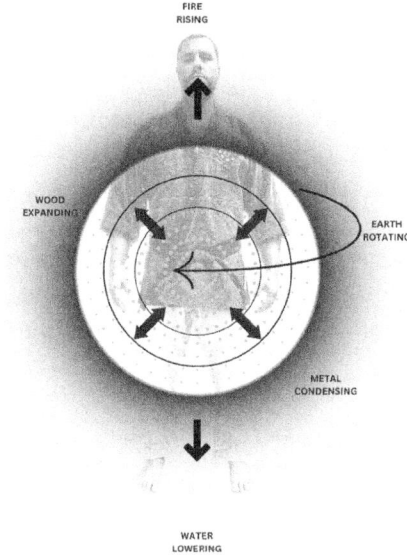

Training kata using each Energy element enables you to become sensitive to these orientations. Over time, this allows you to identify these frequency shifts so that you can select the appropriate attitude to deal with different levels of opposition. For example, say you know your opponent is primarily an Earth energy. Their rotational field is a strong characteristic in their energy makeup.

According to the *Cycle of Destruction*, Wood frequency uproots or cancels Earth frequency. With practice you would focus on expanding or extending your energy field, the prime characteristic of Wood energy, and use that field to cut through the opponent's Biofield. You have to feel these effects to activate them, and you must try out these formulas, that is, experience them for yourself to overcome any skepticism. The proof is in the pushing.

By contrast, the opposite attitude, the *Cycle of Creation*, is applied when engaging friendlies. We want to enhance and uplift our friends, family and allies. This is the empirical reason behind the extension of compassion to others and the core energetic platform underlying the healing arts.

One more explanation held by some internalists merits attention. We can adopt any one of the Five Elemental attitudes for any individual technique. A Water arm parry, for example, might be the best method for subduing a Fire fist strike, or a *Cotton Palm* for penetrating the Iron Shirt. This formula can get quite complicated and is a much larger subject than I can cover in this book. I believe the above insight also throws light on the strange illustrations in the *Bubishi*, once considered the bible of Okinawan karate. The book depicts forty-eight essential Kempo techniques depicting scenarios with two fighters coupled with cryptic, poetic commentary citing who possesses the winning technique, even though, in some cases, neither combatant makes physical contact. Using the Five Element energy formulas may reveal how its author(s) came to their conclusions and strongly suggests a transfer of inner energy.

Winner   Loser

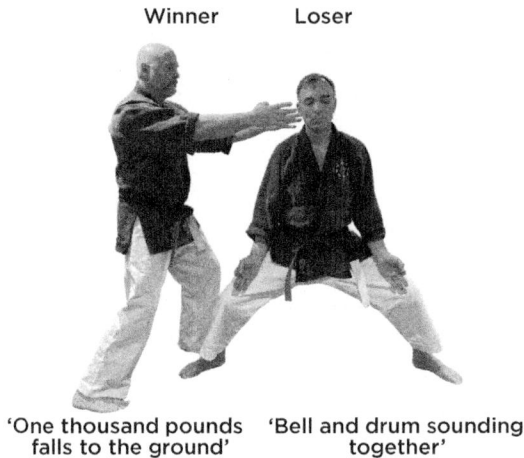

'One thousand pounds   'Bell and drum sounding
falls to the ground'   together'

Unlocking the Bubishi's Mysterious Exchanges

The image above recreates an illustration found in the *Bubishi*, a 14th century treatise on the martial arts. The author points out that the person on the left is the winner. Looking through the Kiko lens we can gain some understanding why the person on the left might be in a superior position. The person on the right is standing in a Water posture (energy flowing strongly downward). By standing with his left foot behind the other's right leg, the victor can catch and redirect the other's falling Ki. The outstretched arms, open hands, and correct visualization, directed at the Great Sun vital points at the temples, dis-regulates the other's Ki flow. A strength test immediately after reveals the loser's weakness.

The 'bell and drum' is likely a reference to the Chinese military tactic of using specific sounds to indicate attack or retreat. Perhaps, the actions of the winner, who sounds bell and drum together via his physical posture, creates chaos in the loser's Biofield, which may be the reason why the author declares him victorious before any physical contact is made.

The Four Universal Training Mediums

To progress in authentic martial practice every engaged student must pass through four universal trainings;

Training of the Physical body.
Training of the Mental body.
Training of the Emotional body.
Training of the Energy Body.

Untrained bodies move by instinct. This can result in either basic, crude actions, or a powerful focus of one's Ki. Because the ordinary mind moves the body in common, ordinary fashion, the first stage of training is to teach the body correct biomechanical rules of engagement. You are shown the proper form for all manner of technique until it can be expressed without awkwardness in a fluid, well-organized fashion.

In the next stage, the student is taught the fundamentals of clear thinking. Practice is oriented to rid oneself of doubt, confusion and lack of confidence. Think of the body as the mind in hard copy. The same rigor applied to conditioning your body is used to sharpen and tone your mind.

In the third stage of training, the student's emotional range is tested through vigorous and intense kumite to measure the three T's; Tempo (including coping with one's adrenalized versus non-adrenalized state). Temper; the ability to positively steer your emotions. And Timing; when to move based upon both obvious and subtle tactical openings in the Biofield. Below is an example of this latter skill."

'Timing is everything'
Anthony Liccione

Two advanced students with thirty-five years' experience between them, square off. One is asked to test the other's resistance to a push. He cannot move his partner. The pusher is then told to sense when the other's energy field recedes. Because our Biofield naturally expands and contracts with the breath, a person will generally test weaker when their field reaches peak expansion (end of an exhale) and markedly stronger during the field's peak contraction (end of an inhale). After a few seconds, he pushes. His partner is flung backward.

The fourth stage is divided into Hard and Soft Gate training. Hard Gate practice acquaints you with the function and feeling of various Ki states when charging or discharging Ki purely through physical motions. Soft Gate training introduces meditative practices to make the mind more pliable, specifically by turning the attention inward to its Energy currents.

More advanced stages beyond the initial four include interfacing the Energy Body with the external Earth Body, and later, the Earth Body and Energy Body with the Cosmic/Heavenly or Divine Body. Consider Newton's Three Laws of Motion under the light of the four universal trainings at this juncture. Could we make similar statements about our mind, emotions and Energy Body?

OBJECTS
Objects will move uniformly in a straight line
Mass of objects plus acceleration equals force
The force given is the force received

MIND
Intention will move uniformly relative to the concentration
held to project it.
Intention plus intensity of projection equals force
The force given is the force received

EMOTIONS
Emotion will move uniformly in waves
Intensity of the emotion equals force
The force given is the force received

ENERGY BODY
Ki will move uniformly in waves.
The Ki wave plus acceleration equals force
The force given is the force received

Here are some simple, sensorial or visual triggers for directing the Energy body to express each of the five Elemental realms:

Fire: Visualize/Feel your energy rising from the ground to beyond your head.

Earth: Visualize/Feel a sphere rotating around your torso clockwise/counterclockwise.

Metal: Visualize/Feel your energy condensing toward your spine.

Water: Visualize/Feel your energy lowering from above you into the ground.

Wood: Visualize/Feel your energy expanding outwards beyond your skin in all directions.

About Earth Element Techniques

I am continually amazed at the results interacting with others using the Five Element formula. Choosing the correct Element gave all of us unusual strength during specific martial tasks. The reason this system works so well likely lies in our subatomic anatomy. Atomic particles have spin, axis, angles of rotation, proximities of proton and electrons, etc. The rough logic that fit for my needs is that we must have the ability to affect others on a molecular level. I had already spent years dialoging about the possible interrelationships of martial technique, kata, mental states, etc. that could explain some of our stunning outcomes.

No matter how fast an atom spins or the direction it spins in, no matter its axis, number of protons or electrons, it always rotates. This is probably why the Horse stance is a foundational technique in so many arts. It is the body's ambassador of Earth Energy. The Horse stance was often taught to students who were expected to stand in this posture daily for hours, extending over several months, before any other technique was taught. Rotation is the quintessential motion of our subatomic anatomy supporting the motive force behind the other four orientations.

42* Okinawa's premiere Form, the Sanchin Kata, presents both a brilliant tactical combat framework and an Energy-cultivating meditation.

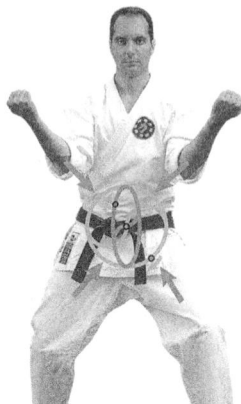

From mid-1960 through the 1970's I never encountered any Hard style martial artists who taught Sanchin as a Ki-cultivating form. They may have been told this was its purpose, but the guts, the internal workings of this formula, were missing. This is evidenced by the manner in which most karate-ka perform the kata today. We see many exquisite exhibitions of its external structure, but my investigations support that the majority remain unaware of Sanchin's internal structure. I am referring specifically to how movement patterns stimulate the Biofield in regard to physical strength.

I was one of those uninformed students. I was only taught Sanchin's outer mechanics. This is not surprising, since most second-generation students never got any significant bunkai for this Form. We were told to practice the kata because it was traditional. Prearranged fight scenarios and kumite provided the bulk of our hands-on experience.

My third teacher, William Russell, had an interesting take on Sanchin, though with hindsight, I feel he was off the mark in one significant regard. Russell felt the primary purpose of the tension-inducing aspect of Sanchin was meant to trigger an adrenaline dump, which was a relatively safe method to acclimate students to the Flight or Fight Response without exposing them to the dangers of a real threat.

In the late 70's, I had a conversation with a neuro-physicist from Manhattan's, New School about the induced tension required while doing Sanchin. She felt the extreme muscular tightening could compress the heart during the tension cycle, increasing blood pressure to a dangerous level. Her quick analysis parallels those Okinawans who anecdotally suspected strokes and heart attacks could be the result of increased strain on the heart from over-tensing.

One of the major problems all combatants initially face is handling the physiological pressures facing a serious threat. Imminent danger sparks the fight, flee (or freeze) response. This latter stage, freeze, plagues a large swath of modern civilization who have lost their instinct to deal with this tumultuous interior response mechanism. The last thing you want is to wage a battle on two fronts, your opponent and your own adrenaline dump.

Russell explained the mechanism of the Sanchin simply and directly if not perhaps, crudely; Tense your body to maximum, hold the tension, then relax as you move from one technique to another. If you tense/relax, enough, you will eventually trick your body into releasing adrenaline. An astute teacher will recognize the phenomenon from the distinct change in body odor as the hormonal pheromone of adrenaline is released out the skin through the sweat glands.

Russell's training perspective had practical value. And for a while it satisfied my quest to not look any deeper into the Form. Years after Russell had passed, the elephant in the room returned more obese than ever. If all I had to do was tense and relax, couldn't I make any kata a Sanchin-style, tension/relaxation form? If so, why were the moves of the Sanchin arranged in their particular sequence? Wouldn't simply standing and tensing satisfy the same objective? At this point, I knew a significant understanding was missing from my teaching about Sanchin. Russell had missed the tress for the forest. I wanted to know about the individual tress, the reason for each of Sanchin's movements. I didn't want to know the move's label as a block, a punch, etc. I wanted to know why its particular sequence was chosen to represent this kata. Why start with a right foot, not a left? Why did the arms cross? Why must the breath be done a certain way?

Right out of the gate, I hit a baffling wall. Sanchin, like other primary kata, has many variations and purposes. There are long and short versions, *Koryu* (old world) versions, Chinese variations.

It was disheartening to think that every kata might boil down to personal preference. I was perplexed. Then in 2007 a rare exhibition by four internationally noted masters demonstrating four Sanchin variants was taped in the UK. I sat riveted to their performances waiting for commentary on their differences. It never came. The only observation offered was how each form varied externally. Not a single interpretation for their contrasts was offered.

Eventually, I learned what was happening to the Energy Body with Sanchin's individual movements. An early takeaway from my research answered why Sanchin begins with a right foot forward in the Sanchin dachi. I believe the masters were looking for a way to draw energy with a right forward crescent the same way the left foot forward did in Seisan dachi, for if you crescent step and turn your heel outward so your foot rotates counter-clockwise at a 45-degree angle, your stepping will match the energy draw-ability of the left foot.

Those who practice Sanchin may offer other rationales for this foot formation. Regardless, this fact is built into the Form to enhance a range of upper limb actions.

Dharma Wheeling

My research has led to many radical ideas about Sanchin's movement sets. For instance, the Sanchin short form, created by Chojun Miyagi, added the second, reward step with the circling arm pattern referred to as the *Dharma Wheel*. Some schools choose to perform large circles. Others, small circles. Some then press outward with fingers open. Others press with fingers bent at the middle knuckles. Some of these presses bring the palms close together. Others spread them apart. We take the position that the two Dharma Wheels must be executed differently to derive maximum power. The first wheel is executed with an inhale on the circle and exhale on the press. Pressing with the middle knuckles bent is an advanced striking concept. By bending the fingers one can draw Ki from the opponent while exhaling. The final retreating step is done with a reversed breath cycle, exhale/inhale with the fingers open on the press. To further amplify the Ki charge we align the palms at the end of the circle to 'spill' into one another, an alternative way to conclude the wheel.

Dharma Wheeling

Having completed the double hand circles (Dharma Wheel) of Sanchin, there are many variations found in different schools for what follows:

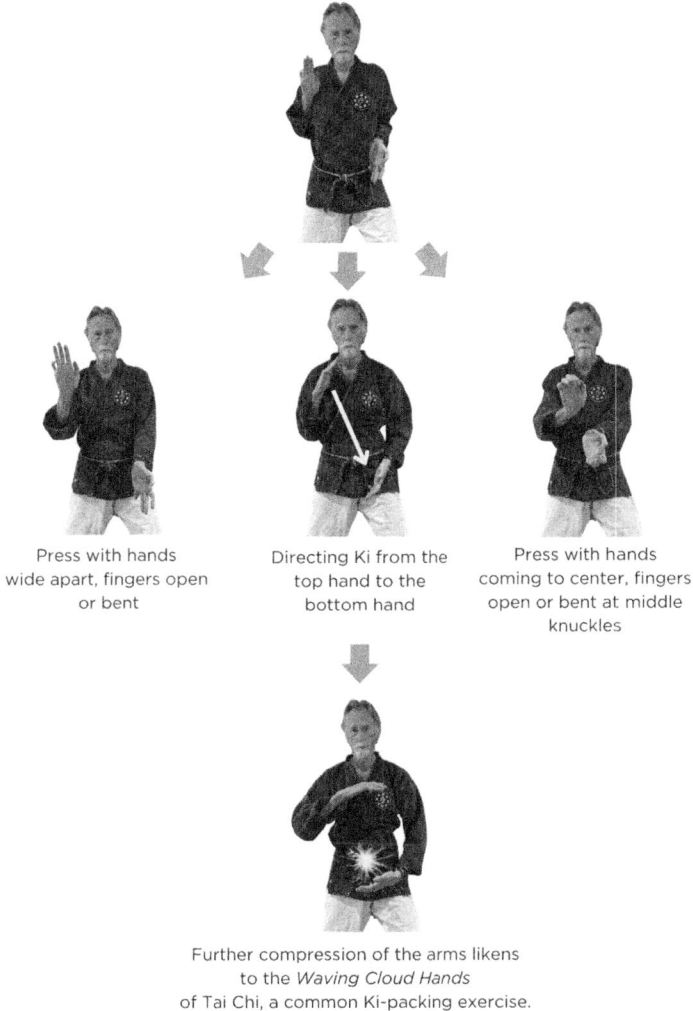

Press with hands wide apart, fingers open or bent

Directing Ki from the top hand to the bottom hand

Press with hands coming to center, fingers open or bent at middle knuckles

Further compression of the arms likens to the *Waving Cloud Hands* of Tai Chi, a common Ki-packing exercise.

Sanchin does not just teach one how to draw and release Ki. Sanchin is an Energy rewiring exercise designed to train the body to run and hold a larger current.

I reached out to Peter Kadar, the first licensed acupuncturist in the state of New Jersey. I wanted Peter to observe my Sanchin and listen to my theory. He commented that Sanchin kata appeared to be doing "in exercise form" what he did with his acupuncture clients, that is, stimulate and balance the body's electrical system.

Acupuncturists are generally unaware of the relationship of Ki

293

flow to martial actions. Given that the degree of charge can great-ly affect muscle contractability, this should be of great interest to martial professionals.

43* Kiko activates Kata's Yantric (sacred) nature.

The language of the Internal, esoteric monastic masters was, and is not, a common parlance in modern dojos. It is acutely for-eign to Western ears and educational upbringing. It is therefore easy to overlook, minimize, misinterpret or disregard its teachings altogether.

In the Esoteric lineages, martial technique is not what it ap-pears on the physical plane. Techniques still retain their outward properties and appearance. A block is still a block, and looks like a block. A punch is still a punch, and looks like a punch, just more so. I have sought for decades to define this 'more so' using my martial skill base, intuitions, historical research, and testing methods.

Authentic martial lineages in Monastic and Internal martial study identify four fundamental roots as their foundation. They are called: *Yantra, Mudra, Mantra*, and *Mandala*. These four roots are linked to Buddhist martial and Yogic practices.

There is no one statement or essay that can contain the breadth and complexity of this field of study, any more than a beginner could have a jiu-jitsu master explain, in a few sentences, the entirety of his or her art. External and Internal training dimen-sions represent interdependent processes that must be lived and directly experienced to be fully grasped.

If you cannot see the practical relevance of a martial concept or technique, you have an activation gap. That is, you cannot acti-vate or properly apply any idea, principle, or technique which you are unaware, do not fully understand, or reject outright.

During my investigation into kata's internal nature, I discov-ered a critical distinction between the embusen and the Yantra, revealing a significant gap of understanding.

Embusen, Yantra, & *Activation Gap*

We do not usually associate a Sanskrit Indian term, like *Yantra* with Asian martial art practices, even though we know historical-ly that Indian martial arts and Buddhism deeply influenced Asian fighting arts. The word Yantra means *Sacred Diagram*. In a literal context, a Yantra is often depicted as a two dimensional, geometrically complex pattern of lines. Yantric patterns are coherent matrixes said to contain mystical or inner teachings within their structure that cause the activation of actual and specific human experience or phenomenon.

When engaging a Yantra you will experience a phenomenon on two distinct levels. 1. when you actually look at the Yantra's visual pattern and 2., when you physically move along its lines with prescribed motions. The experience of a Yantra is not just psychological. What does a Yantric design activate in martial training?

Japanese Karate practitioners are familiar with the concept of the embusen in regard to kata performance. *Embusen* is a Japanese term meaning *performing warrior line* (*Em* = performance, *Bu* = warrior, *Sen* = line). It refers to the spot where a fighting pattern begins and ends, or to its line(s) of movement or floor pattern. Embusen vary for different kata. Let's look at the commonly experienced 'I' or 'H' pattern embusen.

Where the embusen refers to the directions of movement to be followed by the karate practitioner, the Yantra asserts that the direction itself is critical for activating the kata. Where the embusen refers to the kata's superficial pathways, the Yantra refers to the design's 'spiritual' potential. I can easily swap out the term 'spiritual' for the word, 'quantum,' suggesting small, unseen, but vital detail. Most kata are not, or no longer, practiced as Yantra. For example, most karate practitioners are unaware that some historically essential Forms are only activated if they begin facing the correct cardinal direction.

There are instances of Buddhist forms leaving complex floor diagrams that only monastic initiates would be aware of, and whose significance would be reinforced by drawing its Yantra with one's footwork upon the ground. Westerners would likely interpret this design to be of a psychological nature, a cognitive reinforcement of a vital concept or principle. Tracing the symbol of 'compassion' on the ground with your footwork, for example, would reinforce the focus on giving compassion. But this definition doesn't offer any martial insight into the Yantra if such a simple goal as memory recall is intended, for the idea of compassion could simply be chanted or remembered in more direct ways.

Imagine performing a kata that spelled out with your footwork, 'Bend your knees when fighting.' This would be a nonsensical act. There are far easier ways to remind oneself of such.

The value of the Yantra lies in its ability to lead one into a non-cognitive realm, or to say it differently, into non-ordinary mind, into the mind of no-mind, mushin, empty mind. There is a similar concept found in Christian theology first observed by the Ancient Greeks called *Kenosis*, the act of self-emptying, unbinding oneself from desire to open the mind for the entry of Divine will. The Yantra activates a hidden aspect of physical and mental reality whether you are aware of it or not.

A Yantra is an 'event' not an inert visual structure.

What did these martial mystics want us to activate that we multi-decade professionals haven't already seen? What did they activate for themselves?

By simple deduction this activation had to be a property that increased physical and/or mental prowess to give one an advantage in a combative or contentious engagement.

The floor pattern of a Yantra, if begun in the correct cardinal direction, if traced with the appropriate footwork and stances, including breathing patterns, precise upper limb arrangements, and using specific mental foci, would yield an enormous power advantage to the practitioner. This is a feature of kata beyond its common teachings.

This is a rare art, known only to an ever-shrinking martial minority. And this knowledge is disappearing at an increasingly faster rate from the authentic martial lineages as society chooses materialism over spiritualism, the obvious over the subtle. We are creating a cultural momentum that devalues tying up one's time in lengthy, complex 'otherworldly' alternative practices, certainly in methods that empower a person without them having to pay a premium in the consumer marketplace. For enlightenment practices are anti-consumer.

The popular Japanese Taikyoku's (I or H Forms) are Yantric—sacred designs whose inner application and meaning has mostly been lost. The I Form's embusen and Yantra shape an arm of one of the oldest Buddhist symbols, the right-facing *Svastika*, that in conceptual performance would look like this:

A Conceptual diagram of I or H pattern

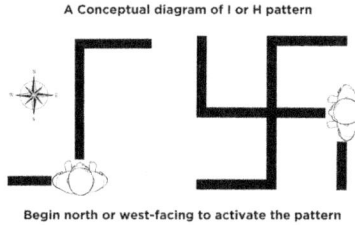

Begin north or west-facing to activate the pattern

The concept of the Yantra may have originated thousands of years ago when early man observed the patterns of the stars in the sky and associated the appearance of certain celestial arrangements with benevolent energy, whether for bountiful crops, surviving hardships like disease, or warfare. According to the research of the Australian martial artist and Chen Yen Buddhist, Kate Marshall, some primitive peoples believed that actually walking those star patterns redrawn on the ground would bestow that same bounty upon the Star Walker, whether it was in good fortune or vitality. If this observation is accurate, it would not be a stretch to see such patterns appearing later in history in elevated martial communities via their fighting forms. Walk this way than that way, and you will activate a heightened awareness, extra-human strength or bountiful harvests. Why else walk the pattern?

In the Isshin Kempo system we have decoded the Yantric pattern of a basic, block/punch I Form to a fine degree. This technical dissection goes far beyond correct biomechanics. We see a clear Yogic-style action of manipulating Source energy for the distinct advantage of significantly more power. However, to move properly along the Yantric track one must become versed in the energetic mechanics of the *Mudra, Mantra* and *Mandala* and their correlation to martial patterns as activating sets following the Yantra's conceptualized lines on the ground.

44* The concepts of Mantra, Mudra and Mandala reveal the intimate interrelationship of Energy Body functioning with all forms and levels of reality.

The 3M's: Mantra, Mudra, Mandala

In his Fire Sermon, the Buddha commented that everything, in reality, is on fire. We can interpret the Buddha's 'fire' to mean that all matter; rocks, birds, people, trees, chairs, pencils, smartphones, eyeballs, mountains, are in various states of transformation. At the subatomic level everything exists in a state of constant flux. Quantum physics hint that this perpetual motion is influencing us on profound levels of health, well-being and, where my research is concerned, strength.

Insights about these effects can be found in the Indian Yogic concepts of the Mantra, Mudra, and Mandala, terms rarely mentioned in modern martial practice. Let's look beyond their yogic attributions and focus on their fundamental nature in relationship to Kiko work.

Mudra

A mudra is commonly understood as a symbolic hand gesture used in Hindu and Buddhist ceremonies, statuary, and traditional Indian dance. A mudra is also considered a movement or pose in yoga.

If we look at this latter definition more closely; a movement or a pose in Yoga, we can extend our mudric definition to include martial movements or poses, and say that:

"A mudra is, in essence, any conscious martial gesture."

This definition might seem a dead-end statement. Any gesture? This isn't going to help a martial practitioner see past the obvious in their arts—until we add the adjectives, sacred or activating gesture. In authentic martial lineages all gestures consist of both a mundane and sacred value. Encased within the mundane teachings lay elevated applications. The mudra was meant to convey this nestled value as superior to its surface attribute when activated. That activation was the wisdom of how specific poses and bodily actions affected Source Energy flow, a parallel aim of the Yogi. The posturing of the body and the movement of the body, was understood as having a specific effect on our covert Energy systems. Covert systems are ones that cannot be perceived by the eyes or ordinary senses. This includes the Chinese Meridian system, the Indian Ayurvedic/Chakric system, the body's fascial communications network and our own mental or cognitive network. You can't see the thoughts in another's mind.

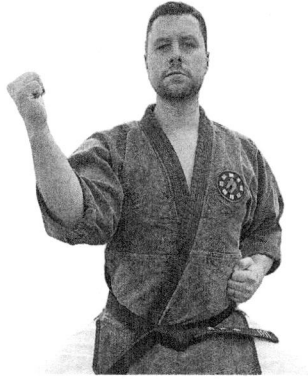

A test: A student performs a traditional middle-blocking action. The resistant strength of the middle block is tested and noted. The test is conducted again. This time the student is instructed to make subtle changes in breath, limb, and torso posturing, possibly even torso direction. During the thousands of tests I conducted, these simple changes often led to a dramatic 50-100% increase in physical strength. This is too significant a difference to ignore in one's training. This is why a whole field of study called Internal martial arts exists and why terms like Ki or Chi came about as the Asian label for this phenomenon.

When the actual effects upon these systems are known, it can be said that one is performing a proper mudra. A physical action performed with less awareness is considered superficial or at best, an action or pose moving toward full mudric potential. This isn't saying superficial actions lack power. It implies that an action's true mudric consequence would go mostly unnoticed, unfelt and therefore not fully in one's possession.

Name it and you claim it.

If the Yantra provides the map of kata's proper directionality, the mudra, through its precise gesturing of body motions and postures, guides us along the Yantric pathways and the activation process gets underway. Therefore, a martial Yantra is useless without its Mudric component and vice versa. This brings us to the third piece completing the activation process, the concept of the *mantra*.

In Hindu and Buddhist culture the conventional definition of a Mantra is a word or sound repeated to assist concentration in meditation, or a statement repeated frequently to calm or empty the mind. This definition however, fails to reveal the Mantra's activation rationale for martial artists, for neither explains exactly why or how a mantra aids in concentration or why one would repeat a martial pattern outside of the obvious.

"Mantra is the soundless sound (quality) of a repeated gesture."

Esoteric Teachings offer us a much broader interpretation of this concept. A mantra is the 'sound,' implying 'quality,' of a mudra (gesture). A mantra is the soundless sound or quality of a repeated gesture. This quality is inaudible to the human ear. But it can be heard by initiates with an awakened *Third Ear*. The more common term Third Eye, suggests the awakening of non-ordinary sensing or sensitivity. This often labelled *Sixth Sense* detects changes in human frequency, as well as shifts in surrounding Energy fields. So, we repeat a high-quality martial gesture because it gives off a higher quality frequency. This higher quality frequency gives us expanded awareness, greater vitality, more strength. And this high-quality frequency has a distinct energy signature that can be detected by others with a cultivated, non-ordinary sensitivity.

No one will argue that a biomechanically correct martial technique is preferred to a biomechanically incorrect martial technique. Likewise, a repeated sacred sound (a bioenergetically correct action) generates a frequency that elevates mundane technique to sacred technique with a practical outcome—it's a lot stronger!

The correct gesture(s) (mudra), following the proper diagram (yantra) gives off the correct aura/frequency (mantra) whose actions will collectively enhance any martial technique. All of these activations form a whole picture of the entire spectrum of martial reality in any given moment, thus forming what could be called the ideal representation of the universe as a microcosmic parallel to the macrocosmic world. When a student is aware of and activates this level of performance, the totality of the parts that make up the kata is understood to be a mandala.

A mandala (Sanskrit: lit, circle) is a ritual symbol in Hinduism and Buddhism representing the Universe or universal reality. In our case, the mandala represents an encircled space—our martial universe—in its entirety, because in principle, this circle has encompassed both its mundane and sacred nature. Under this lens the martial world becomes a projection of the entire cosmos for it contains all dimensions of reality within it.

All animate and inanimate reality possess these qualities. As far as human existence is concerned, the three qualities of mandala, mudra, and mantra can be correlated to the concepts of Light, Love and Law. Light refers to coherence, clarity of mind, clear-mindedness. In martial arts this ideal is found in the term mushin meaning, 'no mind' or 'empty mind,' a mind bereft of filters and distractions. Buddhist martial artists would call this Light state, the *Void*. Meaning, void of the ego mind, no place for mental clutter to accumulate, attach to, or obscure the light.

Love refers to the unconditional self, whose compassion is expressed through allowance. To know your opponent is to embrace all that he, she, or it is. Only then can you see the moment clearly.

Law refers to the immutable forces of the universe. For all its apparent chaos and randomness, the world is held together by the same forces that tear it apart.

Light is the mantra/sound/vibration.
Love is the unconditional gesture (mudra) of the person.
Law is the mandala of fixed natures.

These four interconnecting roots Yantra, Mudra, Mantra and Mandala frame and support esoteric martial practices. They create the foundation for authentic, Martial and Yogic lineages of the world.

When you think of the incredible evolution of the earth and all that has emerged since its conception four billion years ago and realize this universe produced you out of infinite combinations, infinite possibilities, this makes you pretty special. You may have your look-a-likes, but only you occupy the space you are in right now.

45* Kiko gives rise to the Form and No Form schools.

As manipulation of the human subtle energies underwent cod-ification in Asia, two types of internal schools arose, each with distinct methodologies. These were the *Form Schools* and the *No Form Schools*.

The Form Schools go into intricate physical detail to arrange the body into its maximum configurations to derive the most en-ergy from any martial technique. This method was probably the foundation upon which kata was created.

The No Form Schools take a more subjective tact. These lin-eages go straight for mental control of the Biofield. An example used to explain the difference between the two methods is that of water (Ki) pumped through a hose (Body). The Form Schools say if you unkink the hose the water (Ki) will flow with maximum force. The No Form Schools say if the water is a strong enough force, the kinks will straighten the hose from the pressure alone.

One method isn't better than the other. It's more like tunneling from two ends of a mountain toward a single truth.

Form Schools probably emerged as the first teachings. It's more natural to progress from tangible, bodily configurations toward the less tangible reality of what you can't see but might sense—the flow of energy.

The problem with the No Form method is that students need to experience the effects of the Hard Gates, the actual physical as-semblage of the body to initially grasp how the mind controls the physical channels. Kata presents the Hard Gate matrix in pains-taking detail. Kata not only shows us the proper static postures, but how to enter, settle into, and move through these postures correctly. Entry into an adversary's Biofield is an entire sub-art built into kata.

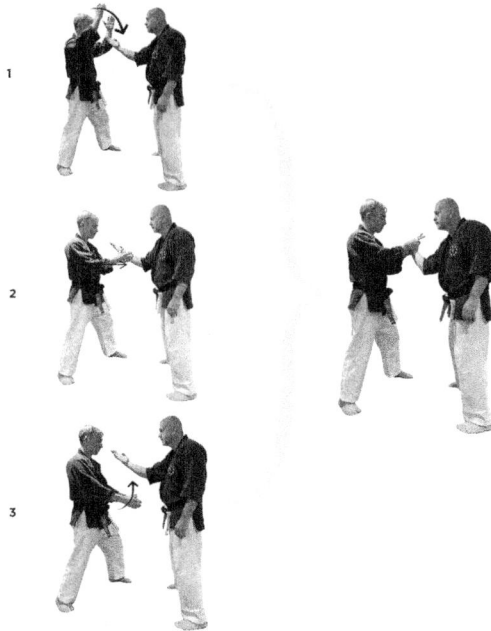

The Art Of Entering

Let's say you are given a choice of three ways to enter into placing a wrist lock on someone whose right arm is extended for you to grab. 1. You can move both your arms downward toward their wrist. 2. You can reach directly forward on a horizontal line, or 3, you can raise your arms upward. In every case your final grip on their wrist must be the same. After hundreds of tests, we observed that the majority of subjects attempting this technique found action 1 strengthened the resistor. Action 2 yielded an expected level of resistance. Action 3, noticeably reduced the resistance, particularly if one inhaled during the motion to grip. How you physically enter into a physical engagement; the stance you chose, the breath pattern you select, the angle of your arms moving toward your target, all create uniquely different outcomes. Traditional fighting forms reveal the optimal way to engage.

I believe the better katas were created as kinesthetic chronicles whose goal was to preserve the intricacies of the Hard Gating system so it could be carried forward and unpacked by succeeding generations. Sadly, Westerners were not given the cipher to unlock this data, nor did they have the awareness that this level of martial art even existed. As a result, we have, in some quarters, an obstructive skepticism that this energy dynamic is not real.

The Form Schools take the position that if the body is correctly postured, Ki will get to the muscles for the required boost in strength. You need not know anything about Ki, internal energy or the Biofield. As long as you execute the proper outer form and your mind remains relatively relaxed or neutral, your Ki should flow respectively.

The No Form Schools take the position that as long as you consciously and correctly direct the flow of Ki, it doesn't matter what outer form your body takes, the Biofield will move accordingly. The distinguishing characteristic of the No Form Schools is their ability to detach the Ki flow from one's external movements.

OBJECTS

46* All objects vibrate and thus possess an Energy Body.

The Mudra, Mantra and Mandala *of Objects*

Similar to my discussion on how our Biofields communicate with one another, I must talk about the influence of objects upon us. This subject came out of left field during a testing session. With the exception of weapon's training, I had no idea of the profound affect that average, everyday common objects can have on our physical strength. Let's visit the concepts of mudra, mantra and mandala in regard to inanimate objects.

Mudra

The mudra of any object is its precise placement in space. Consider the placement of a thing its cosmic gesture. Your favorite chair is placed there, the wall-hanging here, your toothbrush next to the cup. You training bag hangs on the south wall. The tree stands outside to the right of the back door, overhanging the East side of the deck. There may be millions of combs in the world but the one in your bathroom is unique by its *gest* (single gesture) on the right side of the sink. No other comb fills your comb's space in that moment.

An object's gesture is how and where it is positioned relative to you and other objects. The dog's bowl is in the kitchen one day, on the back porch the next. These varied settings for the dog bowl and all the above-mentioned objects each possess a different energy signature and affect.

Where you stand relative to objects around you, whether in the dojo or elsewhere, will influence your training and response to situations. Therefore, objects and the surrounding terrain can be used to your advantage when you understand their vibratory relevance.

Mantra

An object's mantra is its vibratory field or frequency. Described another way, the mantra represents an object's cosmic sound. This is not a sound ears can detect. It is a sound our Energy Body detects. It is the sound of atoms holding a particular structure together. This sound is an object's energetic signature. Every rock, every pebble, every grain of sand, has its own energetic *res* (From Latin, *persona of an object*). No two objects, even if made of the same substance have the same resonance. The fact that no two objects can reside in the same space makes every object unique.

Although inanimate objects cannot move by themselves, they are subjected to natural forces. And we are one of these forces. The pen on your desk makes a different gesture when you change its location or when a strong wind blows it off the desktop onto the floor.

A thing's history is reflected in its spin or emanation. This spin is read by your Biofield and converted into a mental impression revealing degrees of positive, negative or neutral affect.

Who cares about the placement of objects? We can arrange objects around us with the same effect as placing our bodies into certain positions (gestures) to derive more strength. The most relevant objects for martial artists are both natural and man-made weapons.

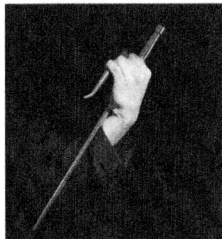

Weapons

The most valuable lessons involving helpful objects for martial artists are found in *Kobudo*, the weapon's arts. An entire book could be written on how the design and composition of different weapon's affect our Biofield. Take the *hanbo* (short staff), as an example, a forte of our school. All wooden staffs have a fixed Yin and Yang end. The Yin side draws Ki. The Yang side discharges Ki. What difference does this make in handling the weapon? A lot. Imagine one end of your staff has been seized by your opponent and you choose to small circle your staff out of the grip. If the opponent has gripped the Yin side of your weapon you can inhale and circle with much greater ease than if your staff is gripped on its Yang side.

*Sai are like lightning rods in the hands. They draw huge amounts of Ki into the user's body.

*Katana and other edged metal weapons powerfully cut external Ki currents surrounding another's body.

Interior designers create bedroom environments conducive to sleep. Prisons are designed to pacify its prisoners. Your ability to manipulate space by selecting and arranging the objects in it can increase your martial abilities. Your Energy Body does not end at your skin. It stretches outward to things around you. You can add to your victories and successes by arranging your extended body with the same care and attention you bring to arranging your physical body. Below are several radical examples of how inanimate objects weakened test subjects in a small room.

Test 1: We placed a vinyl-covered striking bag along the northwest wall of a rectangular shaped studio. Vinyl has a weakening affect upon most people's Biofields. We were able to deduce (and duplicate) nearly to the second, when the effect of the vinyl bag would weaken our test subjects standing along the south wall.

Test 2: We had subjects walk through a door on the left-hand side and tested their strength. Next, we tested them walking through on the right side with a notable difference. We even saw strength shifts with subjects in a room with the entrance doorway opened versus closed.

Mandala
A mandala could be viewed as the representation of an object's fixed or immutable nature. Objects like stones, combs, pots, pens, your training garb, all have their undeniable natures. The stone isn't going to be a pen or a light bulb. The comb isn't going

to be a pot, and you are not going to be a giraffe. The mandala of every object is the part that defines its essence. You're not exactly the same from day to day, yet, your essential nature remains constant. You might have a tooth pulled, gain or lose weight, grow or cut your hair, change your mood or mind. The constant part of your nature is the mandala. This is similar to science establishing that all matter is composed of molecules forming reality's hard structure, its exoskeleton. All inanimate things possess the qualities of the mandala, mudra, and mantra.

A common trait we share with inanimate objects is that, reduced to its quintessence, everything is pure energy. And science admits to understanding only 5% of this energy's behavior. Though inanimate objects seem to our eyes visually inert, on the subatomic level, objects 'move' by way of their vibration, and we are affected by these frequencies. The vibrations of things imbue them with an 'energy personality' that either draws or repels us when near them. It is for this reason that animists attribute a 'soul' to plants, inanimate objects and natural phenomenon and why a discussion of objects should be included in every martial artist's curriculum.

Some people are attracted to bodies of water, or desert, or stone versus wood, to dark training uniforms versus light colored ones, to rash guards versus gis, to round objects versus square ones, to Judo, Jiujitsu, Karate, Tae Kwon Do, Muay Thai or MMA. They vibe with us. Their vibe forms our personal Energy tribe. A Tribe or Order is a collection of individuals, events and objects strongly bound by a common denominator—like frequency. Do you have a favorite shirt, pen, color, friend, song, place, etc.? As a martial artist, do you have a favorite technique, kata, training partner, training routine, training gear, place where you stand in the dojo?

We are attracted to things in sync with us. This is why we attach to certain people and objects and engage in certain events, like martial arts. If you accept the theory that other humans send Biofield signals to us, it's not difficult to see that inanimate objects radiate signals of their own. 'I am nail! I am hammer,' come use me.

I was curious if the vibration of different objects added to or deleted from a person's physical strength? If so, could objects be cataloged on a subjective scale of weak to strong? My interest was to narrow down the effects of these vibes to the strongest signals that either increased or decreased my physical power.

It turned out, to no surprise, that objects comprised of natural materials; soil, stone, wood, water, grass, sunshine, fresh air, add to, enhance, and support our Biofield. Objects of a synthetic composition like plastics or toxic chemicals, despite their practicality, subtract from, diminish our Biofield.

Why do you think the majority of students of the Japanese arts wore cotton and the Chinese wore silk training garb? The concentrated vibes of these natural substances magnified their physical strength. If you don't believe me, try a strength test with a friend and note your level of resistance. Put on a leather jacket and try the test again.

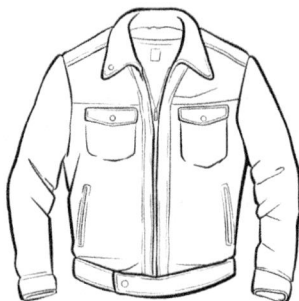

Invisible Leather Jacket

Years ago, I was contacted by a West coast, career Tai Chi expert named Robert. Robert had become familiar with my work and was curious about the Ki side of my training. A long-distance friendship ensued. Robert tells the story:

"During a conversation with Hayashi, I related a recent difficulty in holding my stance against a particularly strong partner in push-hands. Hayashi offered a piece of advice that at first sounded counter-intuitive, if not downright fanciful: he suggested that in my next encounter with this person, I simply visualize myself wearing a leather jacket. No further details were given, nor did I question the logic of this maneuver. When the opportunity finally arose to test this theory under real conditions, I was surprised to find that it worked. My root had indeed improved markedly as a result of Hayashi's casual-seeming 'suggestion'."

The overall strength decline we see amongst the populace is not just due to our more passive activities like the rise in digital screen time, but also the fact we surround ourselves with synthetic clothing, rubber-soled shoes, plastics, oil-based carpets,

EMF emitting mobile phones, toxic chemicals, electronic tablets, computers, walls with formaldehyde, chemicals in our health care products, cleaning products, pesticides on our lawns, nutrient deficient foods, and god knows how much negative thinking people engage in each day.

47* Everyone and everything in proximity is involved in an ongoing, dynamic communication by means of their radiant Energy fields.

In the early 2000's, during a session with a senior student, his mobile phone rang. I had the sudden curiosity to test the effects of his cell phone on his physical strength. I had only strength-tested martial postures. I had never considered testing a subject holding a mobile phone. Would someone's proximity to a mobile phone affect their strength? Remarkably, placing his mobile phone in his pocket, his hand, or at his ear, caused a noticeable drop in his strength. I've since tested many subjects with and without a mobile phone nearby, at various locations around their body. Ninety-five percent of subjects I tested showed a minimum 30-50% decrease in their overall strength.

My theory for this outcome is simple. Whenever our Biofield encounters clashing or divergent frequencies from our own, it must redirect its inner resources away from it central tasks to restore its Biofield homeostasis. This redirect siphons Ki from the muscles for everyday tasks to fight the invasive negative fields entangling us.

Prolonged exposure to negative fields produces anxiety, restlessness, irritation, fatigue, and illness and can perpetuate a pervasive, numbing ambivalence, what I call the devitalizing 'whatever' attitude.

Left Spin/Right Spin Objects

After the mobile phone test, I began to evaluate and classify common objects as *Right* or *Left* spin. A Right spin object was anything that resonated with my Energy Body. Right Spin objects are generally made of natural substances. Conversely, Left Spin objects caused an energy loss, evidenced by a test subject's instant drop in strength. I am not talking about the psychological effects of objects near or on your person, as in, not liking that color, those shoes, that hair style," etc. The effects on the psyche versus Energy Body are not mutually exclusive. Ki effects however, are often beyond one's senses. You might like bleach for its ease in removing dirt from your clothes, but the fluid is toxic to be around. Our Energy Body reacts to toxicity way before our psyche does. Cell phones provide a good example. Carrying a mobile phone causes a condition called *Rouleau* or *Sticky Blood* Syndrome. The EMF (electro-magnetic frequency) from our mobile phones causes red blood cells to stick or clump together, making our phones more like tiny electronic assassins in our pockets. Who feels this affect in their body? Where's your self-protection against mobile phone frequencies? Likewise, I never heard a smoker admit they can feel the toxic effects of inhaling cigarette smoke. The monastics were right. Our enemies can be anywhere, insidious, and often invisible. Why shouldn't our martial arts give us the skills to vanquish opponent's wherever we find them?

My experience with the mobile phone gave me a glimpse into the essence of Feng Shui (wind and water), the Chinese system of arranging objects to optimize Ki flow. This led me to look into if, and how, I could use the environment to increase my strength.

48* Kiko includes the Feng Shui of the immediate environment.

The first time I became aware of the concept of *Feng Shui*, I suffered the impression this Chinese art was a purely psychological phenomenon. The arrangements affected the mind, nothing else. I had incorrectly assumed that *Feng Shui* affects were non-existent if no one was in the room. It was quite a revelation to discover that I could manipulate objects in a room to cause Ki to flow differently such that when you entered you could be stronger with one room layout and weaker with another. Feng Shui wasn't just a compartmentalized impression upon my psyche. My physical body was reacting as well. I believe the vibrations of objects send signals to our receptors that are decoded by our Energy Body leading to reactive shifts in strength.

I began testing the effects of all kinds of inanimate objects with subjects in close proximity, either holding, wearing, or simply looking at them. We found the more synthetic the object, the weaker the person. Conversely, the more natural the object, the stronger one became. We then tested martial art training apparel and equipment. 100% cotton and silk uniforms tested very strong, but cotton-poly blends, despite their practicality and cost effectiveness, tested weak. Striking and protective gear made of poly-substances reduced striking power. Leather gloves increased it.

Some subjects could override degrees of Left Spin, weakening affects, but we felt this might come at a longer-term cost.

At one point I even expanded our strength testing to different types of water; tap water, bottled waters, reverse osmosis, filtered waters. The cleaner and fresher the water, the stronger our subjects tested. Why is water important to martial artists? We are on average 60% water. The cleaner the water the better the conductivity of Ki.

What you wear, how you wear it, the type and placement of objects around you, factor into your overall strength and well-being. Our surroundings are an extension and reflection of our own level of personal integration. Kiko externalized is martial Feng Shui. That is, we can extend our energy reach beyond our skin similar to the way a weapon is an extension of our arms by the calculated placement of key objects surrounding us. Where you train, when you train, what you wear, the materials making up your training garb, objects in your training space, are all variables to consider. All characteristics possessed and expressed by objects; their shape, size, color, substance, even history, exert subliminal influence reaching every level of our being; mental, physical, emotional and subatomic.

Sealing Against the Negative

Whenever you experience or detect an energetic trespass upon your person, you want to immediately halt, or minimize the intrusive frequency. It is possible to 'seal', condense, or protect yourself against weakening Left Spin vibrations from both objects and people. Asian sorcerers like the Taoist Magical Alchemists developed supra-normal means to seal off the effects of negative spirits using magical incantations, mudras and mystical star-stepping patterns. Whether you call unwanted intrusions negative or toxic energy, evil spirits, left spin, the work of the devil, or weakening forces, there are many means to halt such attacks.

Training Garb and Gear

Objects, like our training garb and equipment play their role in your martial success. Kiko takes a deep look into the composition and design of your accoutrements. The earliest martial art uniforms were simply designed and constructed of undyed, natural materials. Today, to reduce costs, modern training uniforms are being made with ever-more synthetic materials, along with our protective gear and training equipment. Regardless of its practicality, synthetic materials do not vibe with the human Biofield. In all our tests, synthetic substances caused a reduction in physical strength. You will likely not feel these effects unless you possess strong sensitivities. Synthetic materials make it harder to maintain Biofield homeostasis. I believe this is why we are seeing so many people suffering from vague illnesses.

KIKO & THE KARATE GI

The traditional karate gi and obi have an esoteric design tradition that promotes the free flow of Ki

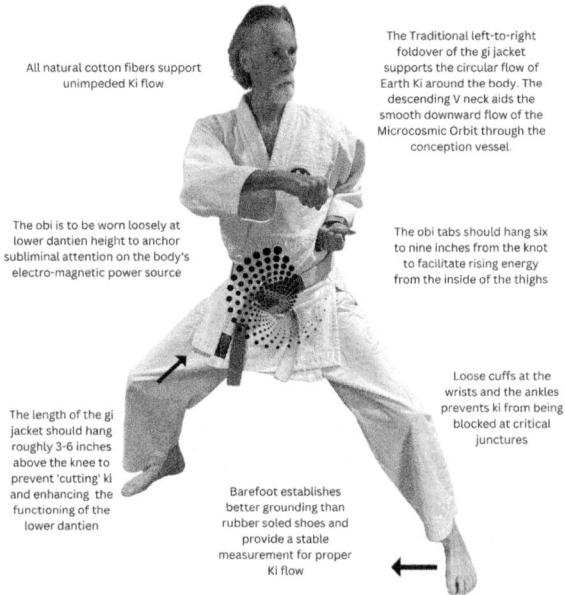

All natural cotton fibers support unimpeded Ki flow

The Traditional left-to-right foldover of the gi jacket supports the circular flow of Earth Ki around the body. The descending V neck aids the smooth downward flow of the Microcosmic Orbit through the conception vessel.

The obi is to be worn loosely at lower dantien height to anchor subliminal attention on the body's electro-magnetic power source

The obi tabs should hang six to nine inches from the knot to facilitate rising energy from the inside of the thighs

The length of the gi jacket should hang roughly 3-6 inches above the knee to prevent 'cutting' ki and enhancing the functioning of the lower dantien

Loose cuffs at the wrists and the ankles prevents ki from being blocked at critical junctures

Barefoot establishes better grounding than rubber soled shoes and provide a stable measurement for proper Ki flow

The Esoteric Nature of Gi and Obi Wearing.

There is more going on with martial garb than students are aware. Take the traditional karate gi and its obi. Putting aside the gi's obvious practical value, let's examine its esoteric nature. Everything possesses a front and a back, that is, an outer and inner character. One overlooked function of the obi is to bring focus to the lower dantien, as attention has a general tendency to wander. Awarding students different color belts helps them maintain a continual mind-anchor on their belly, for as the eyes move to the belt knot, or the awareness of the belt knot, Ki pools there. Secondly, anyone who dons a proper cut cotton or silk training uniform will have an immediate expansion in Ki flow. The gi jacket, crossing left to right, accentuates the body's natural rotational flow of energy. The Japanese consider overlaying the jacket right to left symbolic of death, in our case, a diminished, left spin, counter flow. The length of the gi jacket, when it extends to mid-thigh, gives the wearer enhanced strength because the lower dantien (central electrical nexus/field) extends from just below the navel to the solar plexus and mid-thigh. As the jacket shortens in length, it cuts into the lower dantien's subtle energy field, reducing its charge. The obi worn loosely, with the knot falling precisely over the dantien will also add strength to the wearer, particularly if the belt tabs hang down the inside of the thighs. This facilitates rising Yin, Earth energy.

Tae Kwon Do's shift to a tunic style jacket, dobock (way clothing) in the mid-80's, and the general movement away from traditional Asian training wear to the introduction of rash guards, waist tops, no gis, multi-colored training garments etc., reflect deep cultural shifts in regard to Ki flow. Some of you will likely assert that the practicality and cost effectiveness of these items outweigh the suppression of subtle Biofield vibrations. I think the opposite. Despite all our medical advances, the overall health, strength, and even lifespan of Western populations is in decline. Something's akilter. Devitalizing clothing is another indicator of our culture's degrade.

Correlating to my observations of the weakening effects of synthetic clothing is the work of Dr. Heidi Yellen who, through her scientific research into the frequency of cloth fabrics, made a similar observation in 2003 that the human frequency, measured by means of an Ag-Environ machine, determined that organic cotton had the same frequency as the human frequency of 100 mhz. Her conclusion was that any fabric with a frequency lower than 100 mhz strains our biological system. According to Yellen, polyester, rayon and silk [my research disagrees about silk's effect on the body] registered at the same frequency as a diseased, nearly dead, person. Linen, on the other hand, had a frequency of 5,000, providing energy and healing properties to the body.

313

The world suffers from a lack of vibrancy.

My advice is to seek out the most natural, loose, unrestrictive training wear and unadulterated materials for all your gear. Organic cotton uniforms will give you added, testable strength. Choose leather whenever you can for your hand and foot protection. Avoid all synthetic gear like vinyl and foam materials. Train with the most natural equipment you can find and afford. Most importantly, listen to your Energy Body when making these choices.

Many early cultures trained barefoot to instinctively maintain connection with rising Earth energy. Despite their practicality, modern rubber-soled footwear creates blockages in the meridians in the feet and ankles, preventing us from grounding our own Biofield.

The popular Japanese house declutterer, Marie Conte, states it simply, "If it doesn't feel good, get rid of it." Listen to your Energy Body to boil down your decision what martial gear and objects to keep or toss.

Training Space

What kind of space do you train in? Where do you stand? What direction do you face? Consider these questions from an Energy standpoint. The radiant fields of objects and people in proximity to you are streaming continuous waves of influence, affecting your motivation and bodily expressions.

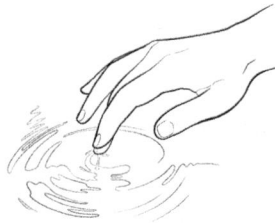

A finger stirring the south end of the pond will send its ripples to the north end. That same action will also affect the air currents above the surface, convey signals to the creatures below the surface, and the neighborhood across the way.

An agitated student at the back of the dojo will stir the energy fields of the senior students standing at the head of the line, might raise the eyebrow of the sensei. The group's reactions will also ripple back to the source. A great cosmic communication courses like invisible blood through the space around and inside all of us at every moment.

If there is an object in your way, impeding your practice, you will move it. What of less obvious, negative energy fields, will you adjust? No one has a problem tossing out their garbage, but few people step away from disturbing, weakening and toxic energy fields.

We never move through empty space. Rivers of energy dance in the space around us. The full orchestration of this dance is muted to most, filtered by an ego that compresses and distills all this potential dynamism to a limited significance, constrained by degrees of sensitivity and an acculturation of what 'should be' perceived as necessary from what is deemed superfluous. Modern culture has blunted its antennae of sensitivity, evidenced by our abject split of matter from Spirit. Martial Dō mends this schism. Weaving matter and spirit together reawakens, heals, recharges, refreshes and restores.

Consider your training space like an intimate partner. There are two qualities we want in a training area; freedom to move physically and emotionally without obstruction, and an atmosphere conducive for practice. Externally, this means an appropriate temperature with proper ventilation and minimal distraction and obstruction. You should feel internally unthreatened; not condescended too, demeaned, embarrassed, ridiculed or suppressed in any way. You should feel comfortable and secure. All space possesses degrees of stimulative, arousing, motivational energy or its opposite; sedative, dampening, constrictive energy.

Choose a clutter free, clean, well-ventilated, and open training environment. Arrange your training space to match or elevate your desire to be potent.

The training atmosphere will also change depending on the attributes of the space. Is the space too cold, too hot, too dry, too humid, emotionally as well? Training space is also altered by activities that have occurred in the past and are occurring in the present. Just as there is an aftereffect left in our memory of prior events in a training space, there are experiences left in the space by others. For example; This is where Eric broke his leg. 'I hope I don't break my leg,' or where Tom decided to marry Andrea, or where Joe had a technical breakthrough, etc.

As you train in the same location week after week, your brain will map out and cue learned movement sequences with objects in that space, your orientation to these objects, and the facility's physical structure. Familiarity with your training area will relax your mind's instinctive vigilance. It should give you a sense of calm knowing the area is secure for spilling out your authentic nature.

An ideal group training space must be adaptable to changing class and curriculum content and conditions. For example, the energy of a small class is often diffused or diluted by a room too big, whereas a large class is restricted by a room too small. The sensei, as 'sensitive', must regulate the energetic atmosphere of the dojo as befits the lesson. This reality will vary by the time of day, season, earth's electro-magnetic field influence, the shape of the room, the positioning of objects in the room, the moods and personalities of its present members, the prevailing consciousness of the dojo's social milieu within the larger social culture. Even the direction a class faces has Biofield consequences.

If the internal masters knew and availed themselves of these nuances, the average person wouldn't have the slightest clue why they felt stronger training in such spaces. These teachers would be using their environment with a tactical awareness way outside the conventional box. Sun Tzu's brilliant commentary on tactics in his *Art of War*, evidences the potency of these factors. We martial artists should embrace the possibility that we can maximize our achievements by including our surrounding environment as an extension of our bodies.

Had the Brazillian jujitsu master, Helio Gracie, on October 23, 1951, not softened the mats and changed the rules in his favor when confronting the Japanese master Masahiko Kimura, considered the greatest judo hero and strongest fighter in Japan in the *Showa* era (1926-1989), the Gracie Jujitsu story might have been entirely different.

49* The relationship of your Energy Body to the living and non-living can be reduced to three core affects; positive, neutral or negative.

In Biofield or Ki work we want to expand our awareness and raise our sensitivity to evaluate our interactions for better outcomes. All relationships are transactions with sought for outcomes. Every moment becomes an engagement either adding to, debasing, or maintaining our neutrality with the world. Everyone and everything you come into contact will, by degrees, either add to you, take from you, or maintain your Biofield's status quo.

Symbols

50* The Chinese Bagua symbol may have been a visual diagram for understanding aspects of Biofield/Ki functioning.

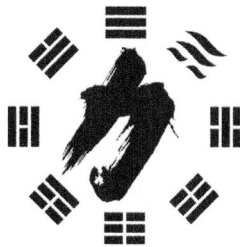

One day, I found myself musing on the cryptic design of the large custom Bagua banner hanging in my studio (image above). I coupled this image to my theory of Ki's sine wave action. I felt the Bagua may have been a symbolic illustration of Biofield functioning. I believe that the Chinese Bagua, in addition to its function as a divinatory formula also provides a visual formula for understanding the energy dynamics behind all transformative reality and phenomena.

Symbols are visual representations of reality. We could say they act as micro realities. The better symbols convey more accurate information. Martial art schools aware of this choose logos that succinctly express their teachings. Some symbols are deep and mysterious. They beg a lengthy explanation to unlock their many layers. Others are the epitome of simplicity, elegance, power and formidability in their directness. Few symbols contain the depth and complexity of the Bagua. This eight-sided symbol is one of the oldest images in Chinese antiquity. It reminds me of some kind of alien high intelligence. I could imagine it on the side of a UFO. I have returned time and again to its design to point out complexities in our fighting system.

The formulaic nature of the Bagua gave me insight into body/

energy sidedness. At a quick glance, the image seems balanced with an equal number of trigrams (three-line images) on both halves. This Bagu design is called the *Greater Heavenly Sequence*. It represents a universe in balance. Another Bagua of similar nature is called the *Lesser Heavenly Sequence*. This symbol, with its tri-grams placed elsewhere on the circle, depicts the transformational states of reality moving toward the ideal of perfect equilibrium. In the Greater Heavenly sequence, the right and left side trigrams are not mirror images. The right side displays a total of four unbroken and five broken lines. The left side displays the reverse, four broken and five unbroken. What significance does this hold for a martial artist?

Decades ago, I came across a trade article revealing a debate amongst several Chinese Tai Chi experts regarding the nuances of executing certain hand technique on the right versus left side of the body. I had not yet crossed into Kiko territory at this time and figured the differences were due to the eccentric preferences of the teachers. Today, looking at this symbol I understand why there are nuances. Every 45-degree arc of a limb, relative to the center of your body, represents shifts in energy polarity within muscle chains.

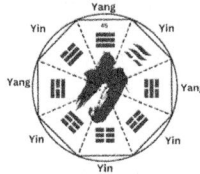

SCIENCE

51* It is theorized that atomic and subatomic communication takes place via electro-magnetic, acoustic and photonic signaling.

I tell all novice students of Kiko that they will be learning, in part, to manipulate their body's electro-magnetic fields. I contend that our Energy Body demonstrates distinct properties similar, but not limited, to electro-magnetism, acoustical and photonic expression.

Through this manipulation these students will not only be able to direct a greater or lesser charge into their muscles to improve or impair their contractability, but can cause the same in others as well. Every martial artist possesses the ability to amplify or dampen their Biofield currents.

A test: A subject's wrist strength is measured to establish their baseline resistance. Next, I ask the person to rub his or her arm in one direction, either from the shoulder to the hand or the opposite, hand to shoulder (contact with the arm is not necessary). I test their wrist strength again. I then have them reverse the direction of the rub and retest. Most subjects notice a remarkable increase or decrease in their ability to resist the move. Why would a light arm rubbing with or without skin contact change our muscle's ability to contract unless some invisible field was at play?

52* Electro-Magnetism and/or Biophotonic communication likely defines one of Ki's many dimensions.

Two theories merit attention as possible scientific underpinnings behind the practical application of Ki. One deals with the function of biophotons or biological light emitted from living organisms. The other, equally pervasive in life forms, is the property of electro-magnetism.

Ki as Biophotonic Energy

We are still on the threshold of fully understanding the complex relationship between light and life, but we can now say emphatically, that the function of our entire metabolism is dependent on light.

Dr. Fritz-Albert Popp

The German physicist, Fritz-Albert Popp's proposed the theory of *Biophotonic* communication. Popp asserted that every cell in the body communicates key electromagnetic bioinformation by means of biophotons or biological light. Biological light is not the same as light given off from the sun or a light bulb. These latter sources are not coherent forms of light. Biological light vibrates at billions of hertz per second. Behind the hundreds of thousands

319

of reactions that take place in each living cell every second is an electromagnetic pattern of energy, carried by the photonic light instructing the cell what to do with each other, at what time, and what place, both non-physically and non-chemically.

Our cells are light-conductive. They emit over 100,000 light impulses (photons) per second. Our bodies are filled with fiber optic structures. All tissue; nerve, fascia, collagen, contain light conductive tubulin structures that comprise an impressive fiber optic system moving at the speed of light. Cells piggyback information to every corner of our body by way of photons. Popp postulated that our DNA stores and emits this light to our entire structure which influences all our physiological processes as the possible steering mechanisms behind all our biochemical reactions.

When we are in coherence, our form is self-regulating, self-healing [and my assertion, self-strengthening]. Ki masters, martial artists, yogis, and others have claimed such abilities for centuries. Unhealthy cells, witnessed by Popp, do not admit coherent light. He believed that a loss of coherence results in a loss of vitality and eventually leads to illness.

The Rhine Bio-energy Lab in southeastern U.S. is one organization claiming that people can manipulate the flow of Energy, prana, or Ki as biophotonic energy. Using a multiphasic ultra-violet light detector designed to measure individual photons, the Rhine Lab has established evidence that Ki exists in the form of bio-photons. Rhine researchers have recorded dramatic increases in the number of photons emitted by people meditating, performing healings, or claiming to manipulate subtle energy. The biophysicist, Beverly Rubic, shared with me that using delicate testing instruments she recorded a Chinese Chi-Gong master emitting photons through his hands at will.

Popp proved that intention alone can emit photons, which interestingly, emits only from the brain's right hemisphere, our intuitive side. Apparently, the higher one's IQ, the more colorful the light emitted on the visible spectrum.

If, as proven through multiple sources, we can control the flow of this inner coherent light then perhaps, this is one of the mechanisms by which fight masters magnify their strength and control their opponents. Our biophotons are also in touch with the quantum world beyond our skin for as this light encounters people and objects around us, it also receives transmissions from them.

Every protein produced by our genes contains light detectors regulating every bodily function. When stimulated properly, our metabolism works well and health emerges. Proper light has been proven to stop inflammation, activate stem cells, detox toxic metals, and more. I'd like to add my theory that when this system works well, we optimize our martial practices. When disturbed, our Biofield dis-regulates, likely leading to states of weakness.

Ki as Electro-magnetic Energy

In 1985, two researchers, Robert Becker and Gary Selden, found electrical currents and their associated magnetic fields in the human body. Today, we know these complex fields are linked to heart and brain function, blood and lymph flow, ion transport across cell membranes, and other biologic processes on many different scales. In addition, a broad spectrum of radiant, electromagnetic waves emanates from the body, ranging from ultra-low, to very high–frequency broadcast waves; microwaves; infrared rays; visible light rays; and ultraviolet radiation. The peak intensity of this electromagnetic radiation in the human biofield falls in the infrared region of the electromagnetic spectrum. These phenomena contribute various field components to the Biofield.

It makes sense to me that Ki is partially electro-magnetic in nature. All living interactions are about charge. Changing electric fields produce magnetic fields, and changing magnetic fields produce electric fields giving our cells electromagnetic character. Life force may be the ability to attract in a self-organized charge.

Because our bodies are electromagnetically connected to everything, the electromagnetic quality of environmental factors affects our genetic expression. This aspect of electromagnetism is so inherent, so primary, so all encompassing, nothing escapes its influence. Emotions, perception, bodily healing, fluctuations in physical strength, all use electromagnetic processes. The contraction of muscle cells obeys electromagnetic laws. Our body's fascia system, that extensive network of connective tissue throughout our structure, appears to convey information by means of electro-magnetic signaling. This signaling includes the charging and discharging of specific muscle groups by the combined means of mental and physical controls, a practice unknown to most of Western society. In addition, there appears to be a link between traditional Chinese Medical meridians and the fascia system.

Helene Langevin, Professor in Neurology at the University of Vermont and her team found that most Ki points lie along the fascia planes between muscles or between a muscle, tendon and bone, or where networks converge. Langevin hypothesized that Ki blockages can be viewed as alterations in the composition of the fascia.

Science stands at a nascent stage measuring the various frequencies of electromagnetic radiation from our bodies. It remains unknown how this energy is used, or its value to human life. I think the answer is staring us in the face. The internal skill sets of the Kiko masters have actualized their Biofields as part of their underlying strength/health system. They just didn't use this particular language.

It has been suggested that the reason Western civilization hasn't looked at this subject is because it is filled with souls too young to advance beyond their own self-motivations for external power and dominance, and so we remain stubbornly anchored to the physical world.

53* Some people are naturally more attuned to Ki's linear, electrical flow while others are more connected to its spiraling magnetic flow.

Emotional, body-grounded, gut driven individuals appear to be more connected to their Ki's spiraling, magnetic field. Such individuals seem more aligned to the big picture, a circular comprehension attributed more so to Right Brain hemispheric action. Head-centric, intellectual types, by contrast, may find a natural focus on Ki's linear flow, correlating to the linear nature of logic and left brain thinking. Either way, Ki can be effectively pushed through the body by visualizing either a linear or spiraling flow through the limbs.

54* Not all meridians function equally.

According to traditional Chinese medical theory, our bodies possess meridians, what I call, Strength Channels, coursing through us. In our testing, we witnessed that some meridian channels can carry a much stronger charge than others.

Traditional Chinese medical charts indicate that the meridians are bilateral, the same on each side of the body. What the charts don't show is how the meridians carry variable currents, or how, for example, when facing north or west, from our testing, the left side of the body takes in more energy than the right side. I surmised the meridians must carry a range of charge similar to how a light bulb can handle a range of voltage. A 75 watt bulb will still light up with 50 watts of energy. It might even be able to exceed 75 watts for a period before its filament burns out. During testing, I discovered that in a normal resting individual facing north, the left side of the body's Yin channels carry a greater energy-in charge then the right or Yang side. The opposite holds true on the right side of the body. The Yang channels carry a greater energy-out charge and a lesser energy-in charge. This is simple to prove.

Too much or too little Energy messes with the body's homeostatic parameters. To continually take in Ki requires an ability to store or use the charge somewhere. Something would have to change in the physical structure to handle or retain more energy. I believe the meridian's volume-carrying capacity changes depending upon a host of factors. Our system is geared to deal with a modicum of Ki flow irregularities. Beyond that, we may experience crisis mode. I believe internal practices like Okinawa's, Sanchin kata were designed to bolster heightened states of metabolic arousal like the Fight or Flight response.

55* An exchange of electrons between people may explain the strength differential when Biofields interact.

Whenever one postures near another, martially or casually, I have witnessed during testing, an energy exchange taking place, oddly similar to the way an atom gains or loses an electron.

Every atom or molecule we are made of is comprised of electrons, protons, a nucleus, and their oscillating energy fields. Atoms include charge, spin, speed of spin, axis, directionality and orientation to other structures. There is also gravity and spacing between particles. There are enough possible combinations of factors to produce an atomic 'signature' unique to each human structure. I believe our Energy Body or Biofield reads these signatures via biological light, electromagnetism, or a combination of both, to organize our energy flow to keep us functioning within our bandwidth of being. Furthermore, we remember the energy signatures of both living and non-living structures, like the taste of an almond, a task well done, the intentions of a competitor, the sound of flowing water. Our mental circuits flow best with coherency, order and understanding. We are constantly encountering higher and lower orders of interactions, higher and lower orders of understanding. Progress carries us into higher states of being.

A normal atom is electrically neutral with an equal number of protons and electrons. An atom gains or loses electrons when it collides with other atoms. Atoms that gain or lose electrons are called *ions*. Ions have an electric charge. Atoms that lose electrons become positive ions; atoms that win electrons become negative ions.

Since we are all walking bundles of atomic charge, I theorize that when we come into contact with one another, radiating our personal atomic signatures (physically) and intentions (mentally) we gain or lose electrons as soon contact is made. I believe these gains or losses of electrons on the subatomic level manifest on the physical plane as an immediate increase or decrease in strength and can be perceived by certain sensitive individuals as shifts in physical strength.

Humans naturally emit photons in the form of thermal radiation, primarily in the infrared spectrum. However, this emission is not consciously detectable by other humans in the course of ordinary interactions. Because the intensity of this interaction is quite low and not within the visible spectrum it is believed there is no established mechanism for humans to sense or perceive these emissions as a form of direct communication or interaction. However, we have complex sensory systems that allow us to perceive various stimuli from our environment, including visual, auditory, olfactory, tactile and other sensory cues. These senses enable communication, social interaction, and the interpretation of environmental signals but don't encompass direct perception of another's person's photonic emissions in the conventional understanding of human perception.

Some scientific research is exploring the potential for subtle electromagnetic interactions between living organisms, such as bioelectromagnetism and Biofields. Still concrete evidence supporting the conscious perception or sensing of others photonic emissions in a meaningful way, distinct from conventional senses, remains elusive and largely speculative.

The relationship between biophotonic emission and the body's electromagnetic field is complex and not fully understood. However, some hypotheses suggest that these ultra-weak photo emissions might be linked to the body's electromagnetic activity. It is theorized that biological processes generating biophotons may also involve bioelectric interactions, possibly impacting cellular communication, regulation, and overall health.

We are not just light-producing creatures. We are light! And thus, it may turn out that we have the ability to emit and receive photonic emissions from one another in a manner altering each other's electromagnetic fields. Many Kiko practitioners have told me they feel like they are transmitting or receiving 'something' words cannot describe.

I believe two people standing within close range will alter one another on a subatomic level, affecting each another's electron orbits, axis or spin. Hypothetically, when I give you energy, I might be prodding your electrons to take a quantum jump to the next excited state. That jump might be what gives a person increased power. I do not believe this postulate has been scientifically tested.

According to atomic energy physics, the electron will shed that increase in photonic voltage (decay) and revert back to its previous state. Coincidentally, we noticed during strength testing that our subjects could initially only hold a charge for approximately three seconds in a sine wave cycle that falls and rises for about 30 seconds before reverting to its homeostatic status. (Observation 68)

In your day-to-day, should you find yourself over-energized and need to release energy, you might notice standing to the left side of another. If you are under-energized and need a boost, you might find yourself standing on the right side of that person. If you don't want a person to alter your energy field you might turn askew, cross your arms, cover your dantien, or perhaps rotate a foot inward to prevent further energy drain or discharge. People exhibit unconscious actions that appear to protect them from a siphoning of their vital energy reservoir in the lower dantien.

Two fighters square off. With the exception of southpaws (lefties), both parties choose a left foot lead. From a Ki standpoint, this posturing is an inbuilt function to prevent individuals from initially drawing Ki from one another as the right side of the body tends to emit a stronger Ki field, which could be more easily drained if the combatants stood with right leads.

56* Your Energy Body has five primary orientations or attitudes which the Chinese refer to as Elements or *Phases*.

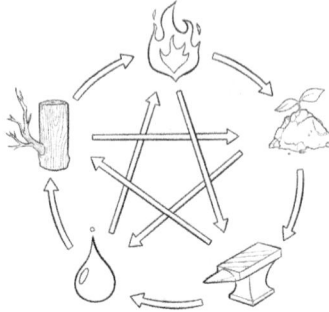

Cycle of Creation
(clockwise outer circle)

Fire Generates Earth
Earth Generates Metal
Metal Obtains Water
Water Produces Wood
Wood Fuels Fire

Cycle of Destruction
(inside arrows)

Water Puts Out Fire
Fire Destroys Metal
Metal Cuts Down Wood
Wood Covers Earth
Earth Absorbs Water

The five elemental orientations are called phases because they are not fixed events. They represent cyclical, ever-shifting, trans-formative attributes. Each phase exerts an influence upon the others. These influences fall into two primary Cycles: *The Cycle of Creation* and *The Cycle of Destruction*. The Cycle of Creation consists of actions that uplift, integrate or generate. The Cycle of Destruction comprises actions that release, downgrade, degrade or destroy. We need both cycles to get traction as living beings. Degrees of acquired positivity parallel the shedding of measures of degradation. Simply put, to become more positive, you have to give up or release some measure of negativity. To become stronger, you have to give up or release some level of weakness. To become healthy, you have to give up or release some level of ill health. Strange as it may sound, all our interactions lead either to the replacement of something better or worse. What is your martial training replacing?

57* Your Energy Body is always attempting to synchronize with the Energy fields of your immediate environment and the Universal Cosmic System.

At any given moment, your nature is always trying to do the best thing for you, to make the best decisions in your favor, even if those decisions lead to your demise. Sounds contradictory, doesn't it? Consider that some alcoholics will go into an unconscious stupor to avoid the debilitating pain of their life condition. It is their way to evade being overwhelmed. To the alcoholic, drinking feels like the right idea—escape the pain. But it is the wrong means. It is an attempt to steer oneself toward a better destination by choosing the low road, the wrong path. How many times do we see a confident fighter choose the wrong tactics and lose? He thought he was making the right choice. How many sensei have witnessed the student who seeks to prove his own self-worth by blatantly hurting other students?

The therapeutic side of martial arts is directed toward balanced training, otherwise you may gain terrific combative skills but still find yourself off-center and, like the alcoholic, end up at the wrong destination.

58* We live in two worlds.

As Within, So Without. As Above, So Below!
Hermes Trismegistus

We live in two martial worlds; an immaterium, composed of mind, thought, feelings, consciousness, dark matter and hidden energy waves, and a materium, our hard to the touch, form-filled, substantive world. Martial arts function in both of these dimensions. Western culture has focused on the external world, its see and touch reality—punch, kick, block, lock. The invisible side, the receipt and transmission of Ki-mustering quantum forces, is mostly absent in training. Focusing only in the material realm has dispossessed the majority of half their martial tool kit.

In his book, *The Case Against Reality*, the author, Donald Hoffman, states that Quantum physicists conclude, there is no objective reality. Your reality, my reality, is a projection of our beliefs.

Your interior reflects your outside world. Thus, what you believe is what you receive. You only see what you are looking for. Your inner (microcosm) and outer (macrocosm) worlds are polarized reflections, mirror images, of each other expressed in different mediums of energy (waves) and matter (particles).

59* The mezzocosm (middle world) is the junction between matter and spirit. It reveals the entanglement and complimentary nature of particle and wave, and marks a critical threshold of awareness in one's training.

Play with the following thought. How much do you know about the external world? By contrast, how much do you know about your inner world, the interior of yourself? I am not referring just to your physical anatomy but to everything that comprises the entity you call 'self'? Could you hazard a percentage guesstimate of knowledge between your outer and inner worlds? 70/30, 60/40, 50/50?

In Western cultures this percentage is heavily skewed in favor of external knowledge. It might be 80/20. The Chinese refer to the West as a Yang culture—outwardly focused to the point of lopsidedness.

Internal training is the effort to equalize this imbalance. Internal training is the practice of building interiority. Using Kiko, we attempt to expand our knowledge and sensitivity of our own inner functioning to bring it up to par with our external knowledge. Another way to put this is that Western culture is matter dominant. Spiritual practice is a means to level this dominance, to even out this bias by investing in your etheric nature.

Most of you are familiar with the terms, microcosm and macrocosm. Spiritual teachers tell us that the larger (macro) world is reflected in the smaller (micro) world. Conversely, within the small is contained the large. These two vastly different terrains reflect one another. The microcosm is a projection of the macrocosm. The macrocosm is a mirror of the microcosm.

This is near impossible for most to see, no less comprehend. If your interior world is only a quarter of what you know of the external world, you won't have enough grasp of the vastness of your interior to see how these two worlds interface. You must go inward if you wish to build interiority. A term used to describe moving inward is transliminal, literally crossing a threshold between the outer and inner worlds.

There is one more concept to add to this mix—the *mezzocosm*, the middle world. The mezzocosm is the midpoint between the micro and macrocosms. This midpoint is arrived at when your interior and exterior worlds find equilibrium. One goal of internal training is to bring these two worlds into balance, into accord. This union is important if one is to restore their power legacy.

When your knowledge of the external world far exceeds that of your inner world, you will blame all your failures and defeats on events outside of yourself, beyond your control.

When these two worlds are in balance (I'm not talking about your daily life going okay. I'm referring to your knowledge of how these two worlds relate) you will realize you have far more power than you thought over your life circumstances. Empowerment comes from the knowledge that you, as a self-organizing microcosm, can project whatever you choose onto the macrocosmic screen. You may feel your opponent or Life, is out to get you, until you choose to think differently.

As long as you remain under the spell that your outside world exerts a greater influence upon you than you exert upon it, you will not realize the truth of this statement. The aim of Kiko training is not just a faster, stronger martial technique, but a more resilient, vital and powerful self.

The quest to find the mezzocosm begins by building interiority. Learning how to control your body is the first stage. Body control is the most tangible of the developmental stages for building interiority because the results are both observable and measurable and thus motivational. The next stage is learning to control your Ki.

It is an error in judgement to think that you are solely a matter form and anything immaterial is inconsequential, an illusory substance accidentally stuck to you by happenchance with no influence over your life activities or direction.

According to Shifu Nagaboshi, even the most serious and diligent practitioners will never achieve higher levels of their art well within reach. The problem is a lack of understanding how physical practices relate to breathing exercises and concentration techniques. Once this hurdle is cleared, other levels of training can advance. In his opinion, a martial art is greatly enhanced by structuring it correctly with respect to meditation practices. He believed the archetypal image of a Kempo master was one of rapture in seated meditation. Understanding your internal processes puts new levels of achievement within your reach. Shifu Nagaboshi outlined seven meditative stages to provide the internalist with a guideline to follow. The Eight Levels of Meditation are; Self-Restraint/*Yama*, Observance/*Niyama*, Physical Practice/*Asana,* Breathing Exercise, Sense Withdrawal, Concentration, Meditation, and Superconsciousness. See: isshinkempo.com/wp-content/uploads/2019/05/the-eight-levels-of-meditation.pdf

60* Kiko practice is oriented toward three interlocking goals; heightened practical use, enhanced therapeutic effect, spiritual and evolutionary advance.

Not everyone's purpose for martial study aims at the same target or even the same arena. Reasons for engaging a martial art can be incredibly diverse; sport, competition, socialization, weight loss, philosophical expansion, conflict resolution. These goals can range from the superficial to the profound. One's initial purpose can also radically change midstream. You might have started purely for self-defense then became enamored by its athleticism. You might have entered martial arts hearing about its philosophy for mastering your mind, or purely as a competitive outlet. The monastic masters determined that there were three primary, interlinked reasons for taking up any martial study; You do it for its practical value, whether for self-protection, fitness, self-development, competitive release, enhanced concentration etc., you take it up for better health, or you join the thinner ranks of those who train for spiritual growth.

Regardless of your reasons, the longer you train with an open mind, the greater the chance you will see the interlinked value of these three primary fields of knowledge. If you are pushing hard on your physical workouts but neglecting to eat properly, don't get enough sleep, aren't reducing your overall life frictions or stresses, you are undermining your training goals.

When you remove the limitations that maintain a narrow perimeter of your inner dojo, as these walls drop away, you enter the Dō of martial study.

TECHNIQUE

61* Directing the mind to systematically attend to micro and macro orbits around the body vitalizes the Energy Body for more potent movement.

Orbiting

Nearly every internal martial art practitioner will encounter the concept of the *Microcosmic Orbit*. This orbit is described as an unbroken elliptical current flowing from head to tail around everyone's body. (There are varying degrees of depth one can work with). This grand current is active whether you are aware of it or not. It can become blocked, constricted, or reversed. Understanding, attending to, or controlling this current will improve the quality of your Ki flow.

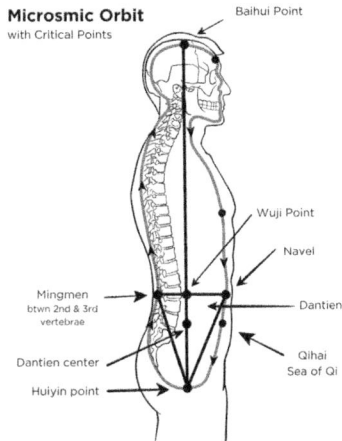

Microsmic Orbit with Critical Points

Baihui Point

Wuji Point

Navel

Mingmen btwn 2nd & 3rd vertebrae

Dantien

Dantien center

Qihai Sea of Qi

Huiyin point

This particular clockwise orbital direction is called the *Fire Path*. It stimulates the body, producing energy and enhanced strength. I've indicated significant points along the current for further investigation. The *Water Path* reverses the direction of Ki flow and is practiced for its calming effects on the body. Other variants exist, each with unique effects.

Think of the Microcosmic Orbit as a river supplying its tributaries, the limbs, and your lower abdomen act as a catch basin or grand reservoir, or what the Okinawans call *Kikai*, sea of Ki. You quickly get the idea of its significance.

You could also think of the Microcosmic Orbit in a more scientific manner as the flow of electrons around the torso and through its four limb conduits to light up the musculature of our arms and legs. Ki as voltage (potential) determines how fast the Ki is moving. Or, you could think of a muscle as voltage. When you limit the current, you limit the muscle's output.

What I find interesting about this orbital practice is how Western culture, is never taught to systematically attend to our Energy Body. People, for the most part eat, think and engage their world with a fair amount of randomness in various states of semi-consciousness. Take your average day; What draws your attention to your body? Maybe you get an itch, an internal buildup of gas in your stomach makes your belly uncomfortable, or your waist belt is too tight, dust gets into your eye, or you get a tingling in your elbow when you bang it. Some stimulus draws you inward, holding your mind there until you can make sense of what, if anything, you need to do. There is no set pattern to the stimuli that constantly bombards us, or our reactions to these stimuli. It's all very arbitrary. When you practice a Fighting Art you will also be drawn inward. You mind will focus on three objectives; the feel of a technique, the look of a technique (does it match up to what you are being shown?), and the outcome when applying the technique—does it work? You will look at, feel, and evaluate your movements as the cross hairs for achieving proper technique. Stepping back from this process, something else occurs, something many professionals don't talk about—the value of holding your attention on your physical actions.

Internal practice takes technical refinement to a whole new level. The act of systematically attending to your Energy Body builds up a charge in the entire system, evidenced by the significant uptick in muscular output.

Practicing the Microcosmic Orbit is the act of directing and feeling your mind move along this elliptical path. That is, you guide your attention to move over the surface of your body in the direction of the Orbit's flow while simultaneously observing and allowing feedback from your body as you do so. This results in a brilliant braiding of the mind with your Energy Body. It reminds me of a bladesmith forging different steels together to create one cohesive billet.

There is no western practice in existence that asks us to direct and hold our attention to any prescribed internal energy pattern to systematically optimize our performance.

The Orbit moves with or without your attention, in the same way your breathing moves with or without your awareness. However, when you switch from involuntary to voluntary, you gain conscious control over a process previously unconscious.

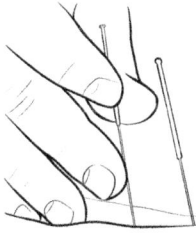

During an acupuncture treatment, the therapist noted that my Microcosmic Orbit had reversed. I told him to wait a moment then retest. On his retest, he commented, "Okay it's flowing correctly." I had mentally reversed the flow. With conscious intent you can clear your subtle channels of obstructions. This leads to increased body charge and more vitality. Here is a simple test that works for most:

A Test: Stand in a neutral posture and relax for nine seconds. Let your mind draw an imaginary line around your body, starting from your tongue lightly adhered to the roof of your mouth, flowing downward over your throat, your chest, down the belly, under and around the perineum, up the back, neck, over the top of your head and back to the tongue. Consider this one orbit. Let your imagination choose the speed of flow. Do this visualization three times. Try a strength test again after completing three cycles.

Attending to better nourishment leads to more tissue integrity and performance. Consistent martial practice builds stronger muscle, coordination, reaction time, balance and endurance. When you meditate, you sweep the mind clean of useless and negative thoughts and calm the nervous system. When you systematically attend to strengthening your Energy Body, your bodily tissues get more juice, more charge. All of these attendances lead to a synchronization toward increasing levels of potency. I call these systematic engagements, the Four Nourishments. When each practice is approached and acted upon intelligently and systematically, they link up to form one overarching system. Throughout history there have been various martial arts, Yogic disciplines, Qigong systems, and Asian temple practices that have recognized the importance of this quaternion engagement. However, modern times has dismantled many of these systems by reducing them to trendy, fragmented, boutique practices with minimal vitalization.

The Four Nourishments

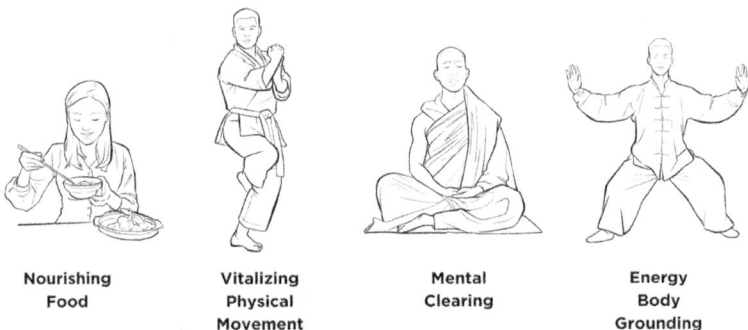

| Nourishing Food | Vitalizing Physical Movement | Mental Clearing | Energy Body Grounding |

Next time you get a moment, take your Energy Body out for a spin, literally. Do fifteen minutes of Orbiting. Give your electrical system a fine tuning. You will not be disappointed.

62* Correct proportionality in limb positioning is part of the Energy Body equation.

The Polarity/Proportionality Relationship

To derive maximum power from your limbs, it is necessary to understand the relationship of polarity to proportionality. All stances and stance work possess both a Yin cycle proportionality and Yang cycle proportionality. Slight external changes to a stance's length or width can switch the polarity from yin to yang or yang to yin. These changes can be done consciously following a Kiko formula. This story will illustrate:

I began Kiko testing the katas of my system by evaluating each movement sequences for maximum Ki charge. The work was slow and painstaking. One sequence in the Seisan kata ends with a downward chop to the side of the body as performed by the system's founder. Oddly, I arrived at a different conclusion. The proper placement of my arm and hand was not to the side but slightly rounded in front of my thigh. I passed this change along to my instructors to present to their students.

One sensei, White Tiger, was about to announce the change to his adult class when he was approached by his student, Tony, a former Wing Chun practitioner. Tony questioned why the hand was placed at the side. White Tiger explained coincidentally, that it was no longer to be placed at the side but in front of the thigh. Tony demonstrated a similar Wing Chun posture and asked why the move was not done like this. White Tiger wasn't sure. When he got the chance, he pulled me aside and related his conversation and showed me the posture Tony had shown him. To his bewilderment I said, "He did not show you that posture."

My response surprised him. How could I possibly know what posture Tony had shown him? I had a pretty good idea from the extensive testing I had done. "This is what he showed you," I said. I took the posture White Tiger conveyed to me and rotated my torso slightly.

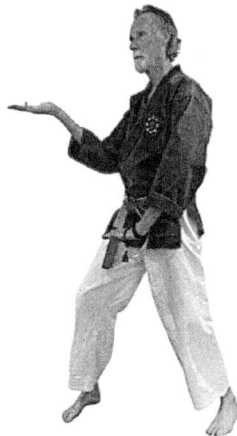

The next time White Tiger saw Tony, he asked him to repeat the Wing Chun posture from the prior week. Tony assumed the exact posture I had demonstrated.

I was however, perplexed later when testing that very move from the Seisan kata, for it did not align with the founder's form. The founder held his hand to the side, while my hand worked best placed in front of my thigh. I soon realized the difference. The hand placement had to do with the width of my stance. Isshin Kempo's Seisan dachi is one foot-width wider than the traditional Seisan dachi. And this made all the difference. Both actions are correct. The lesson is not to mix and match moves amongst different Fighting systems. This alters the Energy equation and outcome. For example, if you stand in the narrower Seisan dachi and place you hand in front of your thigh, you will lose strength. Conversely, if you stand in the wider posture and place your hand at your side you get the same weakening result.

63* Each limb can move up to a maximum of four primary directions simultaneously, out of a total eight directions.

During my research, I noted eight primary directions any limb can move. This understanding gave me sharper insight into how Ki distributes throughout the body. At first, it was hard to see the arms moving in an eight-directional framework. The breakthrough came when I imagined myself a four-legged creature. I bent over, placed my hands on the ground and asked, how many primary directions could I now move my arms? The answer is eight, same for the legs.

1. Up
2. Down
3. Forward
4. Backward
5. Toward the center
6. Away from the center
7. Clockwise
8. Counter-clockwise

Of these eight moves, one alone for the legs, not the arms, is central to the remaining seven. Before you can move a leg, you need to lift it slightly off the ground to overcome any friction.

64* The eight limb directions can be combined into four paired sets.

Of the eight directions, four motions are opposite the other. This gives us four paired movement sets consisting of one direction and its reverse action. Classifying limb motions into primary moves helped me to understand Ki flow as a signaling mechanism to the muscles. The moment you intend to reach forward, a charge is sent to the muscles supporting that motion. This biocurrent reverses when you retract your arm. Knowing the direction Ki flowed gave me greater control over my Biofield and that of an adversary. When you know your adversary's Ki is coming toward you, you can grab hold of it.

Knowing the direction of another's Ki flow also enables a Kiko practitioner to choose the optimum block, strike, or lock to draw it further out of them. Ki flowing down someone's arm toward you also reveals how it is moving in the rest of their body. Because the Biofield system is interconnected, like a circuit board, you gain access to a wider variety of technique and tactics. For example, knowing there is a large flow moving down an attacker's right arm tells me the inside of his left leg is vulnerable. By analogy, if you've ever been to an acupuncturist, you might be baffled when you complain of a toothache and a needle is inserted into your ankle. A strong action in one limb can cause weakness in another.

Four Pairs of Limb Motions
1. Up/down
2. Backward/forward
3. Lateral left/lateral right
4. Clockwise/counter clockwise

65* Four of the eight limb actions are Yin. Four of the eight are Yang actions. One of the four is a primary function fueling the remaining three.

One action in each paired set is a Yin action, meaning, the movement activates the body's Yin channels. An example of a Yin channel activator is pulling or withdrawing your arm toward your center. An example of a Yang Channel activator is extending an arm away from your body for pushing or punching

I am oversimplifying to make a point. On an advanced level, someone can withdraw their arm and still have it be a Yang action as a result of a Soft Gate override. To go any deeper into this aspect of energy manipulation requires in-depth, hands-on explanation. For the purpose of this work, I leave the above trail marker for your further investigation.

66 *Understanding how to overcome any one of the four Yin or four Yang pairs allows you to identify and overcome the other three.

The prime reason for understanding the eight directions and the paired sets is to identify the bioenergetic nature of a move or posture as either Yin or Yang so you can more readily choose the correct formula for weakening your opponent, strengthening yourself, or a combination of the two goals. Let's now look at the two primary formulas for disrupting another's Energy Body/Biofield/Ki.

67* The two major formulas for diminishing another's Energy Body are underwhelming, drawing the charge off someone, or overwhelming, sending a fast, increased charge into them.

The above two formulas frame out the central goal of martial Kiko. We maximize our success by using our own malleable Biofield. I have established that physical or mental actions can project or receive Ki, weakening an opponent unaware of this tactic. Either formula can make an adversary susceptible to greater damage when struck, and less able or unable to resist locks placed upon them.

To achieve a contact or contactless projection or reception of Ki involves a multi-stage process. First, you must learn the fundamentals of Hard and Soft Gating and what distinguishes the two modes from one another. You must also train to rewire your system to hold and run a stronger current. This requires freeing up any blocked or closed Ki channels. Meditation is an excellent base practice for opening both the psychic and physical channels. You can also directly address physical imbalances in your musculoskeletal system with a proper stretching or yogic regime. Next, you need partnered work to sense how Ki flows between people. You can't learn this skill in a vacuum, solo. Finally, you will need concrete, affirming practices that you have successfully sent or received Ki from one another. One effective method is to follow this rule; Overwhelm another's Biofield by a fast projection of Ki from your right side into their left side. A fast projection of Ki will instantly disrupt their field. A slow projection will give them strength.

You can underwhelm an opponent by receiving from their right into your left side. Here, the speed can be fast or slow. Again, I'm oversimplifying and it's a bit premature if you have no skill in moving energy, but this will be a useful piece of information down the road.

68* Duration (the time a limb or the body can hold a charge) is part of Energy Body functioning.

Correlating Strength and Time

At the early stages of Ki work, everyone we tested experienced a three second strength burst. That is, Hard and Soft Gates worked best if acted upon within a three second time frame from the initiation of the Gate to the actual task or test required. Thereafter, every limb change appeared to initiate a re-regulation or rerouting of the Biofield to one's normal vibrational frequency. I believe this involuntary adjustment is designed to keep us within a bioenergetic comfort zone. That is, your body wants to stay within its established bandwidth. This vibratory comfort zone varies for each person.

As the original mystery of the effortless escape from Stone's grip garnered more insights, it also drew in a wider circle of interested martial artists. Our expanded group think tank has accelerated our knowledge of the Biofield's behavior allowing us to catalog many postures and movement sets that charge the body for specific tasks.

I recognize how difficult it is for many people to enter or hold a neutral mind space. Letting go of our individual biases is a separate study and challenge in itself. Even two of my senior yudansha had difficulty relinquishing their need to be strong when we were testing ways to release Energy. This was further complicated by the fact all of us were evolving how we held and moved our Ki. A similar affect can be observed in external training. Things you were ultra-conscious of initially, like throwing your first side kick, snap punch, or trying your first submission hold, get taken for granted years later. As you ingrain your techniques into muscle memory, more of their functioning is given over to the unconscious, freeing up Ki to be directed elsewhere. We had to factor this moving progression into our later tests.

We reached a point where by assembling the limbs in traditional martial configurations, holding a neutral mental state, we could be reasonably assured of positive results. A Yin posture weakened most of us when a Yang posture or action was called for. A Yang posture weakened most of us when a Yin posture or action was called for. Sometimes we would get results opposite of what we expected, but later figured out the missing variable(s); directionality, time of day, lunar cycle, type of clothing, unconscious agendas, etc.

During one test, a thought arose which I had never considered. I had asked someone to stand in a Sanchin stance, exhaling, while executing a Yang (sending) mid-body block. I expected the subject to test strong, which he did, when a flash of curiosity hit me. How long would his strength from Hard Gating last? It could not be indefinite. That would go against all known science. So, I began taking time measurements. The answer turned out to be a remarkably consistent, three seconds across almost all subjects. On seconds 4,5,6, our test subjects went weak. What really blew my mind was testing on seconds 7,8,9. Subjects tested strong again! This ebb and flow current ran for roughly six to ten cycles or 30 seconds before subjects tested neutral—as if they had not Gated at all.

Three seconds is more than enough time to place or resist a forceful joint lock, parry, or strike. This three second 'on' function can be a life saver. Gating will give you a burst of Herculean strength long enough to apply or overcome most locks at their initial stage of application.

A student's inability to hold a continuous charge returns us to the automatic presets of our homeostatic Biofield circuitry. In the beginning, none of us could hold a charge longer than three seconds because we had not rewired sufficiently to run a continuously strong current. The body does not operate like a light switch; flick on, flick off. It adjusts gradually, like the example of the sloshing water tub I used earlier in the book. Once vigorously stirred, our Biofield can only settle gradually.

The other side of Hard and Soft Gating we had to consider was the distinct drop in strength after a Ki surge. I had never considered that physical strength increased and decreased in a sine wave cycle. The Energy Body functions in pulses with peak Yang or Yin strength cycles occurring in timed intervals of three seconds 'on,' three seconds 'off'. Polarity keeps flipping to its opposite until Biofield equilibrium is established, like tapping a car brake to gradually stop.

As the years passed, another side of the Kiko equation loomed. The more advanced practitioners were able to generate a more continuous charge. This shifted the training focus to increasing our mental permeability. A porous mind is more receptive to a free-flowing Energy state that fills as it empties, where the body stays as strong as long as you like with continuous replenishment. My understanding of the term Karate-te (empty hand) morphed. I began to think of my art less as a sought after static empty state, but rather as a vigorous emptying and filling of my being.

In Japanese arts such of Aikido or Judo, the word for "emptying hand" is "*kote osu*" (こておす) or "*kote kaeshi*" (こてかえし). "Kote" (こて) refers to the wrist and "*osu*" (おす) or "*kaeshi*" (かえし) means to release or redirect the opponent's attack by emptying one's hand or wrist. The Japanese for "filling hand" is "*tenbin nage*" (てんびんなげ) "*Tenbin*" (てんびん) refers to the balance scale and "*nage*" (なげ) means to throw or toss. "*Tenbin nage*" is a technique where one fills their hand with the opponent's energy and then throws them off balance like a balance scale.

69* We are the world. The world is shifting.
We are the essence of this shift.

We exist in an expansive sea of cyclical energies coursing through the universe as we enter what some historians call, the

Fourth Turning, the end of a saeculum, an intense generational cycle of crisis and awakening. To borrow a term from the aikidoist, Cliff High, the martial "narradigm" is changing. The narrative we've been told about traditional martial arts that forms our beliefs about their value is reconfiguring. By opening our arts up to the quantum realities discussed in this book practitioners have the potential to enter a new frontier. Choose a balanced martial path and you contribute to vitality, steadiness, equanimity, balance and peace in the world. Quelling even one enemy, inner or outer, brings the world one step closer to harmony.

I believe our mind is the conscious part of our Energy Body. The ego stakes out a smaller parcel of psychic territory with the task of filtering information solely to preserve its identity. Because our egos possess limited awareness of our Biofield, it's easy to find our unconscious mind antagonistic to our conscious desires and thus, get in our own way. A number of pioneering scientists from diverse fields argue that the mind is not just in our brain but also happens between us, that consciousness is the result of our relating.

Failure and success, victory and defeat, loss and gain, is the normal pulse of life. Beyond these natural occurrences, I use a simple template to assess all the meaningful gains from my training. I strive for, and teach others to strive for, three powers; clarity of mind, joyfulness of the heart, and vitality of the body. These attributes optimize one of the three dantiens and lead to lightness and buoyancy of Spirit. If you can achieve and maintain this state of being every day you have reached the pinnacle of inner contentment and success as a natural human being, supportive of a cohesive society in harmony with the natural world.

PART 4

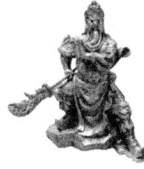

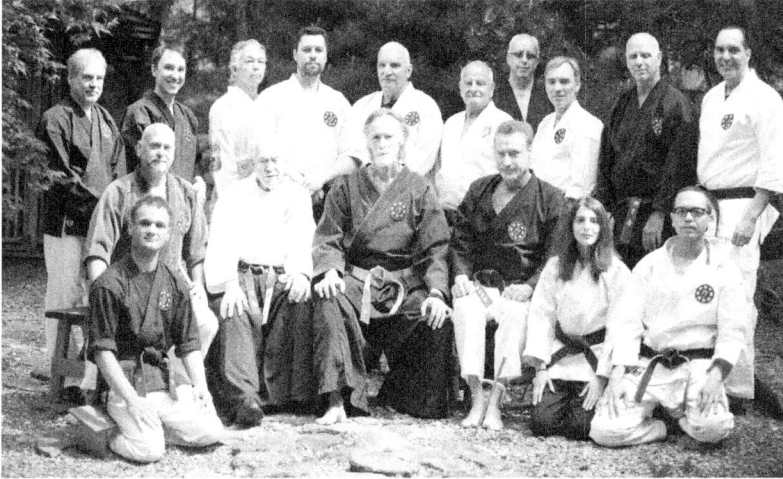

Senior yudansha of Isshin Kempo collectively representing over
550 years of martial experience. May 2023

Questing for Answers

*Live the questions now. Perhaps then, someday far in
the future, you will gradually, without even noticing it, live
your way into the answer.*

Maria Rilke Rainer

*"When the student is ready the teacher appears. When the
question is asked then the answer is heard. When we are truly
ready to receive then what we need will become available."*

John Gray

*"In some cases,' he said, 'we learn more by looking for the
answer to a question and not finding it than we do from
learning the answer itself."*

Lloyd Alexander, Book of Three

Return Fire

Shifu Hayashi answers pertinent questions.

Q. You claim that Kiko is a revolutionary approach to traditional martial art understanding, but aren't you just repackaging Qigong in a fancy new rapper?

Initially, I thought I had arrived late on the bandwagon to something all Soft stylists were well acquainted with. I incorrectly assumed that every internalist had a firm grasp about Kiko principles in their arts, though by different terms and methods. It was just us hard-headed stylists in the dark. I discovered this was far from the truth. There is very little agreement about the nuts and bolts of internal work once you get beyond the fundamentals. Soft stylists do not train with the understanding they are likely manipulating their electro-magnetic biocurrents. On Okinawa, Kiko focused primarily on *Iron Shirt* or *Golden Bell* practices to withstand gross body blows and pressure point attacks. Additionally, because internal principles were often learned by feel, a huge gap exists in Kiko's workings outside of the *kyusho* (pressure point) and Iron Shirt practices. It is the conscious, logical, and progressive interlinking of the subtle energies of the body/mind complex into fighting technique and Forms that distinguishes Kiko from other training platforms. I am not redesigning the wrapper as much as redefining the contents of the package. I am expanding the current model of Energy work by introducing Kiko as an instant foundational strength enhancement. I am not the only one discussing this subject, nor do I have all the answers. The time is ripe for this information to reach a wider audience. To date, there have simply not been enough voices loud and clear enough to grab the ears of the broader martial community about Kiko's value.

Q. How does Kiko function in a traditional fighting form?

Most teachers expect their students to perform a kata with speed, power and precision, and/or demonstrate its practical applications. Kiko addresses a kata's specific configuration in terms of its ability to generate what I believe is an electromagnetic charge/discharge cycle to maintain physical power throughout performance and to disrupt another's energy field during its application. It is not whether a kata is done in the proper surface manner that determines whether one is using Kiko. It is the *meta*-precision inherent in a Form's configuration, how the Energy Body is organized, that makes the difference. It's not what feels right to the performer but what is right for the Biofield. It is the refined, calculated, rhythmic pulsing and pacing, brought about by the careful and conscious entwinement of the breath, body positioning, and a synchronous mindset that defines Kiko-based fighting forms. This dimension is currently lacking in modern kata performance because our rationalist, materialist culture has devalued Ki's subjective basis. If we continue to hold to this current martial mindset, we will lose sight of Kiko's revelatory threshold altogether.

Q. Can you talk specifically about your research into kata?

We know from historical evidence that kata served a vital role in Asian fighting systems. But when it comes to explaining why the specific arrangement of these kata sets were created, things quickly become murky. I define a kata set as a Form's suggested remedy to an explicit action against you. Only after divining the factors of how and why we gained impressive strengths from Kiko did I dial my attention to kata and begin some earnest research. If I told you that performing a movement sequence correctly, would increase your strength by 50% or more, would that draw your attention? If kata possessed this hidden quality, as I contend, my research led to a means to test and validate whether any kata contained this information. I initially tested only individual technique and later advanced to testing short sequences of kata moves. However, I was presented with a major hurdle from the start. Many kata today have decoupled from any internal principles that may have been planted in them. I label these patterns, degraded. Nevertheless, I began testing kata sequences the way I had been taught. Later, I compared the results to Shimabuku's video performances and other variations of the Form. At this stage, I made no attempt to determine the kata's bunkai. That focus came later.

The results were intriguing. First, I discovered there are many Kiko formulas. Second, reviewing Shimabuku's videos, I could not say if the casual manner of his performances represented his most exacting exhibition, because in some cases his moves did not stand up to our testing. Kata detail needs to be very exact to get the proper surge of energy. Since Shimabuku is not here to defend his knowledge, we will never know. Here's an example of what I was up against. In Chinto kata there is a sequence where you about-face into a reverse Cat stance, put up a high cover with both hands, then step into a Horse stance and elbow (at least, that's what it looks like). Shimabuku's version tested weak if we held our hands one fist above our shoulders. If we lowered the hands by one fist width, or raised them by the same proportion, the set gained impressive strength. How many martial artists are adhering to such strict posturing? Even Shimabuku's stances did not always fall into the standard definitions of these postures.

Any fight sequence done correctly should lead to a major surge of energy. When applied to a kata's bunkai, it will give one unusual grip control or striking power. Our ongoing research has revealed other dimensions and value to kata work beyond the current purview practiced today.

Q. How is anyone to remember the optimal direction to turn or what breathing pattern to adopt in the midst of a physical crisis or competition? Aren't you asking the impossible?

Imagine I asked a similar question of a novice viewing a traditional fighting system for the first time. I can hear the lament. 'How am I supposed to remember all these blocking, kicking, punching and controlling manipulations and put them together in a fluid response?' This question is no different. Kiko is another skill set, another layer. The only way to become adept at Kiko is to practice and develop the sensitivity to feel the correct moves once you have absorbed their underlying principles.

Q. Is Kiko applicable to ground grappling?

My research has focused primarily on traditional standing disciplines and their fighting forms. I have seen significant strength shifts in standing grappling technique with Kiko applied. The evidence to date strongly suggests we should see a difference applying Kiko to ground technique. I am particularly interested in the entering tactics chosen to take someone to the ground. In the future we would love to work with some ground experts to explore Kiko's potential in this arena.

Q. What do you say to people who think kata performance is a wasted effort and that one should just stick to hands-on moves?

You don't need kata to become a good fighter. That's been proven. But this attitude doesn't answer the question why older, refined cultures like India or China, arrived at the creation, perpetuation and performance of fighting patterns. Sociologists have defined Western societies as a low context culture. We want to get right to the point. 'You want to learn how to fight? Screw kata. Glove up; punch, kick and roll.' This method however, tosses out any vital history, penetrating philosophies, centuries long trial and error results, and the subtlety of body dynamics. Do we really want to start from scratch? Okay, to each his own. I think we can find as many examples of kata performance done incorrectly, or for the wrong reasons, as done for the right ones. In this regard, it's probably best to stick with a kata's bunkai.

There is another perspective to consider. Treatises on military strategy and tactics are highly sought after works because they give the militarist a grand picture. They put the combatant's goals into sharper perspective. This helps commanding warriors to understand the forest in relationship to the trees, unless you are in the infantry and just take orders. But no martial art removes its combative trees for the remaining barren field. You would not have a martial art. In a similar manner, nobody with intelligence, about to engage a large enemy force, would chuck the insights of a Clausewitz, Sun Tzu, his counterpart in the West, Hannibal, or Hammurabi, Alexander the Great or a J.C. Wylie, because their works weren't in the trench experiences. These works are read because they organize the mind to the core concerns of any battle. These strategists codified the entire battlefield experience. A fight between two people is a war on small scale, utilizing all the same principles. Kata are treatises for the martial art student, written in the gritty action of sweat, blood and tears training. Rather than appealing to the literary minded, the ancient masters presented their lessons directly to the kinesthetic, touch-and-feel, gut senses. You learn through rehearsal. You 'read' by moving your body through ideas encoded in the kata's preset patterns. When you have comprehended what you have read, you put it to the test. Kata without bunkai is a shallow warrior dance.

A long-term teacher told me he never asks his students to perform kata. He prefers to immediately practicalize its moves. His point is valid. However, from my neighboring side of the fence, I ask students to perform kata. Control over oneself leads to better control over others. Also, knowing why a movement sequence is being done in the manner shown reinforces the particular tactics and techniques in muscle memory. I rarely encounter teachers who understand kata as a tactical manual or how it builds internal strength through its rehearsed patterns. So naturally, the practical-minded prefer to dispense with solo kata performance. A kata's bunkai conveys technical controls that we then subject to our own further analysis and testing. Kata analysis is our attempt to ground what is being taught. The problem emerges when kata is taught in a vacuum, where one thinks that sheer rote performance of a kata alone is enough to magically produce ace combat skills. That formula is incorrect.

Let's put martial training into proper context. The vast majority of active students do not have access to round-the-clock training partners. So, when alone, they condition. Kata is one type of conditioning exercise. Any martial artist who rehearses their technique, or a series of techniques by themselves, is essentially practicing Kata.

Also, anyone who tells you there is only one way up the martial mountain should be listened to with a grain of salt. Martial champions and victors have hailed by many routes. New ones are being paved as I write. The one thing all champions have in common however, is immersion in their craft. Train in a manner relevant to your goals and in sync with your nature. Whichever method you prefer, understand how it fits into your overall pursuits.

Q. You say that kata or formwork was the general means by which Kiko principles were conveyed. Were the Asian kata perfect transmissions of this knowledge?

No. They were not perfect transmissions because the critical explanations for why the katas were so precisely constructed were not passed along. Kata for those early Westerners was like being handed a document in a foreign language without much explanation other than its contents were important to understand. In addition, knowledge of Kiko, or any other term referring to subtle energy work, was neither common nor widespread in Asia. The subject was known only to small groups of Asian masters and passed to an even smaller group of Westerners. Even after having rooted into Western culture, now over seventy years, we are just beginning to breach the depth of Asia's fighting forms. Kata's outer nature appears to have been passed mostly intact. My personal opinion, however, is that many kata were degrading even in Asia as a result of the art's commercialization at the beginning of the Industrial Revolution in the mid-18th century. We must also consider the reluctance of vanquished cultures like Okinawa and Japan wanting or willing to share their cultural treasures with their conquerors.

To make disciplines like Karate, Tae Kwon Do or Jiu-jitsu commercially viable, you have to streamline the teaching curriculum, otherwise you lose the average person's attention. Only a minority of the populace have the capacity to understand and appreciate the rich technical diversity the Asian kata offer. You can't easily sell complexity to the mainstream but you can sell the mysterious, as people are naturally curious. The martial arts were mythologized and mysticized to lure more people into their study. Ankoh Itosu and Gichin Funakoshi recognized this when they introduced karate to the public. They diluted their arts to make them more palatable to a wider audience because martial subtlety is lost on most practitioners. Add to this the faulty transmission to first generation Western practitioners, the majority of whom were never exposed to Kiko or spent enough time to get its nuts and bolts, and most are left with stripped-down disciplines.

Q. How would a Kiko practitioner stand up against fighters from other styles?

Kiko is not a fighting style. Kiko is a subset of principles that can be implemented in any standing or ground fighting system. It would be more pertinent to ask, 'How would a fighter with a refined understanding of technique fare against a fighter with less refined technique? Outside of heart and grit, I think the answer is self-evident. Consider Kiko an 'inside' art. External and internal technique are meant to be interlocking. If I showed you how a slight change in your stance with the correct respiratory pattern added significant power to your techniques, would you want to take that knowledge into your next match? Most traditional arts already have strong biomechanical foundations. Kiko reinforces this foundation by adding a sturdy, bioenergetic sub-flooring.

Q. Is it possible for someone to be attuned to their Ki flow without formal training in Kiko?

Yes. In the physical arena, such people are called natural athletes. But this kind of person is a rarity, even though I feel many people slip in and out of higher connectivity under the right conditions. My broader answer however, comes in shades of gray. Most of us find that we ride upon Life's seas sometimes in sync with the waves, other times not. Intuition and logic can either help or hinder our progress. Kiko challenges our current paradigm. How much are we actually aware of? Are we as organized as we could be? Are we being effective? Is this the best performance we are capable? Over decades investigating martial Kiko, I never came across a single person who demonstrated a firm grasp on the subject. Regardless how gifted, strong, and intelligent, most benefited from Kiko work. I consider Kiko a rarely used rung on the human evolutionary ladder. Although Kiko can lead a disciple to unexplored territory, sadly, it is missing from most martial tool boxes.

Q. As a Buddhist, aren't you practicing and teaching violence while contradicting your practice with a vow not to harm life?

Martial art is neither the practice of, nor support for, violent behavior. At their core, these arts were meant to quell violence, not encourage or glorify it. Buddhist martial discipline is the practice of non-violence. My martial practice has placed the concept of conflict under a mental microscope to better understand aggression, violence, and my personal role in reducing it. Since my Buddhist indoctrination, I have focused my training on ways to defuse or neutralize oppositions rather than vanquish by injury or death when less lethal methods are available. I've sought to give others not just defensive technique but the means to control their emotions to avoid losing their moral compass to an animal impulse that could lead to a regrettable outcome.

There is always the possibility in a violent exchange that your actions come down to your life or another's. In such a circumstance, you will have to choose—live or die? Only you can make that choice. Better to work through the thorniness of this question now than in the midst of such a struggle.

There is another feature to the question that regards the ego.

Psychologists use the term 'ego' to describe a part of our mind that identifies us as unique and separate from everything outside us. This aspect of our mind can find itself in a protracted tension between belonging and defending its separateness. Threats to its boundary can trigger insecurity and the false belief that aggression is the only means to defend oneself. But the only way to develop a balanced state of mind, whether a defense against illness, undesirable characteristics, or literal opponents, is not to rid yourself of the undesirable experience, but rather, to embrace it. This action is found in the concept of *Ahimsa*, non-violence. Ahimsa is a non-violent way of dealing with opposition.

If you think forces exist to destroy you, you will want to rid yourself of them. Instead of assuming a defensive or aggressive posture, you can develop and extend *metta*, in Sanskrit, *maitri*—loving kindness. All our root problems and difficulties actually generate from the concept of duality or separateness which creates a gap between others and 'I'.

When you do not think in terms of fighting against your problems or an enemy, you will see that the martial arts, from a transcendental point of view, deals with, and exercises, the art of war in a very different manner than the popular concept of 'enemy' conjures.

Three things cause us imbalance; ignorance, hatred and desire. Unbalanced behavior will always deal with a situation by acting improperly. This leads to an incomplete action, the result of not being fully aware of the situation, of not feeling present. When a present action is not handled properly, the fundamental imbalance remains unresolved. One will drift to the next problem igniting a series of cyclical conflicts, like eating unripe fruits. You may put one piece down and seek another fruit that seems to taste better. But if your taste buds are impaired, you will be unable to avoid eating unripe produce, causing you endless indigestion.

Ignorance means ignoring the present. Someone who ignores what is, creates a situation of never being in the now. Instead, their mind is occupied by experiences either of the past, or expectations of the future. Such a person will be unable to accomplish present work thoroughly.

To think of overcoming or challenging issues with aggressiveness is imbalanced and will always lead to some level of violence. The real way of the warrior is to avoid being aggressive. Move instead from a foundation of loving kindness. Solving problems through aggression versus compassion are very different actions.

Reacting against, or being hostile to, other people will prevent you from dealing with a problem in a clear, intelligent manner. When you are emotionally aggressive, you are defending yourself in a clumsy way and not at all developing your full strength. A mind over-occupied with defending against an opponent in the fear something might happen to you or your ego if you do not, is missing the power of a positive attitude. This positivity has nothing to do with the pacifistic idea of 'not fighting, or turning the other cheek.

Chinese Buddhist monastics practiced martial arts to deal with situations without triggering hatred, ego panic, or the false security of the ego. To an outsider, their action might appear to be aggressive, but it is not fundamentally aggressive. When you are fully present, fully confident, fully knowing who you are and what you are doing, it is possible to fight with positivity.

A balanced response can only come from understanding the other side of a problem from a non-dual viewpoint. Maitri suggests we must fully embrace our opponent or problem in order to see the issue with clarity. Only when you strive to be one with the situation can you truly understand your opponents and their tactics.

If you do not challenge aggressively, at least theoretically, you should not have combative feelings of any kind. This point of view trains one to dissolve the blinding effect of ignorance. This results in seeing the situation clearly and dealing with it more effectively.

Though it may sound contrarian, the most effective way to challenge anything is to develop loving-kindness. Maitri is not the same as the popular concept of charity or sentimental kindness to your neighbors. It is not just being kind or nice alone. It is the understanding that you have to become one with a situation. To do this you must promote a level of loving kindness within yourself. You don't need to be without personality or feelings and just accept whatever someone does. Your goal is to overcome the barrier your ego has formed between yourself and others. When you dissolve this self-created perimeter and open yourself, you will automatically develop real understanding and mental clarity. To engage problems from a posture of balance, you must develop loving-kindness, openness, a feeling of longing for oneness, so there is no aggressive desire in your actions at all.

Two examples from dojo members illustrate metta: A husband

commits a sexual crime against an innocent child. He is sent to prison. While in prison, the wife discovers her husband abused her own child. Family members and friends are horrified. Anger is stoked. People want to see the husband suffer. The wife, refuses to harbor any feelings of revenge or hatred. She extends metta to her husband. Of course, she is angry, but she recognizes he is still human, someone who himself may have been abused and is now imbalanced. Her metta looks past his poisonous acts to the hurting person beneath. Disappointment, anger, and fear, still flow through her, but beneath these emotions, she extends metta. She never sought to get back at or even with her husband. As his sentence pended, she prayed for his repentance even though she can never be with him again.

A mishap in the dojo during kumite between two advanced practitioners led to one man getting a concussion. In his concussed state his anger rose to a dangerous near uncontrollable level. His mind could think of nothing but revenge. For weeks he struggled with waves of anger, convinced the blow was purposefully done. Everyone tried to calm him. He eventually realized that he must reign in his aggressive feelings before they became destructive. He finally made peace with the event and with his training partner.

If he had extended loving kindness from the beginning, he would have felt a natural, primitive upwelling of anger, but his metta would have allowed him to see past the pain and anger, that accidents happen. And even if his sparring partner had intentionally hit him, violence met with violence would only create further turbulence between the two, leading to either one or both quitting the dojo and preventing the solution for any other transgressions with more violence in a continuous destructive cycle. Metta in this situation would have come with the following realization; I was hit. I am hurt. I am angry. I recognize my partner was either out of control or gunning for me. Either way, he must be suffering. If the latter, he suffers from imbalance. If the former, he must suffer from seeing me hurt.

When a situation is so severe that the only way to stop violence against you is to terminate the person causing it, this must be done with the full knowledge and presence of mind that this person must be dispatched to save oneself and or others from further suffering.

This is what is meant as the *challenge of no-challenge*. A desire to challenge with force against force prevents a proper engagement. This understanding lies behind the Chinese, Tibetan and Japanese art of war tradition. Such warriors do not think in aggressive terms, nor would their minds be occupied with the battlefield, or with the past or future consequences. The awakened warrior is completely one with bravery in the moment. He is fully concentrated because he knows the art of war. He is entirely skilled in his tactics so he does not have to refer to past events, or develop his strength by thinking about future consequences and victory. Being fully aware in the moment, one can challenge a problem from a whole and balanced perspective.

When a warrior develops maitri the oppositional force becomes one with him. The opponent who approaches expects our strength to come towards him. Oppositional force relies on this counter strength to fuel itself. When that strength is not there, the opponent will collapse. He will miss. His force will become self-defeating. It is like someone fighting his own hallucinations. The harder he tries to hit, the faster he falls. If you do not produce a counter hatred the level of opposing force collapses.

Maîtri can also be connected to your thoughts in meditation. When meditating, do not try to resist or express your thoughts, just accept them. Avoid getting entangled with them. In this way the whole structure of thought becomes one with you and is no longer disturbing.

There are other ways of using thoughts, other connections with this art. For instance, yoga as taught through the Indian tradition, is based on the concept of developing inner strength. When we talk of strength or power, we generally think of over-coming or controlling someone, or strength developed to challenge or to defeat someone. I am talking about strength in its own right, the strength of fearlessness, *Jigme*, in Tibetan. To be without fear is to have great strength. If you can connect to the origin of the existing strength within yourself, developing new strength becomes unnecessary, whereas, if you had to develop new strength through gymnastic training, without the mental strength to reinforce it, such strength tends to collapse.

This is how the martial arts are related to developing a balanced state of mind in combat. This is why I neither teach nor embrace violence as a viable solution.

Q. With five and a half decades of experience, can you comment on aging and martial practice?

There are two foundations upon which all learning progresses; *building skills* and *expanding awareness*. These two factors function best when balanced. Since I took up formal martial study in 1968, I've not only observed my own aging and learning process but have witnessed thousands of students passing through their own life stages.

Very young children up to age seven just want to have fun. They want to explore and express freely wielding their own innate biological sensitivities. Our very young students are eager to move using their instinctive guidance systems. Highly structured movements like kata do not appeal to young children's natural instincts for spontaneous play.

At ages roughly 7-12, there is a shift in expressive focus. This group wants to see and do the spectacular. This is mostly because they still retain childhood vestiges of the imaginal realms where anything is still possible until proven otherwise. They want to break boards, do sky-high flying kicks, flip their friends, and twirl weapons. They also want their teachers to demonstrate superhuman, superhero skills. A young boy once asked me with a dead-eye seriousness when I was going to teach him how to shoot fireballs. Essentially, this age group wants validation about power. They want to know how to get, hold onto, and express real power. They have an intuition that power is something good that can both protect them and give them what they want in life.

Ages roughly 13-40's want to test their abilities with their peers. This age group is all about comparison and conquest. Their art becomes a proving ground for how they differ from others and for what they will become in the future. Such experiences will shape their adult persona. They are all about the *how* of their arts. They will test their limits amongst their peers. Most strive overtly or covertly for some measure of alpha status. They can be highly competitive, enter tournaments to win trophies, collect affirmations and confirmations that they matter both to themselves and others.

At ages roughly 40-60 I see a gradual shift in training emphasis. This group becomes more curious about the *why* of their arts. They may want to know more about the differences between other styles and ways of executing technique. This age group tends to veer from the need to prove themselves to others to proving something to oneself. Where the prior age group needed to prove themselves by challenging others, this age group wants to advance for a wider variety of personal reasons; to overcome deep-seated fears, feelings of inadequacy, a genuine curiosity about martial art and philosophy. They will search for greater self-confidence, a feeling of satisfaction and personal accomplishment. They also lay the groundwork for a more fulfilling future and a healthier lifestyle. I see a slow transition amongst them to broaden their study toward the Dō of martial arts rather than the technique of martial arts. The transition to better health is often made during this period.

Those aged 60-and up look for greater levels of integration and meaning in their arts. For some, this is a time when spiritual instincts awaken and a more Yin, or inner quiescence and conservatism is sought. These practitioners will seek out meditation, ritual practice, and the deeper meanings behind their arts as they relate to the rest of their life. At this stage, the walls of the dojo melt away. Practice and expression become a microcosm of the everyday world with its myriad challenges, struggles, losses and gains.

Q. How do you weigh the need for street-practical value against the complexities and nuance found in Kiko training?

I'd like to hear more experts weigh in on this question. First, I need to disentangle some key variables in this question. No street practical value versus Kiko equation exists. Kiko is just another training tier. There are many paths up the martial mountain. As teachers, it is our job to clearly define the purpose and value of our kihon, kumite and kata. Were the traditional Forms of Asia designed to be amended or edited at will, or were they to be interpreted exactly as shown? Amongst the world's fighting schools this answer has historically sloshed from one side or the other as sociocultural values, needs and perspectives change with the times. We have to further ask; are the world's fighting forms to be viewed as a basket of random technique or a carefully constructed tactical approach to personal, civilian defense? If katas were consciously constructed to convey any other lessons outside of combative skills, such as for meditative and therapeutic purpose, how were these aspects to be accessed and applied?

Next, we have to look at the individual needs and predilections of the student and the culture which produced this student. Cultures exposed to constant or imminent threats of violence will seek practical techniques and disregard other dimensions as fluff. In the face of a pending threat, complexity will be shunned. Nuances are shucked in favor of simple, direct and forceful methods of resolution. On the other hand, an educated culture, free of survival or self-protective needs, will seek further levels of refinement. Also, the long term, ten plus year, martial artist will be looking to broaden and deepen their knowledge base for thriving in life at large. They will not be sustained by repetition of the 'same ole stuff'.

Some time ago I watched a *Youtube* video of a prominent U.S. expert demonstrate combative applications for every kata in his system. His applications were believable and effective. However, he took broad liberties with his Forms. His stances and footwork were radically different from his solo kata demonstration. The kata's arm motions were exchanged for other novel technique. A step to the right in the kata might be performed by his stepping to the left instead. Clearly his understanding of kata bunkai was an open and free expression of well-understood biomechanical principles. But he showed a poor grasp of internal principles. For we have Kiko principles that would challenge this expert's change of footwork and arm motions as possibly reducing his effectiveness. Most experts demonstrating bunkai are not actually fighting. Their remedies are prearranged. Though we can clearly see a potential in these exhibitions, real strengths are not tested in their full and proper context. Fights can get very messy. For this reason, the biggest challenge to traditional martial training has come from the full contact fighters.

You can see how the initial question flowers into more questions. In our School we consider all these inquiries part of our conceptual evolution. Concepts need to advance along with technical skills because the more you know why you are doing something, the better your odds of doing it correctly. Confidence generates power. Confidence is part of Kiko's Soft Gating system because it removes inhibition, doubt, and ambiguity from the mind, freeing up Ki. Of two men physically and technically matched in a fight, who do you think has the best chance of prevailing, one confident or one lacking confidence?

Kiko gives us a means by which to test the power of any set of kata moves. If it charges and strengthens you and/or draws down the adversary's strength, we have a solid technique. All my years of testing point toward kata moves being taught within a tight tactical blueprint. Once mastered, these principles can open to creative applications aligned with appropriate biomechanical and bioenergetic principles.

Q. Is the primary focus of Kiko training solely about gaining more power, defeating opponents, and becoming the dominant alpha?

Kiko is a tool, not a philosophy. You would not ask this question about a hammer. Each practitioner must choose how to use this tool to best suit their needs. If you wish to gain more power, Kiko will provide an abundance. If you need to release energy, Kiko will enable you to do so. As a martial artist, we want maximum engagement strength. But I want to share an observation about a long term, twenty-plus year karate-dō student named, Eric. As Eric immersed himself in the study of Sanchin and became more adept at moving his energy, he would take in so much energy his eyes would literally bug out of his head and he would become uncomfortably restless. Eric is a rare breed whose family lineage consists of individuals who could absorb copious Ki from the environment. Eric has no problem drawing Ki. Letting it go proved difficult. He was like an overfilled balloon with little to no release valve for the over-abundant charge he gathered. Eric was the first student whose reactions to Ki training made me realize that Sanchin could not possibly be directed solely toward gathering Ki, but discharging it as well. Years later, during the Covid pandemic lockdown, Eric showed me what he was doing with his kata. His kata had morphed. His movements had drifted away from what I was teaching. He performed slowly and deliberately, more like a Tai Chi practitioner. He exaggerated moves by overextending his limbs. I asked him to tell me what he was doing. He said he was trying to get more connected to his body, "even himself out."

I knew he would not test strong by Kiko standards. But he wasn't trying to test strong. He had transformed his Sanchin into a natural, personalized, Qigong practice to balance his overly Yang Energy Body. He didn't want to be maxed out. He wanted a full but balanced charge throughout his system. This is a valuable lesson for anyone working with power-generating principles and techniques. Be mindful of what you seek. Too much energy is no better than too little. Choose your goals carefully for they often come with unexpected consequences.

Q. Does everyone get the same results from Kiko training? If not, why not?

Not everyone gets the same results because anomalies exist amongst certain individuals that can cause different, even opposite results. This latter group, however, based upon our testing so far, appears in the minority. Psychological and physical blockages initially hamper students to get the same degree of positive results at the outset.

More than 95% of the subjects we tested showed strength increases using Kiko over a broad range of trials, though there were variations in the percentage of the strength increases they experienced. Increases ranged between 30-100%. Some reasons for marginal strength increases were obvious: mental or physical blockages, misunderstanding of the moves or test being performed, an unconscious agenda distorting the outcome, low level fatigue or illness that had depleted the person's energy prior to the test. Sexual release within twenty-four hours of testing can show a strength decrease while certain full moons resulted in across the board strength increases. The affecting variables are quite extensive; A failure to understand the effects of directionality, synthetic vs natural testing environment, proximity to weakening objects, clothing too tight, wrong colors, an innocent ignorance of the effects of the Five Elemental energy organizations, etc. Prince Five Weapons, one of our senior members and acupuncturist, shared that, similar to his acupuncture clients, some people are low responders to treatment while others are hyper-responders. This is true with Kiko application as well.

One breakthrough came from observing a senior karateka who often got the opposite results from the rest of us. The reason turned out to be a postural anomaly, a forward-sloped neck that reorganized his Biofield to generate Ki differently. Another student had long slender monkey-like hands, which altered the way he absorbed and discharged Ki.

Until you are versed in Kiko principles, these anomalies will not be apparent. It is imperative you find a qualified teacher who can unravel your unique energy system.

Q. How is it that so many martial artists and teachers have missed the relevance of Kiko in their own fighting systems?

The reason for the missive is the nuance involved in Kiko study. People do not enter martial arts for shades of distinction. They want immediate, see-and-touch, up front, direct, practical and potent technique. Off the top of my head, here is a list of reasons martial students don't see Kiko:

1. The bulk of Western martial culture remain unaware that this dimension exists within their arts.

2. Most martial students don't stay in their disciplines long enough to cross into Kiko territory. The average martial student is in their art for less than 2.5 years. The arc of the average career professional rarely extends beyond twenty-five years. Consider also that the average martial art teacher is a part timer accounting for 75% of Western teachers.

3. The amount of time deemed to become an expert has been shortening for decades. People in popularized styles are earning black belts in under two years.

4. Ego-centricity limits martial artists who feel they have arrived at some personal or collectively determined peak. They develop no further, erroneously thinking there is nothing left to see and thus create false ceilings within their arts.

5. Over-commercialization has forced many teachers to teach to the mean. As a result, they do not have the time or energy to probe deeper into their own disciplines.

6. You can't develop Kiko in a vacuum. You need to work with partners. The more variety the better. It's also difficult, if not impossible, to convey this information virtually/online. You have to have at least one other person of like or open mind to develop your internal sensitivities, someone to give you candid, unbiased feedback.

7. Cultural pressures distract from this study. We are being assailed by endless superficial attractions competing for our attention.

8. A lack of general sensitivity to one's own Biofield and its affects have created a wall of disbelief. If you don't see it, or can't see Ki, does it actually exist?

9. Martial orthodoxy has established fixed systems to the point where it is not easy to suddenly teach differently from what has previously been taught, in some cases, for hundreds of years. Old,

entrenched dogmatic networks are hard to dismantle. Some even have punitive consequences for those who ask too many questions. It's been said that doctrine is the corpse of revelation.

Q. Why are there so many variations of kata? Are some kata better than others?

Many kata formulas generate impressive power, which is why we see variety in the world's fighting forms. Though most Western martial artists are not aware of Kiko principles within their own arts, this does not mean their kata were transmitted imperfectly. The hurdle Westerners have faced is the lack of guidance to fully activate all the inner principles contained in these kata.

Imagine that two men are challenged to craft a unique kata of their own. Each is given a handicap. One man must always face North. The other, South. I contend they will come up with different ways to express their technique, even though they discover the same principles. The Earth's geomagnetic fields and contour of their immediate terrain will compel them to shape their technique in a manner that works for their particular orientations.

Try slowly placing an arm bar on someone while you are facing north while they resist. Try the move facing south. Did you get the identical outcomes? Most testers will not. Energy moving through the body is altered by the direction you face. This is just one of many factors influencing movement and strength.

Sometimes the kata is not the problem, it's the person expressing what he or she believes is the essence of the Form. You do not want to miss the forest for the trees or the trees for the forest. Afterall, we are all ultimately students searching for deeper connections and truths about our arts.

Q. Why is Ki such a gray area of discussion?

The subject of Ki has been a gray area for centuries, mostly because its understanding has changed throughout time. Archeological records indicate that Neolithic cavemen practiced a type of QiGong. The Indians called QiGong, *Yoga*. The Egyptians, *The Mysteries*, The Tibetans, *The Art of Wisdom*. From the 4th century on Chi was viewed dualistically, as an opposing force. Its earliest version derived from Chinese oracles who prophesized using a binary, yes/no response. In the Yellow Emperor's Classic, the word

Qi meant a type of matter like the steam emitting off rice, suggesting a nourishing essence. In some cases, it was referred to as *Ethers*. In Egypt and Greece, Chi was called *Ouroboros*, the snake biting its tail, and understood as a unity phenomenon. The earliest translation of Chi in the West appeared in 1600 with the concept of *Spiritus Sanctus* (sacred spirit). Later, the psychologist, Carl Jung, wrote about *Mind Chi* or psychic energy. In China, Mao Zedong asserted Chi had a material reality when it was proven with electromagnetic waves, infrared rays, static electricity, magnetism, and flow of subatomic particles. According to some, the best definition of Chi today is *Vital Energy*.

So, you see we have wide ranging ideas about what martial Ki is and isn't. Most lay notions about Ki in regard to martial practice are too superficial to be taken seriously. This has presented a confusing face to students hoping for a clear explanation of the subject. Hard and Soft stylists also lay claim to a middle-ground of technique. Hard stylists assert that additional power comes from subtle shifts in body angles. The Soft style community claims this same ground is the result of the enigmatic Ki. Both positions are right to some extent and this is where the confusion sets in. Finding a consensus and a common language seems nearly impossible at this juncture. This gray area has given wiggle room for charlatans to pull the wool over gullible student's eyes. Since neither the scientific nor the martial community at large has succinctly defined Ki technique, the debates, skepticism, and wishful thinking will persist.

Hopefully, I have shed light into these shadows to ground some of Ki's internal concepts. We need to demystify the concept of Ki and show its practical face to the everyday martial artist.

Eventually, the only explanation for the strength increases we could surmise early on was that we had freed or activated a store of previously unavailable muscular energy. If this were something we were doing unconsciously, we were unaware of what it was or of the factors supporting it.

We hypothesized that we had tapped into and or activated some kind of internal, alchemical activating force or forces happening in the body/mind complex, not commonly perceived. If Ki was the catchall term used by the Asians to describe this subtle energy, or phenomenon currently unexplainable by modern science, that's the term we settled upon. We had experienced a 'Ki' event.

I felt that solving this mystery merited attention because the technique defied the amount of effort expended. This is why some aptly refer to internal power as 'effortless power.' It does not match the effort the common practitioner expects of good technique.

I don't think the martial skeptics past or present have grasped that the Asians themselves did not understand the science behind this phenomenon. The more astute old-world masters did however, appear to understand the behavior of subtle energies in their technique, although I believe they grasped it mostly on a gut level. Nevertheless, we have their kinesthetic treatises on the subject in their Fighting Forms. This behavior appears to have been carefully cataloged and passed along for hundreds of years within the esoteric monastic martial community, of which I am a member, and also within the key or essential kata of Okinawa.

Q. Is martial life on the whole advancing or declining?

It's difficult to give a definitive answer as the martial arts industry is not a homogenous entity. Its growth or decline depends on factors such as region, type of martial art, and target audience.

Since the turn of the century, the martial arts have entered an emerging, redefining reality. Just as quantum physics upended the thinking of the biological sciences, it appears to be redefining the future of our arts. Martial arts have entered the Quantum Age. Overall, the industry has been growing steadily in recent years. According to a report by Global Industry Analysts, the global martial arts equipment market is expected to reach $2.9 billion by 2025. This is driven by increasing interest in combat sports and fitness. In addition, the popularity of mixed martial arts (MMA) and the Ultimate Fighting Championship (UFC) has led to a surge of interest in martial training. The pandemic accelerated the growth of online martial arts training, allowing people to practice from their homes. Many martial arts teachers have pivoted to online instruction. Some have even seen an increase in enrollment as a result. But not all martial arts are experiencing the same level of growth. Traditional martial arts, such as Karate and Tae Kwon Do, have faced challenges in attracting new students, as they may be perceived as outdated or not as practical for self-defense in comparison to MMA or Brazilian Jiu-Jitsu.

Overall, the martial arts industry is complex. Its growth or decline depends on many factors. However, the industry is generally expanding, with growing interest in combat sports, fitness, and online training.

In my opinion, the martial arts, as a Way of Life in the modern world, has become harder to live. I feel it is inclining toward major contraction and could easily be extinct a hundred years from now. There are lots of martial schools out there, but their curriculums have been growing sparser and more superficial, paralleling our nutrient-deficient foods. Big egos, financial agendas, business trumping art, frenetic life pace, less discretionary income, competition with a rich digital world, children dominating the industry, the propping of mental pursuits over physical endeavors, the mad pursuit of the material over the spiritual, all these factors are eroding a once venerable Way. Rooting into our physical bodies in pursuit of wisdom is becoming a more difficult challenge. Our materialistic pursuits have tamped down spiritual growth, curiosity about inner life, and threshold-crossing experiences overall. Western youth are opting for a more sedentary, highly cerebral existence. We have become a leveling and superficializing society. Our over-headiness is part of the problem. These new age variables are challenging both our public and private worlds to meet what is unfolding as a very insecure future for the martial arts.

Western culture's over-emphasis on materialism has not only distorted and diminished the martial art's spiritual nature, it is diffusing and dissolving it. For as our outer life strengthens, our inner life weakens. I am reminded of the windy mountaintop that twists and contorts the trees that dare jut out, toppling the weaker ones. Nowhere is this truer than in Asia, the birthplace of martial culture. The internal arts in particular are being denuded/declawed by the Chinese government for the simple reason they can lead to a radicalized, free mind.

Another reason for our current martial degradation is a lack of authentic teachers. Martial teachers, yoga teachers, fitness teachers are reproducing offspring much too fast. In this shortened timespan we are passing along a weaker teaching DNA. Disciples are given less time to mature into their arts. Some black belts are teaching after a year and half experience. Yoga certifications are given out within three months. You can become a Reiki 'master' in two years. If the term master is given out in ever-shorter time frames, what does one become after sixty years; a super-duper, hyper Granddaddy of Grandmasters?

Sadly, many immature teachers, despite their right intent, lack substance, even if they possess novel viewpoints or talents. They do not compare to old-world masters who honed their craft over an entire lifetime. There are enormous hurdles to becoming at peace with oneself, even to those hungry minds yearning for true clearing. We are halted or slowed by confusion, fear, anxiety and doubt trying to wade through a suffocating tsunami of information. The cost of long-term training alone, alongside a transient, anxious clientele, prohibits most from deep, meaningful advance. The spirit of the peaceful life some seek, itself retreats along with our once organic environment. I fear a spiritual winter may blanket great swaths of the Western world.

The advanced, aging, martial herd is starving. Most long-term practitioners have picked dry the low-hanging technical foliage of their landscape. When you can no longer derive sustenance from your traditional sources, you will either seek another system, find a more adrenalized experience like the MMA, shift your focus to a fitness-style workout, or quit the arts all together. When you drink from the half-empty part of the glass, you will always be thirsty.

Many of us have witnessed the continued degradation and slow extinction of old-world martial principles. Granted, if something is outdated, or tired, doesn't fit the culture, then it has to go. Cultures advance when they husk truth from its old shell and reorganize it to fit the new times. Truth never ages! Mainstream martial artists need to grow stronger legs to reach the higher hanging fruits. Unfortunately, those who cannot see this fruit mistakenly clutch the fool's gold of the traditional arts baffling ambiguities? The spineless path says, 'Come in, get a great workout, learn a little self-defense and a little Asian tradition. You're amazing!'

Q. What did the idea of 'spirit' mean to Asian martial culture?

What spirit meant to early Asian martial cultures, I believe Quantum physics, on an empirical plane, means to the modern Western martial artist, with one major difference. In the former there appeared a vitalizing intelligence behind the concept while in the latter, such intelligence is completely absent. The Asian spirit appeared as dragons, entities, ghosts, ancestors, or just intangible and unexplainable spiritual presence experiences or forces, sometimes having a profound influence upon one's actions. For centuries, the Asians revered this Spirit in its many manifestations. But to see, catch, or feel it one had to open their senses to the imagistic world. In the West we have the invisible world of unseen fields, waves, tiny particles, perhaps even Dark Matter whizzing about in mystifying ways, but the notion of this world is completely devoid of any animate qualities.

When someone remarks about the spirit of a Fighting move or art, they may be talking about motivation, mental psych, a religious or moral high ground, or a God principal? Things get dicey when we ask where this spirit resides or what it is made of. Some well-grounded answers have been offered up on this subject. But far too many explanations regarding its martial implications remain sketchy, and thus have thrown well-intentioned seekers off the scent of deeper truths.

A Chinese, Hung Gar master once stated that only after you practice a Form 4,000 times can you call it your own. The first thousand you are trying to get the external moves down. The second thousand you are learning to apply your moves in a practical, self-defense manner. The third thousand you are learning to control your Ki. The last thousand you have entered the spirit of the Form. Your art becomes a moving meditation.

People get the concept of 'spirit' on a gut level. You are 'in the spirit' when you feel connected to your actions or tasks. I assert that most of the world's katas were created on the basis of strong intuitions connecting the developers to the spirit of their moves, rather than their kata being created by means of deliberate, conscious, brick and mortar assembly. Excessive mental involvement is more of a Greek-inspired, Western concept.

According to the authors, Bruce Rosenbaum and Fred Kuttner, in their book, *Quantum Enigma*, once any two objects have interacted, they become forever entangled and begin to influence everything else entangled. They concede, that though such complex engagements become wildly complex and undetectable, there appears to be a principle of 'universal connectedness' science has yet to understand.

This entanglement of 'influences' exerted upon seemingly random objects, whose meaning we have yet to understand, is exactly what I believe the Kiko masters keenly observed, or felt, and addressed in their forms and other practices. These acutely sensitive experts must have felt something else transpiring, something out of sight to the general populace that led to their unusual strength, speed and control over others. I've experienced this quality for myself many times as have a substantial number of my advanced students.

From the very outset, when I noticed an influence outside of my own conventional thinking, my attention was riveted looking for it to occur again, and whether I could observe a consistent behavior. This inquiry turned out to be the most exciting era of my entire martial arts career.

To the Asians, these so called 'barely detectable influences' were attributed to the intrinsic, vital interplay of chi.

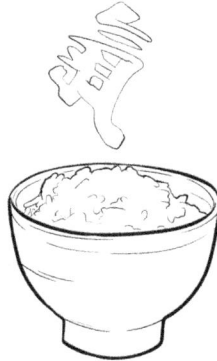

The original Chinese calligraphy for Qi was a pictograph showing steam emitting from a bowl of rice. This is a clear analogy of a collectively recognized ethereal substance, emitted by all forms of life. This 'steam' wasn't a temperature, an off gas, or scent. It was related to vibration, and involved the deepest activities of the mind. It could cause mind-bending, mind-boggling events to occur, particularly in areas related to physical strength.

The Chinese may not have known what comprised Qi, but they had carefully recorded its behavior. Modern science has yet to determine the exact composition of Qi. Scientists do not deny the existence of hidden influences as the above quote suggests, but they don't fully understand what these influences or energies are totally comprised of. The scientist, Neils Bohr, raised Einstein's ire when he suggested these energies be called *influences*. Einstein didn't deny such energy existed. He thought science could do better to uncover the nature of these mysteries.

We are in the same predicament with the concept of Ki today as the ancient Chinese a thousand years ago. They didn't know what comprised it either.

I've been studying the behavior of Ki, martial spirit, or the vital breath, for over a quarter of a century, on top of prior quarter century practicing 'regular' karate. I entered this later study when

I started dissecting the patterns of the Okinawan kata. I felt unsatisfied with the mainstream interpretations given for kata. Looking back, some were quite ridiculous. It's embarrassing to think that I believed simultaneously blocking two kicks thrown on either side of me might ever be a reality. So much for the idealism of a twenty-year old in the late 1960's. Even to this day there are martial lessons presented as advanced practices in dojo around the world that seldom go past basic karate 101. It isn't just our TV shows dumbing down. Whole societies are degrading. If you repeatedly train only to look at the surface of life, you will habituate to a superficial life. Worse, you will end up robbing reality of its innate depth.

I didn't see the spirit of karate in my bunkai (applications of kata), or the nuances of kumite (sparring), at first. It arrived well beyond the time the average career teacher lasts in their arts. Very few martial artists, and certainly martial teachers, will spend a half-century continually advancing their craft. Most simply rehearse already acquired skills. I began to see this spirit in the particular configuration of the limbs, breath and directionality in kata, and in the organization of my own mind attending to the kata's patterns, sparking me to ask, 'Why this way, why this foot, this hand, done in this manner?' Had past masters seen what I was just beginning to comprehend?

Q. How do you understand the concept of Dō, in your case, Karate-dō?

There are plenty of people who will have different opinions about what martial Dō is from my viewpoint. I can only account for my own perspective. On my behalf, I ante up a lengthy, half-century career on an evolutionary path using martial arts as my primary vehicle.

Undertaking a Dō or Dao (Tao) art, implies the discipline of advancing yourself physically, emotionally, psychologically, and spiritually, as the focus of training. The martial arts have never been just self-defense or competitive sport systems. Historically, they were dynamic life systems that used the interactions in the dojo; its kata, kumite, bunkai, and participating members, as a grounding and leveraging means for understanding one's authentic nature. Most people are natural seekers. If you seek martial art as a fighting art, that's where you will derive its meaning. If you seek the Martial Ways as a ladder to personal development, you will get the benefits of both its fighting and non-fighting nature.

Framed another way, a martial-Dō is a holistic, educational system. It begins with your physical body as a microcosm of the world at large. Fighting is what I call the first source, the most primal interaction of all living organisms, the struggle to survive in its most naked expression. If you understand the will to survive, you will see martial art as the father of all struggles. The mother of celebrated life movement is dance. We can refer to the 9,000 year old Indian cave paintings depicting scenes of hunting, childbirth, religious rites, burials, communal drinking, and dancing. If karate-dō could be likened to one of the five primary forms of Yoga, it would be a Karma yoga, the study of the cause and effect of our intended (and unintended) actions. Karate-dō was once a venerable, coveted, sacred way, pursued by a few. I consider it a royal path for discovering your true nature.

The concept of a 'true self', versus untrue, or less true self, is not a topic sought by modern, mainstream martial art practitioners. 'Just do it' is the preferred trend. This lack of a clear High-Way into the martial art's elevated principles is the main reason so few people walk it. Most practitioners do not know such a path exists, except in movies or in their imagination. By contrast, when you don't have a basic ability to defend yourself and you feel threatened, you will seek an immediate remedy to find security. In a like manner, because people exist with many divides in their lives; fears, lacks, concerns, doubts and confusions, they may seek out a resolution for those concerns, but lack a clear or intelligent plan toward their remedy.

How many people are fully aware of their own interior divides? Even if they are aware of them, how many will address them at all, or well? Even if they tackle them, it's often with varying degrees of success due to scarce or limited resources. Along with the tools and the time to develop our skills, we can all benefit from some guidance at times.

I believe people compartmentalize their lives with distinctions of value; from 7-9 p.m. they are karate-ka training in the dojo, from 7 a.m. to 5 p.m., employees, 5-7 p.m. husbands, wives, fathers, mothers, lovers, friends, hobbyists, etc. Endless possibilities exist. All these distinctions and divisions of self, come with challenges small and large. We are engaged in conflicts whether we resolve them or not. Conflict is the very essence of life that defines and shapes us.

Wouldn't it be great to have a powerful ally, fresh new tools and perspectives? Wouldn't it be great to have a private sanctuary, a retreat, where you could train toward your own security, peace and serenity? Wouldn't it be great to know that this ally was wise beyond measure, experienced, tested and truly committed to your success? This is the role the martial sensei once played and still plays in the martial journey.

Karate jutsu is the physical side of the art. Karate-dō is its spiritual counterpart. The Dō attempts to cut one loose from mental limitations or internally bound energies. Karate-dō is like a personal mentor who knows how to fight intelligently and fairly for your desires.

The high path in martial arts, its Dō, Tao, or Way, invites one into an organizing process whose goal is to expand, open up, connect you to your authentic nature. A competent sensei can extrapolate and interpret vital life principles and techniques and present them in a logical, even-paced fashion so students can steer their futures confidently, evenly, firmly mirroring the high principles of their own path. Martial art is not just the way of a crisp gi snap, or the road to badassdom. The Dō offers a way of re-forming you into a more dynamic self.

How many people do you know study disciplines whose goal is to empower and balance themselves as a whole person? How many individuals fully commit to such a path? In my opinion—1%. How many people do you know commit themselves to consistent life mentoring? The Dō serves this purpose through directed physical practice. Martial arts should actively engage your whole person, not just your body, but your body/mind/emotions/spirit complex.

Martial Dō must not be confused with a religion in an institutionalized, theistic sense, but rather as a unifying path whose purpose is to reconnect conflicted fragments of the self into a cohesive, high-functioning whole. Karate-dō provides the tools. You choose which pieces to link.

The issues and struggles that confront most people cause them to live fractured lives. They might be happy at work but miserable at home. Lots of people just wing it. How and where does one find, create, or learn the tools to deal with or mend this splintering?

Many mainstream martial arts serve a clear purpose. They offer civilians the means to defend themselves from threats of injury or death. Later, as these practical disciplines interbred with Indian and Chinese monastic spiritual cultures, some of the arts were retooled to embrace a broader reality. If done with certitude, the Dō could lead one out of the din of conflict altogether. This is why some martial paths were regarded as 'venerable'.

Most people shun conflict. They chose to walk the path of least resistance. It's less wear and tear. Yet, many of these individuals lack the skill to walk it without incidence.

Just as a set of martial techniques can be viewed as an organized way of moving against a live opponent, martial Dō evolved the inner tools for transcending broader struggles in relationships and with existence itself.

Both methods suggest intelligent ways to secure peace, whether peace of body, mind, spirit, emotions, soul or heart.

Where one art concerns itself exclusively with the physical realm, the other takes up the concerns with one's role as life steward in the universal scheme of things.

Sadly, I've observed too many people lack any instinct about this larger role, mostly because they cannot see beyond life's superficial value and thus believe there aren't any paths beyond material conquest worth pursuing.

Q. You've talked about the Dō of martial arts being a broader study than the sole acquisition of physical skills. How has this larger sphere of action influenced your life?

I once had a pointed conversation with a gifted healer who candidly asked me what side of life I stood for. Without clarifying, I knew she was asking whether I stood 'for' or 'against' life, not just my individual life, but for the betterment of society and the earth as a whole?

Do you stand for the betterment of the world or not? Are your behaviors and thoughts consistent with your answer? The majority of the world vacillates, sometimes for the better, sometimes not. Many people live a semi-conscious life regardless of their justifications.

The world isn't going to get better unless we strive to make it better. Some people study martial arts to protect themselves, others as a competitive outlet. The Dō's philosophical platform suggests we ask what we need to advance life, not just what we need to protect ourself or how to be a better competitor. This brings one face to face with the elemental question of what side of life we espouse.

This existential question was also a monastic issue in the Asian temples. Are you for the growth and support of your culture, propagation and support of the earth, or do you exist for your own primary benefit and that of your immediate tribe, regardless of the destruction or degradation your behavior might cause? The Buddha wanted to end suffering. He took a stand for life. He advocated for the support of seven spheres of being; right mindfulness, right view, right intention, right effort, right meditative engagement, right speech, right livelihood, and right action. The Sanskrit word *samyak* often translated as "right" or "perfect" can also mean "complete." Being mindful encourages complete engagement with life.

The Buddha did not advocate passivity of self. Buddhist warriors existed in Asian history. They formed armies. They fought. They killed. Every great religion that advocated supporting life confronted broad instances of necessary, and sometimes unnecessary, unfortunate violence.

Q. Can you comment further on the Dō versus the Jutsu of martial arts?

There is no friction between the Jutsu and the Dō of martial arts. They are two vital halves of every fighting system. However, I see a greater lack of awareness about the workings of the Dō side of martial arts in Western cultures.

The jutsu confines its influence exclusively to the material sphere where it restores lower chakric functioning by establishing confidence in the physical world. But practicing kicks, punches, blocks, locks and fighting forms year after year might never address other equally meaningful realms. Of course, since everything is connected, it's impossible for any physical practice not to seep into other life dimensions. But this would be by happenchance for most. The Dō-based martial arts consciously reorient the student's emotional responses to fear, doubt or confusion into a more affirming role against ever more subtle levels of invasion.

Martial jutsu will give you physical strength, balance, timing, leverage, coordination and flexibility, all worthy, prized objectives. Yet, because the jutsu is only half the potential field of study, you could still remain emotionally, mentally and spiritually imbalanced, inflexible, or blocked, in essence, unpotentialized.

First degree black belt in the Okinawan and Japanese arts was only ever considered expert in the *basics* of one's art. Its holder might still go to work the next morning feeling lousy about their job, hating their family responsibilities, feeling worthless, filled with worry, anxiety or fear, concerned about finances, weight, relationships, etc.

Contemporary martial jutsu is concerned only with the immediate and practical issues of an imminent physical threat or competition. Martial-Dō is interested in resolving other harder to pin down agitations, issues and concerns. You might think these other concerns are separate from martial training. They are not. The monastic and spiritual masters believed negative feelings, mental illusions and mental discordances to be just as dangerous as a flesh and blood enemy. We can credit the Shaolin culture for re-orienting martial arts in a way to vanquish these unseen nemeses. The Japanese term, *Masakatsu Agatsu, 'Victory over self'*, sums it up quite well.

Martial Jutsu addresses the Five Physical Barriers

Of the mind – The body you've been given
Physical Superficiality – moving in a limited range
Physical Ignorance – unaware how to move the body intelligently
Physical Confusion – not sure how to move the body
Physical Doubt – lack of confidence to move in the full range of expression

Martial-Dō addresses the Five Mental Barriers

Ego – the self-limiting nature of the mind resulting from an assumed self-identity
Mental Superficiality – cruising life's surface and missing its depth
Mental Ignorance – unaware of higher planes of thought
Mental Confusion – not sure where to direct your mind
Mental Doubt – lacking confidence in your future success

Q. Can you explain the personal mantra you say runs in everyone's head, 'Choose or be chosen?'

Sometimes, I ask students to pair up in the dojo for kumite and tell them, "Choose or be chosen." Which action most defines your life? Do you let others choose for you? Or do you go after what you want? We entered into this world with a seed sound in our spiritual DNA. It echoes the cosmic mantra, 'Choose or be chosen.'

You will not choose wisely if you are semi-asleep to the nature of reality. And just because your eyes are open doesn't mean you are fully awake. There are degrees of human wakefulness. Nagaboshi Tomio laid out seven stages of meditation. These were the Yogi's and kempo master's attempts to highlight that we can have numerous awakenings throughout life. We wake up from more than just a night's slumber. But you won't know this until you experience other waking states. And you are not likely to experience any of these additional states in Western culture unless you engage in higher consciousness practices.

In and off itself, a martial art will not raise your consciousness just because of your physical practice, in the same way exceptional furnishings do not elevate the room if the furniture has been thrown in a heap in the center of the floor. How your art is assembled, presented, assimilated and reassembled by you, is what determines what you get and where you go with it.

Being smart or smarter than someone else doesn't mean you are awake. Some people slumber brilliantly. The difference between smart and wise is that the former is devoid of feeling while the other comes from a place of compassion, from the heart. It's a whole-person-knowing, a realization, waking up to an expanded and compassionate reality.

Shifu Nagaboshi's Four Stages of Learning:

Humbleness (*Reigishao*), openness to new information
Understanding, coordination of mind and body.
Perception, awareness of mind/body/spirit unity.
Realization, complete interaction and flow of mental/physical actions).

Being awake is being mindful of your mental and physical actions. Becoming mindful is the beginning of authentic seeing. Seeing your life clearly fertilizes the soil of wisdom. Don't we all want a bio-friendly inner ecosystem? Don't let hawkers of lesser realities chose their reality for you as we see happening on a global scale today.

No one is saying our choices are easy. It's not the difficulty of choosing between the lesser of two evils, but often the difficulty of choosing between the greater of two goods that throw people into quandary. When you let other people, institutions, or events choose realities that go against your will, your sensitivities, or your intuitions, your spirit will be diminished no matter what your surface gain in the short term. When you are not whole you will find yourself in a struggle with degrees of resistance and doubt and choose a less than whole existence.

Being whole is being wholesome. With consistent wholesomeness comes authenticity. With authenticity comes right action. You will know the right thing to do or say when you are whole and you will always choose the correct reality, the life you want and are meant to live.

We are born to move; freely, fully, powerfully, and to claim our life desires, even if this means claiming the end of desiring itself. Martial art came into existence to fulfill this end. But it started at the lowest of totem values, in dirt and mud, blood and guts, life and death struggles. No one escapes answering the mantra, Choose or be Chosen.

Q. What does kata offer that a non-kata curriculum does not?

I've contemplated this question for decades. I could add; Is kata necessary to be an authentic martial artist? Why are there so many different kata? Wouldn't just one or two suffice? Are some kata better than others? How do you determine such? How long should you practice a kata? Is there a right way to perform a kata or endless possibilities to match the unique characteristics of their exhibitors? Is it kata conundrum or kata doldrums?

Kata was the single most intriguing thing that caught my eye about the martial arts. Kata has held my attention more than any other facet of my study. These power patterns have represented the backbone of the traditional fighting arts for centuries.

Coordinated fighting patterns first emerged in ancient India as Nata. In China they are called, *hsing* or *taolu*, in Korea, *poomse* or *hyung*, in Indoneisa, *jurus*, in Brazilian Capoeira, *sequencia*. These are just a few examples. Many other countries have their own traditional martial arts with distinctive terminologies for their forms or patterns. The specific terminology can vary within different styles and schools of martial arts within a country as well.

Western cultures entered a love/hate relationship with kata since their importation. In all traditional martial systems, you have to marry your kata whether you find them attractive or not, and divorce is out of the question, unless you quit your dojo. Depending who you study with, you might be fortunate to learn some pre-kata forms to ease you into the more complex and exotic fighting dances. In Isshinryu karate you learn eight kata to the first-degree black belt rank. In Shotokan, it's twenty-seven kata. In Tai Chi it's one. The Chinese Liu He Ba Fa is one long form that seems to go on forever. In Bagua, you might just walk the circle for five years.

Although I am a strong Form proponent, there is a lot of propaganda out there that has minimized, distorted, twisted, misrepresented, misinformed, even sought to downright discredit kata's value for a bigger share of the martial market. Kata is a messy subject.

Bruce Lee saw a problem with katas in the West and famously called them "organized despair.' In my opinion, his observation wasn't taken in the proper context by the mainstream community. Western cultures simply did not understand Asian Formwork. Here's some cringeworthy examples:

- The student who asks his Sensei "Why kata?" and gets the sand-blasted, stripped of any sense response, "It's traditional."
- The Sensei who tells his students once they learn a kata to "go figure it out." Or the nationally noted Gojuryu master who told me with a straight face, "Bunkai (kata application) isn't my cup of tea?"
- The wishful thinkers who attribute all kinds of mystical powers to kata, but are never quite able to explain what those powers are, yet they dangle this carrot in front of gullible students, year after year.
- The nit-picking sensei who brings out a ruler and measures the width of your feet or the distance of wrist from shoulder and tells you how critical the postures are, or in one case, the sensei who tells the students in no uncertain terms, "Never, ever pivot on the ball of your foot in a certain move," yet offers zero clarification for his insistence on such detail.

- The sensei who keeps changing his mind about how the kata is to be performed as he or she experiments with what works best for everyone.
- The sensei that lets students accommodate the moves to fit their bodies. If you don't want to do it exactly that way, you don't have to.
- The homogenizing sensei who is happy if your legs are spread out enough, you know, in the general ball park, like the Horse and Seiuchin stances being the same postures, which they are not.
- The sensei who is satisfied with lackluster performances of a kata and moves his students like a rancher leads a herd of cattle to the next Form every three months.
- The sensei who drills students to death on their kata but never corrects their Form or offers any deep insight why the moves are to be done the way they are.
- The sensei who discredits kata altogether and drops the relevance from the curriculum for more, "realistic" fight lessons.
- The sensei who has studied multiple martial arts and creates a hodge-podge hybrid of his Tae Kwon Do and his Shorinryu (real example). Mind you, a young teacher, with maybe ten-year's experience.
- The sensei who misinterprets the kata for having run out of creative teaching ideas and therefore tells his students they must learn to do their katas on the opposite side to become fully balanced.

Is it any wonder why Bruce Lee felt his way about kata? The old-world masters would be turning in their graves if they could see what has become of their arts.

Although Lee did a disservice when his commentary went out to the mainstream community, he issued precisely what the martial arts needed at that time— a bold wake-up call; Lee was basically shouting what I do at the start of every formal class, *Keesho!* (Wake up!) 'What are you doing with your martial art?' Put on your intelligence caps. Aim high, plunge deeper. There's a huge forest of information. Start trekking. Ask questions. That's what Lee and my teacher, Russell, and other martial frontiersmen like these teachers did. These sensei got rewarded for their boldness with real traction in their arts.

The Orthodox kata theory

The Orthodox theory of kata takes the position that the originating masters built such a tight knit kata ship that you cannot add any further wisdom to their compositions. These kata need no changes or modifications whatsoever unless the human body grows a third arm or leg. You just need the manual that tells you what kata's precise movements are designed to do and how to best activate them. Of course, this manual was seldom included.

The Progressive Kata Theory

This theory takes the position that kata was created as a general template allowing others to make meaningful changes to its combative value, as no two people move the same. Analogize this idea to the alphabet. It's a fundamental resource. Once you acquire a working knowledge of it you can select words, ideas, and meaningful narratives, indefinitely. With this free way of understanding kata, you are only limited by your imagination and sense of reality what a fight or self-defense event actually entails.

We do know Kata was created as a kinesthetic dictionary, a virtual-reality combat directory. Kata is ultimately something you do, not something you think about doing. When you perform a kata, you are stepping into the minds of the masters who created them. Of course, not all kata were created equal. Therefore, be forewarned, you may be also stepping into a mental mine field, a murky zone of maybe worthwhile, maybe not worthwhile, patterns.

Intelligent Kata Theory

Imagine you have no martial knowledge whatsoever and you want to learn how to defend yourself. You sign up in a local dojo and discover the school teaches choreographed strings of moves called kata which you innocently and curiously ask, "What are these kata for?" The teacher answers, "We have a half-dozen movement patterns to make it easier for you to remember techniques against common assault scenarios.

The 1st kata pattern teaches you how to deflect and counter all manner of hand strikes aimed at your face and torso.

The 2nd kata teaches you how to escape from single and multiple grabs against your arms, legs, neck and torso.

The 3rd kata teaches you how to apply and to avoid basic throws and other takedown maneuvers.

The 4th kata teaches you how to escape from common grips or holds from behind.

The 5th kata teaches you how to control your adrenaline system and mitigate any fears that might immobilize you....

Who wouldn't be interested in learning such skills when presented in this manner? Kata described like this make perfect sense as a clear and valuable resource. When you don't have a partner, you are going to need some mnemonics to remember all those kicks, locks, strikes, blocks and escape techniques until you can free style them without thought in an organized manner.

Q. You once stated that discovering your art's internal nature felt like a martial rebirth. Could you comment further on this idea?

That one technical anomaly with Stone back in the early 1990's showed me that I had been blind to a vast, unexplored martial frontier. What had been hidden in plain sight every time I donned my gi suddenly presented a flash of virgin terrain. I had witnessed the birth of a mysterious, unrevealed, shadow art. I understand now why Shodan (1st degree black belt in the Japanese arts) means 'new beginning'. With that single discovery I realized I had only been told a half truth about the essence of Okinawan karate-dō.

Years after this revelation, I received a package addressed to Hayashi Tomio, (obviously the wrong person. That wasn't my name), only to discover that I was that stranger being reborn with a spiritual name inviting me into an esoteric lineage for my earnest foray into the ancient heartland of the martial arts.

To my delight I found myself welcoming a new realm of possibility and clarifications of previously unknown, vibrant and vital martial knowledge as seen through the monastic lens. It felt like the making of a movie with me being cast as a local hero. It was a remarkably profound turning point in my teaching career for it validated many of my deepest intuitions about the arts.

You've probably heard, 'There are no coincidences in life'. We all move in a vast, interconnected, oceanic consciousness with occasional, cryptic synchronicities appearing at various twists and turns in the journey. In this cosmic hook-up every moment, every breath, is pregnant with energy and meaning if we are willing to look for it.

My spiritual name, Hayashi Tomio (tall forest seeking the light), became my emerging new identify, which I gratefully adopted as I continue my search for the heart of Karate-dō. My discoveries would not be the karate of the ancient, idealized, white-eyebrowed masters. Their time has come and gone. Old wisdom dons new garb with each generation of Way seekers.

This book is my personal chronicle of the martial arts very alive, vital, in the now, hidden growth forest, which the Okinawans once clothed in the mystical garb of Kiko. Kiko completed for me the full and authentic face of these arts. Kiko awaits anyone aware and open enough to foray into it.

Q. Can you comment on the term, 'The Curse of Knowledge' and its relevancy to martial training?

One of my yudansha pointed out that teaching individuals about Kiko reminded him of a term used in both business and science, 'the curse of knowledge'. The curse is being unable to effectively communicate the relevance of one's knowledge to others.

In a phone interview in 2022 with Bill Pogue, 10th dan in isshin-ryu, Sensei Pogue shared the following perspective. "Many martial art teachers in the 1960's, like myself, had heard of the concept of Ki or Chi, but it was rare to find anyone who could give an intelligent and detailed explanation of how it functioned in their arts—although there were a lot of colorful attempts. One of my teachers, K. Pittaway, 10th dan, tried to get me into this 'stuff' but he could never articulate it convincingly, so I never pursued it. How many other seekers have missed this path for lack of a clear map?

One can go so deep into their craft that they lose the ability to communicate clearly to a beginner or novice and instead, confuse, or lose, their students. There is no shortcut into advanced martial knowledge. Even if you could compress all the trial-and-error effort into a short time span, in the end, one simply confronts a foreign language with Kiko. The subject dwells outside Western awareness. Therefore, it will take time and energy to convince, comprehend and apply.

Q. What do you mean by the statement, The Tai Chi of Karate/ The Yoga of Martial Arts?

People study martial arts for reasons other than, or in addition to, self-protection or competition. Their goals vary. When I reached middle age, I became fascinated with those *other* reasons. That's when I began to see the link between Hard style fighting arts like karate, and the fundamentals of arts like Tai Chi and Yoga. Yoga and Tai Chi are Sourcework disciplines. That is, they work with bodily energies, bodily systems; circulatory, endocrine, nervous, musculoskeletal, toward health, well-being and evolutionary advance.

Interest in Source energy was likely present in the construction of the essential kata of Okinawa. The more I probed, the more I saw the relevancy of yogic practices in our martial patterns. The Tai chi of karate refers to the Soft principles within the Hard. The yoga of martial arts refers to the larger Way of study within the narrower, superficial way, that is, solely for personal combat or competition.

Q. Have you encountered problems with others using the word Ki?

I've encountered three categories of people who have trouble with Ki. Those who think it's a trick for they cannot believe what they saw or experienced. The 'show me the science' people, who cannot accept the term because they cannot find any hard evidence of its existence. And the people who want to believe in Ki but simply cannot wrap their heads around it.

Ki for me is a catchall term for behaviors whose rationale has yet to be scientifically corralled. Because the scientific community does not know what Ki is entirely composed of, they are not sure how to test for it, and thus remain stuck. Science also currently lacks the tools to measure the effect of consciousness on physical strength.

I think it is natural to be critical of unusual or uncommon phenomenon like Ki at first, but it is equally unnatural and unhealthy to be in denial about unexplained events. I was reading through some old correspondences between two Buddhist practitioners. One correspondent stated that his scholarly mentor disliked the use of the word Chi, Ki or Energy as "too sloppy" a term. I suspect he meant the term was too open-ended, too lose-fitting, thus prone to misuse and misinterpretation. Most common examples or definitions for martial Ki in my opinion turn out over-simplified, false or misleading.

In another instance, I visited a well-established, thirty-five year career Tai Chi practitioner who discounted the use of the word Ki for anything to do with his training or teaching.

What label do we ascribe to unexplainable martial events? Flow, luck, God's will, Karma, unknown body dynamics, because there are unexplainable events. I'd like to believe that everything can be explained biomechanically with hard science, but too date, they have not. Quantum physicists bear me out. The best scientific minds in the world remain baffled by unexplained mysteries, the biggest being consciousness. We don't even know what Dark Matter is, yet we are told it accounts for ninety-five percent of our universe.

I've directly experienced many instances where there is no concrete explanation for the martial outcome. Plenty of theories abound, but they are suppositions, conjectures, hypotheses based upon observation. In the wise words of Galileo, "When it comes to a choice between observation or theory, go with observation." After observation comes analysis.

As a result of the many unexplained personal experiences I've had, I began to record my observations of the behaviors of this hidden field of possibility. I concede that using the word Ki is akin to the physicist, Neils Bohr, using the word influences as a catch-all for unexplainable events on the atomic level. Quantum physicists note their existence but don't fully understand the essence of the behaviors. Einstein, who railed at Neils Bohr for his use of this vague term, felt science could do better. Until science does a better job defining Ki, the word will continue to stick as a unique label.

I do feel the word 'Chi or Ki' has been used too cavalierly in the martial arts, in some cases without substantive direction. This misrepresents Ki. However, not everyone is making sloppy strokes choosing this term.

Not surprisingly, the entire history of scientific advance has frequently encountered staunch, closed-minded resistance. Old Science at odds with New Science is an age-old struggle. The die-hards hold tightly to their old ways, whether they brand challenging new insights bullshido or not. We can thank Quantum physics for upending the Cartesian sciences, including our martial science. Just as civilizations advance is inevitable, martial advance follows in lock step.

I am a college educated, well-read, career sensei. I can distinguish between a technique that has a clear biomechanical explanation and one that does not. I wasn't interested in, or looking for, any validation of Ki during my first quarter century of training. I was quite satisfied with the success of my teaching career and curriculum. But like any enthusiastic follower of the arts, I was open and eager to learn more. By happenchance, Ki found me and piqued my curiosity. I didn't seek it out.

Chi, Qi, or Ki is the umbrella term the Asians use to describe a martial singularity that could not be explained by normal scientific means. That's all the term means to me. It does not mean I can fly through the air, levitate people off the ground, send my students aflight without touching them, or flawlessly win any match. Maybe that's possible, but it's not my pursuit. I am not referring to the fantastical when I discuss the use of Ki in martial technique. I have the support and acknowledgement of 3,000 years of Asian culture on the subject in favor of my view. Is Ki any better a term than Einstein's, label of 'Spooky action' for unexplained reality? Does this term make Einstein a pseudo-scientist, a quack?

Are we to eliminate Qigong, internal martial arts, acupuncture and the great success of medical Qigong because of Ki's 'spooky' nature? I don't think so.

Q. How do you account for unexplainable martial phenomena?

People once believed the world was flat. Did it change anyone's day-to-day behavior? No. Unless you were a seafarer worrying about your vessel falling off the end of ocean, or a scientist wondering if you got your theory right, you proceeded as usual. People once believed that the sun revolved around the earth. Did it alter anyone's day-to-day behavior. No. Some early Asian peoples believed that an invisible energy existed around and inside of them. Did it alter society's behavior back then? No. Unless you were a student of the internal alchemies. Up until my forties, I didn't care if Ki existed or not, either in my martial art or my everyday life. I was a successful career teacher with thousands of engaged and satisfied clients.

All that changed the evening I experienced the unexplainable. My parochial paradigm cracked wide open. Today my answer about Ki's existence is an unequivocal 'Yes.' Ask me about the science behind it and I can only produce theories. Ask me about Ki's behavior and I will talk your ear off.

I'm a well-read, seasoned, career sensei. I have broad teaching experiences and many long-term 20 to 40 year students. I've taught with the world's best in terms of actual on-the-mat time: 7 days a week for 22 years, 6 days a week for the next 32 years. 20-35 classes every week, without fail. I've taught and perhaps, more importantly, stood witness in over 50,000 classes.

I leave the hard science of Ki to the pioneering scientists. My interest lies in observing and recording the behavior of these unseen energies in regard to traditional martial practices, like kata, and their applications. If you consider the definition of a scientist as a person studying or who has expert knowledge of one or more of the natural or physical sciences, then consider martial art a natural physical science.

As a healthy critic I don't denigrate something just because I am unfamiliar with it or haven't seen it with my own eyes. I follow the Buddha's advice —disbelieve anything anyone tells you until you can prove it with your own experience. I don't trash people for speaking a different truth from my own. I've tried just as wholeheartedly in experiments involving believers and nonbelievers alike to disprove the existence of Ki as I perceive it. My conclusion: Ki is a real phenomenon and Kiko is the art that demonstrates its effects on other human beings. Today, I look for better questions that can lead me deeper into the how and why of such phenomenon.

Q. Can you comment about the value of kinesthetic maturity?

Years ago, I was vacationing on the remote Monhegan Island, Maine. I had been invited to a small, evening social gathering. One member of the group, an English university professor, whom I had never met, was sharing his knowledge of academics when he commented bluntly on the physical movement arts after I had been introduced as a 'karate teacher'. I was surprised to hear him testily remark, "I don't need anyone to teach me how to move."

Given that I could easily be considered a movement professional, I found his statement curious, if not a bit arrogant. A crazy thought ran through my head that I ought to drag him out the house with a come-along joint lock technique and ask him if he might have wanted to learn an escape antidote, but I bit my tongue and kept things civil. From my vantage, this professor had no idea what he was talking about, for in Asia there was, and is, a profound appreciation, respect for, and a great deal of knowledge about, the essential nature of physical movement, well beyond what we in modern culture, and certainly this professor, understood.

We can all benefit from the right kind of teachers whether through books, videos or live guides. Take away everything we've ever been taught and civilization would be standing back in the Dark Ages. Teachers are a vital backbone in every society.

Western culture has frequently assumed an arrogant stance regarding the wisdom wheel—claiming to be the first to do this and that in regard to physical movement programs. We may be the first to repackage or rebrand ancient information in new and novel ways, (often to better monetize them), but when we look at what the martial and monastic cultures have given us in terms of insight, it's profound.

Less than 1% of the world's martial arts population is aware of the contents of this work. I don't say this to be elitist. I have a passion for martial knowledge. I don't see or hear too much of the esoteric being bandied about. I've devoted half my life studying the inner nature of karate-dō. I simply don't find many aware of a certain level of technique, believe in it, care to discuss, or share it. I have even presented my position to some well-respected masters. They couldn't be bothered, even though I was willing to freely share my insights with them. Baffling, for sure. However, I learned a long time ago that some people just don't want to let in any new information that challenges well-established comfort zones. Others, like the English professor I encountered on vacation, believe they've already 'been there, done that.' I hope I never lose my humility and create such a false ceiling over my head.

Q. Do you believe that Isshinryu Karate's founder, Tatsuo Shimabuku, was aware of Ki manipulations in his kata?

This is a difficult question to answer. The closest I can determine is both a 'yes' and 'no'. In a many hours long private discussions with Master Frank Van Lenten (Isshinryu, 10th dan), who studied with Shimabuku in the 1950's, Van Lenten admitted that Shimabuku was the first Okinawan teacher to discuss Ki with him. The only specifics Van Lenten was willing to share however, were the master's use of breathing to alter his body temperature, a technique referred to as *Tumo* by Tibetan Buddhists. Supporting the 'yes' side, I have found myself occasionally reverting to Shima-buku's kata performance as a more accurate demonstration of proper Ki technique, yet at the same time, his performance does not hold up consistently to what our research reveals. There are instances where Shimabuku is inconsistent in his stances when demonstrating various kata. The problem in determining if any expert is representing proper Ki flow lies in two testable condi-tions—Hard and Soft Gate use. Hard Gate is what you can visually detect in a kata performance. You cannot know Soft Gates unless the performer openly shares his intentions. Since Soft Gates can override Hard Gates, once you know how Energy is meant to flow in your body, the outward physical form becomes less important. Meaning, you can often dispense with the standardized 'correct' external form. We must also consider that any change in compass direction will lead to a change in technical emphasis. I know this does not help answer the question. It leaves kata performance too open ended. But there are lots of factors to weigh. The bottom line is that we cannot assume there has been a perfect transmission or perfect understanding of kata's value. Some of Shimabuku's successors, in my opinion, were also not the best ambassadors of the essence of his art. This is a major problem with Asian Fighting Forms in general. It's rare for a student to surpass their teach-er's grasp of Form. If a teacher's understanding of kata is subpar, everyone subjected to their instruction will be hindered in their advance.

In the Seisan kata there is a short sequence where you turn left 90 degrees into a Seisan stance, do a left middle block, followed by a punch/punch/kick/punch set. According to the American Okinawan Karate Association under the guidance of Steve Arm-strong during the early 70's, this set was taught with a forward slip step. Today, you may or may not see the slip step used. Initially the slip step seemed insignificant, at best, a decision based upon dis-tance; Slip step if you need to get closer. Stay put if you are close enough. But a deeper analysis revealed that a left foot lead slip step adds impressive power to the middle block. The non-slip step does not. But I must point out that the slip step must be a one-foot length forward action, initiated with the lead foot (one can slip-step front foot followed by back foot, or back foot followed by front foot). These two methods lead to energetically opposite outcomes.

Was Shimabuku aware of his inconsistencies? Did they matter

to him? Did he override physical moves with intuitive or conscious Soft Gate controls? There is no way to know. Shimabuku offered little commentary about the specifics of his own kata performance.

Q Can you give an example of a martial technique performed with and without Kiko skill?

Yes. I will use the opening movements from Isshinryu's Seisan kata to point out the difference in a Q & A format. For those unfamiliar with the sequence, it goes like this:

A left foot crescents forward into a Seisan dachi, followed by a left middle block and a right mid-body vertical punch—a typical bread and butter counter. Mainstream, Hard style, ballistic martial artists interpret this set as follows: Someone throws a right or left hand at your face/torso. You block it with the left middle body parry using your forearm and counter strike. (There are many ways to interpret this sequence. I've chosen this one way to illustrate how Kiko works).

A Non-Kiko interpretation

Q. Why crescent step forward?
A. The Crescent step evasively weaves the body. This allows you to slip a strike while moving closer to the attacker.

Q. Isn't a Crescent step slower than a straightforward stepping action?
A. This is empirically true. The shortest distance between two points is a straight line. In this case, however, the Crescent step protects the groin, bisects the opponent's stance breaking his structure, and weaves clear of a strike, so it is worth the effort.

Q. Which part of the blocking arm should make contact with the attacker's punch; Bone edge, flat of the arm, pinky side? Does it matter?
A. Although different martial art styles advocate making contact with different parts of the forearm, hand, or by evading the strike altogether, Shimabuku taught students to block with the flat outside of the forearm. He felt that two forearm bones presented less a chance of injury than a single bone contact.

Q. Why block with the left arm?

A. Generally, the left arm (Yin) is used for blocking and the stronger right arm (Yang) for striking.

Q. Why step into the Seisan dachi?

A. Seisan is a natural body posture. It offers the stability to withstand an unbalancing force without compromising maneuverability.

Q. Why not use Seisan dachi all the time?

A. It's best to have options. This is just one stance that can be used.

Q. Why the left foot forward? Why not a right foot?

A. Generally, you pair the left arm block with a left foot forward action. Blocking off one's rear leg is not supported by the Seisan stance. In many traditional arts you will see blocking off the lead, left leg and to the inside of the attacker's limb.

Q. What about breathing? Should I breathe in or out, nose or mouth? Does it matter?

A: As long as the mechanics of the block are correct, breathing is secondary to deflecting a strike.

All the above answers have merit but they relate exclusively to external martial actions. I will now answer the same questions from the Kiko perspective;

A Kiko Interpretation

Q. Why Crescent step forward?

A. The half-circle step dilates the Yin channels to pump more Ki up the inside of the left leg. Three channels ascend inside each leg. When done correctly the crescent runs a strong electro-magnetic charge that pulls energy from and around the defender's body. A defender that steps forward with a right leg causes the channels to discharge energy. This is a real event occurring in the body invisible to both parties.

Q. Isn't a Crescent step slower than a straightforward step?

A. We are only talking a micro-second difference in speed between a straight versus a crescent step. The crescent is a precise evasion, a bedrock of Kiko understanding. The left foot is used to step forward and outside of the attacker's lead right leg where it will draw the greatest amount of energy from the attack. When anyone moves aggressively toward you, a Ki wave will precede their actual physical body. Stepping with the left foot will draw from this wave.

Q. Which part of the blocking arm should make contact with the attacker's punch; Bone edge, flat of the arm, pinky side? Does it matter?

A. Although you must avoid getting hit regardless of your blocking method, different degrees of skill can be applied to this end. In this case, the ideal is to have the blocking arm retract toward you, rather than extend slightly away from, or perpendicular to, the striking arm. Parrying arm actions should be viewed like crescent stepping. Arcing inward to outward or outward to inward makes a big difference.

One of the reasons we don't see Kiko principles used is that mediocrity rules. Mediocrity battles mediocrity in the mainstream arena. You don't ever have to use or be conscious of any Kiko principles to effectively block a punch if your opponent is working from the same toolbox. Chances are your adversary doesn't know any advanced martial techniques either. Someone who exhibits superior technique may be using Kiko principles unknowingly or intuitively. The ten-thousand hour training principle can fuse body, mind, spirit (energy fields) into proper flow. A primitive versus refined body connection present two levels of awareness and skill. I call them metaphorically, the 'red' and 'white' talents.' Kiko stacks the deck in one's favor, by allowing you to energetically overload or underload the opponent. There are Kiko formulas for achieving a proper energy exchange that advocate making contact with different parts of the forearm.

Q. Why crescent step into the Seisen dachi?
A. It's an open Ki flow foot position.

Q. Why not use it all the time?
A. Diverse stances generate different Biofield formulas with different results. A left foot forward Seisan dachi is ideal for 'stealing' energy from one who attacks with a lead right foot.

Q. Why the left foot forward? Why not a right foot?

A. The left foot crescent is a Yin, energy-in, action. The right foot is a Yang, energy-out action. Although the left foot forward crescent step will take energy in, this only occurs if the defender's left foot is placed to the outside of the opponent's right foot. In this instance a defender can steal, or draw from the opponent's downward Yang flow on the outside of his right leg to increase the charge in his own body.

Q. Why block with the left arm?

A. The left arm generates a stronger Yin current for receiving energy, even if you are left-handed.

Q. How should we breathe; in or out, nose or mouth? Does it matter?

A. The first rule of Kiko practice—everything matters. Breathing matters. The respiratory mechanism is part of the biomechanical Hard Gating system. As a general rule, breathe in when the limbs move toward the center of the body and out as the limbs extend away from the center. We want breath to complement limb action. Breathing in through the nose enables one to maintain the tongue on the roof of the mouth for running the Microcosmic Orbit. You will need to investigate and try out reverse breathing and abdominal breathing methods to see what is the ideal method for you.

A Thought Experiment

If neither the attacker nor defender stood close enough to actually make physical contact, yet still executed their individual actions toward one another, what do think would occur? We've observed that even without physical contact, the attacker will likely experience a pervasive drop in overall body energy and the defender will experience a rise in muscular output. Neither person will be aware of this because most people lack the sensitivity to detect this shift in their Biofields. Yet, it becomes obvious to the players conducting some simple tests afterward. Other operant variables might not lead to producing positive results but, in many cases, they can often be determined, given the explanation of factors as yet discussed.

If you take my statement of the 'no touching effects' at face value, you will surely ask, what just happened? Our Biofields are always and instantly affected before contact, depending upon the intention of the parties involved.

Any two persons standing two to three feet away from one another, though not physically touching, still 'touch' by means of their projected Biofields. Kiko demonstrates this interaction in meaningful and observable ways. Biofield events are never passive.

We need look no farther than the properties of two magnets to see how human fields entangle. If a bar magnet sits far enough away from a second magnet, you will not see any visible evidence of its attracting or repelling influence. But as one magnet nears the other, the magnets will react by moving. If both magnetic fields are pointing north or south, they will repel one another. If north meets south-facing, they will attract and draw together. If you ever played with magnets, you saw this action. The human body generates a similar event. (The magnet's north and south pole are, by correlation, the body's left and right sides). This touching initiates a bio-switching process. When you are 'energy-touched' by another, your own internal currents will either constrict or dilate. The other's electro-magnetic field will instantly stimulate your Ki system. Psychologically, we see a similar action. You are either drawn to, away from, or indifferent to certain people, events, or objects. These same outcomes occur on the subtle energy level. But in this case, the affects either charge or discharge specific muscles. For example, Ki flowing into the deltoids will give a punch more thrust. The internal masters know precisely how to configure their body posture and breathing to maximize every strike, block, stance, lock, and evasion.

Internal experts may use a different vocabulary to describe what is happening but they will be aware of this phenomenon by varying degrees. In kata training we deduce what is affecting what, then duplicate the behaviors in the Kata's lessons. However, you must know exactly what is occurring on the subtle level to avail yourselves of these lessons.

The ideal picture of Kiko-based kata gives us a reliable map of how Energy should flow through the body postures. Unfortunately, in order to understand where your Ki needs to be, you must first have an idea of what you are doing with an opponent. This has been a major problem with kata's exportation to the West. The detailed description of its inner workings in bunkai was not included with the external forms. Critical pages were missing or redacted from its teachings. Western karate-ka get their fill of kata performance, but not their fill of advanced kata understanding. There is a lot of superficial kata bunkai out there. At this juncture, American martial arts got disconnected from their rich Asian heritage. This has forced many Western sensei to reinvent or rediscover the deeper principles in their respective arts.

Not knowing this underlayment exists, large numbers of Westerners have taken their martial arts at their face value and built up an entire language, curriculums, and industry around their art's surface teachings. Westerners are a very visual, results and action-oriented, Yang, society. Asian Fighting (kumite) are dynamic, exciting, adrenaline-pumping. Since we couldn't see the inner nature of these arts, we elevated their topical values to the pinnacle of martial performance. We continue to proceeded full steam ahead praising our art's exoskeletons. With the current dumbing of society, our fighting arts may continue to become more watered down with each passing generation.

Q. Why do you consider Kiko hidden?

Buried might be the better term, as Kiko seems to lie beneath more topical agendas. If left to their own devices, I doubt martial art students will ever discover Kiko technique or its principles on their own. I didn't have the slightest clue this art existed after twenty-five years of professional teaching. Any logical presentation that defines how a biomechanically correct martial move should be done generally discharges further curiosity. This renders any secondary curiosity, like why a technique should be done one way versus another, rarely pursued. When getting clarification on the how, people seldom ask for the why. When the logic for the why is answered, it discharges from your mind and the quest ends. Even our mental actions, on the atomic level, are just a continuous series of energy charges and discharges. Desire, on the quantum level, is a charge that builds up when you want something. Discharge of the desire is what happens after you get it. The entire Hindu Chakric system is a bio-circuitry of charges and discharges occurring throughout the body's electrical system making us all partially self-charging biobatteries. I say partial because we are not closed systems. We need external resources; air, water, food, sunlight, etc, to perpetuate this process.

If you were never taught that the internal nature of your martial art is woven into its external fabric, this most assuredly guarantees this information remains an unclaimed potential.

Q. Could you comment on what you refer to as the Small and Large circles of Life?

The trending concept of mindfulness, of 'waking up' to the present moment, suggests too many people are walking around entranced in their cozy, individual reality bubbles. These states, or paradigms, represent our primary beliefs. A belief is not a static reality like money sitting in the bank. Beliefs are the engines of the will whose intentions are carried out by our bodies. If you don't wake up, you might find yourself moving in one of Life's small circles, making a lot of noise, but covering little distance.

Beliefs function like muscles. They give us mental traction the same way muscles give us physical traction. Our beliefs form our foundational reality, continually creating the world we inhabit and maneuver through.

If you feel that your world is an angry, hostile place, then, by your own projection, you will create and inhabit an angry, hostile world. It has been observed by cultures much older than our own, 'As on the inside, so on the outside. As above, so below.' Hateful inside births hateful out. Peaceful inside, gives rise to peaceful outside. Angry inside is angry out. Hostile inside is hostile out. Fearful inside is fearful outside. Confused inside is confused outside. Our first problem, first challenge, is to weed out our real enemy by asking, do our insides (beliefs) match our outside consequences? When you wake up to this reality you get to choose what kind of world you want.

The big picture, the Large Circle of life, exerts its own kind of pressure on the martial path. Modern cultures worldwide are being disenfranchised from real power, partly due to our own blind drives. When distracted, we pursue the wrong goals. There is value in authentic ways, in what earlier cultures deemed important and sought after.

Most martial artists today have little clue about the narrow and wide paths in their training. The Martial Ways are not just a random collection of fighting techniques. The more holistic systems offer clear ways of looking at life. They present a particular set of eye ware. The martial viewpoint is not a dogma that suggests life must be looked at like a ceaseless battleground or competitive arena. Rather, these disciplines present a specific type of lens to look at anything you desire.

Awareness itself is a constantly shifting attribute. At any given time, you are either looking inward, that is, attending to or addressing the interior of your body or mind, or looking outward, taking in your surroundings. Western culture is so outwardly focused that its talk is mainly of taking it in. Rarely do people consider the reverse, taking their insides out. This has led to a great imbalance of self.

When we invite the Dō of martial arts, we begin a multi-dimensional quest into nature of the self, the nature of our own mind, our own awareness, not just the awareness of our physical power, but of our mental and spiritual strengths. The best place to start looking at this triple nature is in the physical realm, the most concrete part of our earthly journey. How does it feel to be in your body, to move your body, to be your body? The trend over the last several decades has been to shift attention into our heads/minds. Western culture seems intent that we spend most of our time in the head, not in our guts, or in parts of our bodies. We locate in our stomachs when hungry, in our loins when aroused, in our hearts when loving and being loved, and so on. But how much are we really in our bodies, our minds, our emotions? Could we be living with more enriched meaning or feeling if we dwelt more frequently here? We can. As a physical discipline, Karate-dō asks us to embrace these moments for their richness and to challenge and broaden our view.

Why do you think there is such a big movement toward mindfulness today? We're losing the moment. Life is meaningless unless you give it meaning, attribute sense and value to your experiences. Why not maximize that meaning? We don't want to just optimize our headspace. We want to maximize our emotional and physical space, widen it, stretch it.

The majority peer toward their martial art's defensive or competitive practicality, or through an imagined mystic invulnerability imbued by ancient practices, or they live for a fight lust or adrenaline high. Martial Dō breaks these fixations, widens the scope of study, asks why conflict at all? The Buddha taught a way to transcend conflict. His way required you place your full attention and awareness on this subject, that you take time to look and question your life in a positive, forward-thinking manner. When you question your life, you must bring all the parts of yourself into perspective and give them a voice.

Q. In light of your Kiko research have your katas changed?

Yes, my katas have definitely changed. However, they would have changed despite my knowledge of Kiko because all students will naturally progress through three developmental stages as they move from basic to advanced martial skills;

1. Heightened control of the body from solo performance will sharpen one's moves.

2. Partnered bunkai will ground a kata in realistic emphasis and pacing.

3. Resistance training will develop the impacting muscles for increased engagement strength.

Proper kata training should lead to more realistic combat expression, which differs from pure athleticism. Simply being fast and strong doesn't presume either proper Form, pacing, or correct technique. Speed, power and pacing must follow Form. Kiko offers additional refinement of these performance qualities.

Historically, we still do not know many of the exact rationales behind the earliest Asian katas, which leaves us with a fundamental issue. Do we perform a kata exactly as taught or can we amend sequences to fit our body? The answer is not clear. Rationales given for why a kata should be performed one way versus another fall on evaluative scale of weak to strong practicality or realism, and weak to strong Biofield enhancement. Weak being either not very realistic, bunkai unknown, less practical or impractical. Strong being very realistic, practical and probable.

To get an idea of the complexity of the subject, I practice a kata called Sunsu. It is the only kata in the eight forms that make up the weaponless portion of the Isshinryu system created by its founder, Tatsuo Shimabuku. We do not know if Shimabuku drew from other Kata either within or outside his own system to create Sunsu and/or if he purposefully included reversed movement sets found in his other Forms. My theory is that Shimabuku's Sunsu kata was showing others how to properly perform kata sets on the opposite side of the body from his other forms so that the Ki flows in your favor. For this reason, I call Sunsu a Yin kata. The other katas, in my opinion, are Yang oriented.

There is a sequence in Sunsu where you turn, spear and execute what looks like three elbow strikes. This set is repeated three times, each in a different direction. Having learned that directionality influences strength, you can see why I might raise this question. I was taught these moves as identical sets. None of my teachers offered any bunkai for this kata. Common Isshinryu bunkai perform the elbow sets as strikes.

When we tested the three sets as identical patterns, all our subjects tested weak or, at best, neutral in strength. I knew this could not be correct. I tweaked the moves until subjects tested strong for both Yin and Yang actions. It became apparent these moves have been misinterpreted. Kiko revealed that the palm up spear was likely used to roll an opponent's arm. The first elbow is thrown in reverse to lower the opponent's head and the last two elbows conclude a shoulder lock manipulation. This bunkai is realistic, powerful and probable. The height of the spear is also critical for increasing lifting strength when controlling another's arm. Even the timing of the slip step and elbows must align with the correct breath sequence. Under this light, I consider Sunsu worthy of being called a martial 'art'. This level of depth is thoroughly engaging. It has motivated myself and my students to probe deeper.

If you were to compare my 1970's Sunsu kata to today's expression, you would see slight changes in the timing and angles of the limbs. Since breath is seldom emphasized in modern kata, you probably would not pay attention to whether I was breathing in or out, or what significance this would have. But these changes make all the difference between being partially blind (I'm doing it because that's how my teacher told me to do it) or having both eyes wide open, and between reasonable strength versus exceptional and effortless power.

Q. Can you expand on the concept of 'Ka' and its relationship to the martial Way?

I was listening to a life-long Aikido-ka link the Japanese term 'ka' (student) to the Egyptian concept of Ka, for soul, as in dedicated soul student, or one who dedicates his soul to his art and training. It seems that more and more students are dedicating less of themselves to in-depth practices, not because there is no desire to do so, but due to a lack of vitality from many factors. It is the natural course of living things to expand at birth and contract at death. Within this spectrum we are presented with the full cycle of life but not always the full spectrum of our potential within this life.

All of us have the capacity for an astounding dynamism to extend our influence into diverse strata of both our hard (tangible) and soft (intangible) realities. Our being has roots and branches that touch and draw sustenance from both the mundane and the spiritual, the profane and the sacred.

The Enlightenment path of the Martial Ways is one of the venerable disciplines in this world. Its most profound teachings lie buried under topical agendas. It is important that future students understand the difference between the Enlightenment path of the Martial Ways and other lesser goals or ways.

The first distinction is often made with prefix 'Dō' added to the name of a martial style. Karate-dō is used to identify a Life Student of the 'Way' called Dō-ka, or spiritual practitioner of Japanese or Ryukyuan martial arts. The primary goal of this training is to achieve an elevated organization, integration, and authenticity of self. Self-protective skills are inherent in this training but they are peripheral objectives revolving around the idea that when you are truly at peace with yourself you have achieved an unshakable, adamantine, diamond-like security. I offer you this explanation so as not to confuse you about training objectives.

The major difference between studying a purely physical discipline from studying a broader holistic one lies in the attention to larger life patterns that can undermine your health, organization, security and peace of mind, which are sometimes hidden from our own psyches.

Holistic disciplines are far more energy attractive, constructive, and life-altering because they draw forth vital insights about your core nature. Thus, they are more effective for resolving or transcending a wider range of conflicts.

This study is the focus of our dojo's advanced practices. As such, you may find yourself engaged not only in intense body-work but also in intense dialectics and/or directed introspections toward exploring and opening deeper levels of yourself that may have been previously limited, restricted or bound. Our school has over a half century legacy and long-standing place in our community.

We welcome anyone interested in exploring the venerable path of the Martial Ways to join with us to become a Knight of the Bagua.

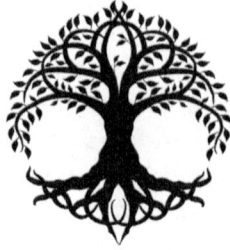

MEDITATION

As the pebble drops into water
so thoughts drop into Body,
Body drops into Earth,
Earth drops into Cosmos,
Cosmos drops into Infinite Spirit

Infinite Spirit is abundant and positive.
Infinite, abundant and positive Spirit drops into my thought

Abundant and positive thoughts drop into my body
My abundant and positive body drops into Earth
Abundant and positive earth drops into Cosmos
Abundant and positive Universe drops into Infinite Spirit

My infinite Spirit is abundant and positive

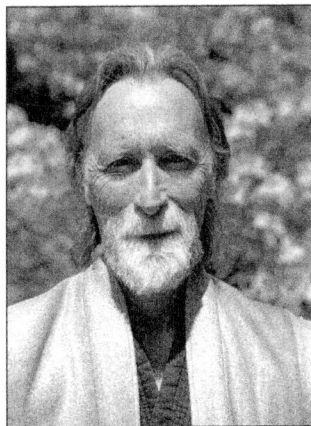

Christopher J. Goedecke (Buddhist, Hayashi Tomio) is a long-time resident of Morristown, New Jersey where he pursues his life-long passion of teaching and writing about traditional martial arts. Learn more about Isshin Kempo and Shifu's Kiko research. Join the dialog. Shifu Hayashi can be contacted at windschool@earthlink.net. He is available for school seminars.

www.isshinkempo.com

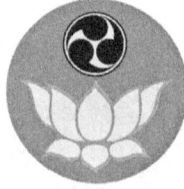

WORKS BY

Hayashi Tomio
(Christopher J. Goedecke)

ADULTS

The Soul Polisher's Apprentice:
A Martial Kumite About Personal Evolution

Internal Karate: *Mind Matters and the Seven Gates of Power*

Rebel Isshinryu: *The 57 Challenges*

CHILDREN & YOUNG ADULTS

The Wind Warrior: *Training of A Karate Champion*
Smart Moves: *A Kid's Guide to Self Defense*
The Unbreakable Board & The Red Dragon Surprise

IN THE WORKS

Sensei & The Flying 'S'

Printed in Great Britain
by Amazon

45186589R00225